RESEARCH METHODS FOR NURSES AND MIDWIVES

SAGE was founded in 1965 by Sara Miller McCune to support the dissemination of usable knowledge by publishing innovative and high-quality research and teaching content. Today, we publish over 900 journals, including those of more than 400 learned societies, more than 800 new books per year, and a growing range of library products including archives, data, case studies, reports, and video. SAGE remains majority-owned by our founder, and after Sara's lifetime will become owned by a charitable trust that secures our continued independence.

Los Angeles | London | New Delhi | Singapore | Washington DC | Melbourne

MERRYL HARVEY • LUCY LAND

RESEARCH METHODS FOR NURSES AND MIDWIVES

THEORY AND PRACTICE

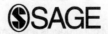

Los Angeles | London | New Delhi
Singapore | Washington DC | Melbourne

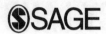

Los Angeles | London | New Delhi
Singapore | Washington DC | Melbourne

SAGE Publications Ltd
1 Oliver's Yard
55 City Road
London EC1Y 1SP

SAGE Publications Inc.
2455 Teller Road
Thousand Oaks, California 91320

SAGE Publications India Pvt Ltd
B 1/I 1 Mohan Cooperative Industrial Area
Mathura Road
New Delhi 110 044

SAGE Publications Asia-Pacific Pte Ltd
3 Church Street
#10-04 Samsung Hub
Singapore 049483

Editor: Jai Seaman
Editorial assistant: Alysha Owen
Production editor: Tom Bedford
Copyeditor: Gemma Marren
Proofreader: Camille Bramall
Indexer: Silvia Benvenuto
Marketing manager: Tamara Navaratnam
Cover design: Shaun Mercier
Typeset by: C&M Digitals (P) Ltd, Chennai, India
Printed by CPI Group (UK) Ltd, Croydon, CR0 4YY

Library of Congress Control Number: 2016938802

British Library Cataloguing in Publication data

A catalogue record for this book is available from the British Library

ISBN 978-1-4462-9849-7
ISBN 978-1-4462-9850-3 (pbk)

At SAGE we take sustainability seriously. Most of our products are printed in the UK using FSC papers and boards. When we print overseas we ensure sustainable papers are used as measured by the PREPS grading system. We undertake an annual audit to monitor our sustainability.

CONTENTS

ABOUT THE AUTHORS

Merryl Harvey qualified as a nurse in 1982. After qualifying as a midwife in 1984, her area of practice was neonatal intensive care. Merryl's clinical career culminated in her working as a clinical teacher and this in turn led her to take up a post at Birmingham City University. Initially this was to run the post-registration neonatal intensive care course. In more recent years Merryl has been seconded to work on a number of large-scale, funded research projects which have focused on aspects of parenting and preterm birth. She secured the Bliss Research Fellow post based at the National Perinatal Epidemiology Unit (2004–2007). Her MSc explored aspects of the neonatal nurse practitioner role and her PhD explored fathers' experiences of the birth and immediate care of their baby. Merryl has a strong journal publication history and co-authored a text on fatherhood in relation to midwifery and neonatal practice which was published in 2012. Merryl is now a Reader in Nursing and her main role at the University is as Chair of the Faculty Academic Ethics Committee. She is also co-lead of the Family Health Research Cluster.

Lucy Land qualified as a nurse in 1980 and worked in haematology, caring for patients with leukaemia, sickle cell anaemia and other blood disorders. Eventually specialising in haemophilia, Lucy was one of the first clinical nurse specialists, supporting a regional outpatient and home treatment service. Following this successful career in practice, she became a clinical nurse teacher and later qualified as a registered nurse tutor. After moving into the University, Lucy has continued to teach and to undertake funded research projects. Lucy's research now focuses on patient experience and she has completed several studies on this subject. In addition to a substantial history of journal publications, Lucy was co-author of an earlier Sage publication – *Resources for Nursing Research: An Annotated Bibliography*. Now, as professor of nursing, Lucy is Director of the Centre for Social Care, Health and Related Research (C-SHaRR) and continues to contribute to the improvement of nursing care through innovative research and teaching.

ABBREVIATIONS

AIDS	acquired immune deficiency syndrome
AR	absolute risk
CAMHS	Child and Adolescent Mental Health Service
CAT	critical appraisal tool
CBT	cognitive behavioural therapy
CCT	controlled clinical trial
CER	control event rate
CI	confidence interval
CINAHL	Cumulative Index to Nursing and Allied Health Literature
CONSORT	Consolidated Standards of Reporting Trials
CRN	Clinical Research Network
DBS	Disclosure and Barring Service
DH	Department of Health
DV	dependent variable
EBP	evidence-based practice
EER	experimental event rate
GCP	Good Clinical Practice
H_0	null hypothesis
H_1	hypothesis
HIV	human immunodeficiency virus
HMIC	Healthcare Management Information Consortium
HRA	Health Research Authority
IPA	interpretative phenomenological analysis
IRAS	Integrated Research Application System
ITT	intention to treat
IV	independent variable
MIDIRS	Midwives Information and Resource Service
MMR Study	Measles Mumps and Rubella Study
NHS	National Health Service
NICE	National Institute for Health Care Excellence
NIHR	National Institute for Health Research
NNH	number needed to harm
NNT	number needed to treat
NRES	National Research Ethics Service
OR	odds ratio
PICO	Population, Intervention, Counter Intervention, Outcome

PICOD   Population, Intervention, Counter Intervention, Outcome, Design
PICU   paediatric intensive care unit
PIL   participant information leaflet
PIO   Population, Intervention, Outcome
PIOD   Population, Intervention, Outcome, Design
PRISMA   Preferred Reporting Items for Systematic Reviews and Meta-Analyses
RAE   Research Assessment Exercise
RCT   randomised controlled trial
REF   Research Excellence Framework
RR   relative risk
SOP   standard operating procedure
SR   systematic review
TENS   Transcutaneous Electronic Nerve Stimulation
TOBY   Total Body Hypothermia Study

HOW TO USE THIS BOOK

This book is written with two distinct groups or readers in mind. Firstly, those encountering research and evidence-based practice for the first time. This group will mainly be undergraduate student nurses and midwives. We anticipate that the other group of readers will be qualified nurses and midwives, who will use this book to refresh their knowledge, clarify meanings and develop their understanding about fundamental issues pertaining to research methods, the research process and evidence-based practice. The book will supplement other resources they will access in their pursuit of further academic study or to undertake other research-related activities. The book is divided into five parts:

- Part I – *Laying the Foundations* – introduces readers to nursing and midwifery research and explores evidence-based practice. The focus of this section is on the ways in which nursing and midwifery knowledge is generated, the principles of evidence-based practice and different research methodologies.
- Part II – *Understanding Research Methods and Designs: The Theory* – explores the theoretical underpinnings of research methods, systematic and Cochrane reviews in detail, and examines different research designs.
- Part III – *Using Research Methods and Design: The Practice* – explores the practicalities of conducting research. This includes the key stages of the research process, generating a research question or hypothesis, undertaking a literature review, sampling, data collection and addressing ethical issues in clinical research.
- Part IV – *Data Analysis and Evaluation* – explores measures of effectiveness (quantitative) and qualitative data analysis, strategies to facilitate rigour and the critical appraisal of research.
- Part V – *Research in Action: Dissemination and Application* – considers the writing up and dissemination of research findings, using research in clinical practice and writing a research proposal. The book concludes by suggesting the significance of research in the future, for individual practitioners, the professions of nursing and midwifery and health care more generally.

As the book progresses we will encounter more challenging terminology, concepts and theories. Throughout the text and on the accompanying website we use examples from midwifery, the four fields of nursing (adult, child, mental health and learning disabilities) and from a range of specialities. Whilst the book has a predominantly UK focus, we anticipate that the key concepts will apply to any setting. To facilitate this application, we have used international sources where appropriate. Throughout the book we include 'think point activities' to help readers consolidate their knowledge and develop their thinking.

The accompanying website also provides additional material and resources to support and complement the text. The website provides contemporary material in a range of formats to suit different learning styles. Inevitably some chapters are longer than other because they address a broader range of issues. Consequently the number of website and think point activities also varies in accordance with the length and nature of the corresponding chapter. In addition on the website there are case studies that run alongside the book. These focus on fictional students and qualified nurses and midwives who are undertaking the activities described in the book. These case studies will take the reader through the various stages of the research process and we anticipate that they will enable the reader to obtain greater insight into the application of research theory, the conduct of research and into the practical and logistical issues that researchers often encounter. We hope you enjoy the book.

USING THE DIGITAL CONTENT AND WEBSITE

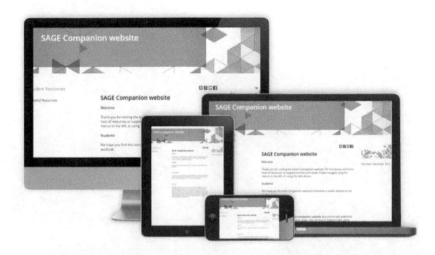

Visit https://study.sagepub.com/harveyandland to find a range of additional resources for students.

Web Activities encourage you to take your learning off the page. These activities will help you apply skills you've already learned, get additional tips from relevant experts, or access the resources and organizations you need to take your research further.

Quizzes give you the chance to test your knowledge through multiple choice questions, short answers, matching activities and other revision tools.

From organizational templates to ethical approval advice, **Checklists and Additional Resources** provide practical guidance every budding researcher needs.

PART I

LAYING THE FOUNDATIONS

INTRODUCTION TO RESEARCH IN NURSING AND MIDWIFERY

Within this chapter we lay the foundations for the topics, concepts and issues that will be explored in more detail in subsequent chapters. In this chapter we will:

- outline the aim and rationale for the book
- establish a definition of research that applies both within and beyond the health care setting
- explore the need for nursing and midwifery research and the reasons why it is imperative that nurses and midwives are 'research-aware'
- introduce the concept of evidence-based practice
- provide an overview of the history of nursing and midwifery research in the UK
- identify the factors and pressures that have influenced nursing and midwifery research to date.

AIMS OF THE BOOK

The word 'research' has become part of our everyday language and most of us will have participated in a consumer survey, the national census or perhaps a health care related study. It is also very likely that we have unknowingly been part of a research study; probably the most likely example of this is a survey of traffic flow, which monitors the number of cars travelling a particular route over a period of time. Research is going on around us in all kinds of settings, whether or not we engage with it. We are also increasingly exposed to information via the Internet, in newspapers and on the radio and television about the findings of the latest research. Sometimes these findings appear obvious and common sense. Consequently we may regard such studies as a pointless exercise and a waste of money. At other times the findings of research studies may seem contradictory or dubious. In other cases such as the Measles, Mumps and Rubella

(MMR) study, research findings that have been widely reported have subsequently been discredited (Wakefield et al., 1998). It is perhaps therefore not surprising that we sometimes regard research with apprehension, caution and suspicion.

However, for those of us involved in health care, research is integral to our clinical and academic work. There are numerous examples of research studies, particularly over the last 50 years, that have led nurses and midwives to question their practice (Stockwell, 1972; Sleep and Grant, 1988). In many cases these studies have instigated important changes in the provision of care. Most programmes of study for nurses and midwives now include modules on **research methods** and **evidence-based practice** (EBP), professional journals contain papers on the latest research studies and books such as this have been written to help practitioners become more research-aware. Nevertheless, it is probably the case that, like the wider public, many nurses and midwives have the same uncertainties and concerns regarding research.

We aim to address these doubts and anxieties in this book. We will introduce readers to evidence-based practice and the research methods that are commonly used in health care. In doing this, we intend to demystify the seemingly complex nature and complicated language of research. We aim to support those who have little prior knowledge about research methods and evidence-based practice. This book will help readers to develop confidence recognising different types of research and establish a solid knowledge base from which they can develop more advanced thinking, use research findings in their practice and successfully complete academic work. We also anticipate that other readers will use the book to refresh their knowledge, clarify meanings and develop their

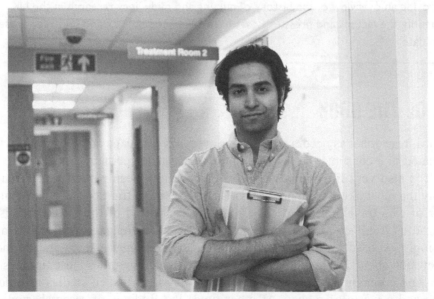

© SolStock / iStock

understanding. The book will support them in their pursuit of further academic study or to undertake other research-based activities.

To facilitate understanding, we will make clear links between research theory and its application to clinical practice. This will provide an insight into how research underpins and develops practice. In this way, we hope that readers will feel more comfortable about research and the use of best evidence to inform their practice and develop the care they give. We anticipate that the book will support students as they undertake academic assessments involving research, whether this is a critical analysis of a specific research study, a work-based project, a proposal for service improvement, a literature review, a **systematic review** (SR) or the development of a research proposal. In the longer term, we hope that the book will also help readers to feel more confident about undertaking and leading research themselves.

WHAT IS RESEARCH?

A logical starting point is to be sure that we understand what research is and to develop a definition that we will use throughout the book. In clarifying what research is, it is important to remember that the word 'research' can be used as a noun, in other words the activity itself: 'the research study'; or it can be used as a verb to denote the process of undertaking the activity: 'to research'.

THINK POINT ACTIVITY   1.1

Make a list of all of the activities that you have taken part in over the last year that might be described as being 'research'. Include health care related research and other studies that you have been involved in. For example, have you participated in a consumer survey? Have you collected data for someone else's study? Or have you taken part in an interview or focus group?

When we think of the word research, we might picture scientists working with chemicals in test tubes in a laboratory or someone standing on the high street with a clipboard asking shoppers questions about the washing powder they use. However, are these accurate examples of research? It probably is the case that the label 'research' is an overused term. In some cases it has been used to legitimise or raise the profile of what might otherwise be regarded as being questionable activities. In other situations the term research has been used misguidedly to describe other types of activity such as **audit**.

Website activity 1.1

According to the *Concise Oxford Dictionary* the word 'research' originates from sixteenth-century French and is derived from two components, 're, expressing intensive force' and 'cerchier, to search' (Stevenson and Waite, 2011: 1222). A definition of research must therefore allude in some way to the activity of 'intense searching'. However, as we will see in later chapters, there are a number of different research methods and designs, and the ways in which they are carried out can vary considerably. We therefore need to develop a general definition that will be appropriate for all the different types of research. Some of the words and phrases that we identified in Website activity 1.2 are specific to particular methods and designs and they would not therefore be appropriate for our general definition of research. However, it is important that whatever the method or design, when research is carried out the researcher must adhere to the key elements or principles of that particular method or design. The researcher should also make every attempt to minimise any flaws or weaknesses in the study. Therefore whatever method or design is used, the research must be carried out in a rigorous, thorough and organised way. Whilst we acknowledge that other definitions of research have been offered, our preferred definition is given below. This applies for research both within and beyond the health care setting and this is the definition of research that we will use throughout the book.

RESEARCH

A study that is carried out in a systematic and credible way in order to answer questions, find solutions to problems, generate new knowledge or confirm existing knowledge.

Website activity 1.2

RESEARCH: WHAT'S IT GOT TO DO WITH ME?

Having identified at the beginning of this chapter that research is an increasingly prominent feature in all aspects of our lives, we must acknowledge that some nurses and midwives regard research in a negative way (Morse, 2006). We might be tempted to think that research is 'someone else's business' and perhaps understandably workload pressures may mean that nurses and midwives do not see research as being their priority (O'Byrne and Smith, 2010; Bohman et al., 2013). As a consequence, nurses and midwives, particularly those working clinically, may view research as being the territory of an elite few, principally doctors and those working in academic institutions. To some extent this view is fuelled and perpetuated by the relatively few clinical research opportunities available for nurses and midwives and a lack of forward planning to build research capacity (O'Byrne and Smith, 2010). We might also think about research as being a means to an end; something that has to be done as part of a module or programme of study that can then be put aside when an assignment or a course is completed. However, understanding research has far-reaching benefits. It is not just about being able to 'do' research. It is also about knowing how to access current research findings, being able to discriminate between sound and flawed research and identifying research that should be implemented in practice (Coughlan et al., 2007; Ryan et al., 2007). Being research-aware therefore enables nurses and midwives to deliver safe, effective and high quality patient care (Nursing and Midwifery Council, 2015a), and is a skill to be utilised by nurses and midwives throughout their professional practice (Fothergill and Lipp, 2014).

THINK POINT ACTIVITY   1.2

Write down your thoughts and feelings about research. Do you regard research in a positive or negative way? What is your current level of knowledge about research?

In health care, research is everyone's business, whatever their role. Having knowledge and understanding of research and evidence-based practice is as important as knowing about other key subject areas such as physiology, psychology and pharmacology. Indeed, it could be argued that research is the most important subject of all. It is not a stand-alone subject; it is integral to and in many cases is at the foundation of all other types of nursing and midwifery knowledge (Figure 1.1). Research should therefore be at the heart of care.

We acknowledge that there can be uncertainty amongst some nurses and midwives regarding research and evidence-based practice. This may be for a number of reasons. The nature of education has evolved considerably over the last decade and nurses and midwives undertaking pre-registration programmes in recent years will almost certainly have studied evidence-based practice or research methods. However, for those who qualified longer ago, these subjects may be unfamiliar territory, which in turn may lead to a lack of confidence (Bohman et al., 2013; Evans et al., 2014). Conversely, those who have studied evidence-based practice or research methods in more recent years may still feel uncertain about them because of the way they were originally taught or because of the seemingly over-complex nature of research and the complicated language that it can involve. It is also possible that some nurses and midwives are suspicious of research (Morse, 2006). To some extent, this view may arise from the widespread reporting of research that is subsequently found to be erroneous (Wakefield et al., 1998). Alternatively some may regard research as being a threat to traditional nursing and midwifery knowledge, values and ways of working and see it

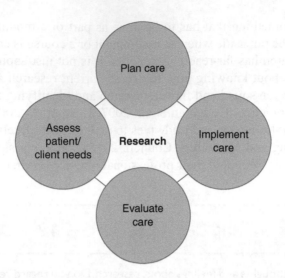

Figure 1.1   Research underpinning patient/client care

as something that is imposed by others in positions of authority. These attitudes may impact upon the attempts of others to use research in their practice. For example, a recent Scandinavian study has shown that whilst newly qualified nurses had a positive approach to research, their use of research findings in their practice was limited (Wangensteen et al., 2011). The importance of strong leadership and a supportive clinical environment in the facilitation of evidence-based practice has been identified (Wangensteen et al., 2011; Bohman et al., 2013).

Website activity 1.3

Whatever the case, it seems that some nurses and midwives feel uncomfortable about research and may try to avoid it as much as possible. Whilst one of the key aims of this book is to demystify the concepts and principles of research methods and evidence-based practice, we also believe that we all know more about research than we perhaps realise. We would suggest that we are all, albeit perhaps unknowingly, 'everyday researchers'. We will have all, at some point in our lives, found ourselves in a new situation; for example, think about a time when, as part of your nursing or midwifery education, you were allocated to a placement where you had not previously worked. In the time leading up to your first day there, you will have carried out a range of 'research' activities to find out about the placement. You might have investigated the best way to get there, your objective being to find the shortest, easiest, quickest or cheapest route. You might have asked others who had previously been on placement there, 'what are the staff like?' in an attempt to find out how you will be treated or how the staff will expect you to behave. You might also have found out about the illnesses, problems or needs that the patients or clients in that care setting have, to increase your level of knowledge so that you felt more confident about the placement. You probably did not regard any of these activities as being research at the time and these activities almost certainly will not completely match our definition of research. Nevertheless, you will have used some of the principles and elements of research in your investigations. When we come to review research methods and designs in later chapters (7, 8, 9 and 11) there will be some aspects with which you are already familiar.

THINK POINT ACTIVITY   1.3

Think of other examples where you have been an 'everyday' researcher. Try to think of examples away from the health care setting. What was it that you wanted to find out? How did you go about finding the required information? Did you find out what you wanted to know?

WHY DO WE NEED NURSING AND MIDWIFERY RESEARCH?

Nursing and midwifery practice must be underpinned by the best evidence that is available. Wherever possible, this evidence should be research-based. Some of the reasons why we need nursing and midwifery research are identified here; these will be explored in greater depth in the following chapter:

- to ensure the delivery of safe, effective, high quality care
- to provide a rationale and justification for decisions about care delivery
- to enable patients, clients and families to make informed decisions about their care
- to maximise patient and client outcomes
- to facilitate patient and client satisfaction
- to support the development, evaluation and on-going improvement of care
- to meet clinical governance requirements
- to ensure the delivery of cost-effective care
- to ensure that the ethical, moral and professional responsibilities of nurses and midwives are addressed
- to reduce the risk of litigation for individual practitioners and the wider service
- to ensure nurses and midwives retain a professional identity within the provision of health care
- to facilitate the autonomy of nurses and midwives.

EVIDENCE-BASED PRACTICE

Evidence-based practice is a structured and objective approach to determine the best evidence upon which care should be based. The best research evidence is one of the four essential components of evidence-based practice (see Figure 1.2). The other three elements are the values and preferences of the patient or client about their care, the knowledge and expertise of the practitioner and the resources available (see Chapter 2).

To ensure that the needs of patients, clients and their families are met, nurses and midwives must be able to identify actual and potential problems and through negotiation with the patient or client implement care that minimises, solves or averts

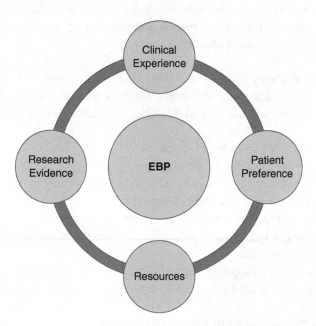

Figure 1.2   The essential components of evidence-based practice

those problems, utilising resources as appropriate. In order to ensure that they are using the best research evidence to inform appropriate decisions about care, nurses and midwives must be 'research-aware'. They must be able to access and understand research, discriminate between sound and flawed research and identify the best research evidence available.

NURSING AND MIDWIFERY RESEARCH: WHERE WE STARTED AND WHERE WE ARE NOW

The history of the development of nursing and midwifery research in the UK is intertwined with the gradual move towards the recognition of their professional status, developments in nursing and midwifery education and the move away from medical dominance over all aspects of nursing and midwifery practice (Bohman et al., 2013). In order to understand where we have come from and where we are now regarding nursing and midwifery research, we need to explore the impact of these other factors over time.

Much health care research over the last century consisted of medically orientated studies that involved numbers, measurement and statistics. These studies were undertaken by doctors to determine the underlying causes of disease and the most effective forms of treatments. Similarly nursing and midwifery curricula in the early part of the twentieth century were developed in an era of medical dominance whereby nurses and midwives were taught predominantly by doctors, and knowledge of any value to them was regarded as being simplified medical knowledge (Yuill, 2012).

Those who led the drive for nursing and midwifery to be accepted as professions at the beginning of the twentieth century recognised the need for nurses and midwives to take control of their education (Hull and Jones, 2012). Fundamental to this was the need for a unique body of knowledge that would be recognised by others, particularly medicine and academia. In the pursuit of this knowledge, early nursing and midwifery research was almost exclusively undertaken following the methods and designs used by medicine. Indeed, Florence Nightingale is often credited with being one of the first proponents of using 'scientific data' to inform nursing and midwifery practice (Attewell, 2005). She collected information about the impact of the environment on mortality and morbidity, analysed this information and used the statistics she produced to support her recommendations for changes to the delivery of care and service provision. Nightingale's work was not confined to nursing. For example, she identified the link between infection, disease and higher maternal mortality rates. To facilitate the further development of nursing and midwifery care, Nightingale advocated the collection and analysis of patient **data**. As a consequence of this early adoption of the 'scientific' approach, it has been suggested that the female professions of nursing and midwifery had to comply with male dominated medical ideology in order to be accepted, albeit as an adjunct to medicine (Rees, 2012). This gender argument is often used when the nursing and midwifery professions attempt to explain their history, subservience to medicine, their relatively slow development as profession and limited research base (Loke et al., 2014).

At the beginning of the twentieth century, nurses and midwives began to assume control of their professional identity and education. Landmark events in this journey include the 1902 Midwives Act (Hunter and Borsay, 2012), which secured the education and regulation of midwives. For nurses this occurred in 1919 with the Nurses Registration Act (Hunter and Borsay, 2012). The Second World War (1939–1945) and the establishment of the National Health Service (NHS) in 1948 brought further changes in attitudes. This included rapid development in technologies, treatments and interventions, and increasing numbers of patients and clients who more readily expressed knowledge and views about their care and challenged opinions (van Bekkum and Hilton, 2013). These changes meant that nurses and midwives had to be well informed about developments in health care and the ways in which care delivery impacted on patients, clients and their families. Role boundaries also began to blur as nurses and midwives began to take over some activities previously performed by doctors (Sleep, 1992). However, they continued to be responsible to doctors and so the medical profession retained its control over nursing and midwifery practice (Keyzer, 1988).

NURSING AND MIDWIFERY RESEARCH: DEVELOPMENTS OVER THE LAST 50 YEARS

Over the last 50 years the professional identifies of nursing and midwifery have evolved and this is reflected in the changes in the configuration and development of new clinical roles, demands placed on the health service and the nature of nursing and midwifery education. The Salmon Report (Ministry of Health and Scottish Home and Health Department, 1966) advocated that nursing, midwifery and medicine should be regarded as independent professions of equal standing (Walby et al., 1994). This was followed by the Briggs Report (Department of Health and Social Security, 1972), which identified that nursing and midwifery needed a research base in order to assume control of its future. More recent decades have seen an increasing number of specialities within health care (Waller, 1998), which have provided nurses and midwives with greater opportunities to focus their career. At the same time, the introduction of the internal market has led to the need to reduce health care expenditure and increase effectiveness (Naughton and Nolan, 1998).

The move away from the hospital-based apprenticeship model pre-registration education to colleges in the 1980s and then to universities in the 1990s has seen the academic level of nursing and midwifery pre-registration programmes rise to Bachelor degree and in some universities, Master's level (Loke et al., 2014). This in turn has impacted in a positive way on the credibility of the professions (Yuill, 2012). In accordance with the directives from the statutory body governing nursing and midwifery education these programmes now include modules on research methods and evidence-based practice, and require students to develop critical thinking and critical appraisal skills. Students are taught to challenge ideas and provide a rationale for the care they provide. Recognition of the notion of life-long learning and the qualified practitioner's professional responsibilities to ensure their practice is evidence-based has also been influential in the development of post-registration education at Bachelor, Master's and PhD level. Research and evidence-based practice are integral to these programmes of study and clinical practice (Bohman et al., 2013). An increasing number of nurses and midwives now have higher degrees and most of these programmes require the student to undertake their own research.

From the 1970s onwards the volume of nursing and midwifery research has increased albeit that initially this was mostly undertaken by those in academia and studies focused on the professions themselves rather than patient care (English, 1994). Nevertheless, as research-based knowledge developed during the 1990s it was recognised that nursing and midwifery research needed to move away from the medical model and use a broader range of research methods and designs (Walsh and Downe, 2006; Van Bekkum and Hilton, 2013). This was partly because of the perceived need to move away from medical control and also because it was realised that much of the nature of nursing and midwifery does not lend itself to the quantifiable measurement that is generally associated with medical research (Jennings, 1986; Sleep, 1992).

Other factors have also been influential in the development of nursing and midwifery research over the last few decades. During the 1970s and 1980s social scientists such as Oakley and Kitzinger began to explore issues that impinged upon nursing and midwifery practice and these gave an insight into not only what research could show us but also ways in which the provision of care could be improved (Allotey et al., 2012). Key nursing and midwifery researchers of the 1970s and 1980s such as Norton, Hockey, Sleep and Romney became the pioneers and role models that other would-be researchers have subsequently followed. The 1990s saw the start of the upward trend in the appointment of professors of nursing and midwifery and a key remit of these chairs was, and continues to be, to build research capacity (Allotey et al., 2012). The drive towards the generation and implementation of research findings in health care has also been influenced by government directives and initiatives (O'Byrne and Smith, 2010; van Bekkum and Hilton, 2013).

There have also gradually become more opportunities for nurses and midwives to become involved in clinical research albeit that initially this was usually being the data collector for medically focused research. Whilst for some, this reflected the continued dominance of medicine (Sleep, 1992; Loke et al., 2014) it at least meant that nurses and midwives had the opportunity to develop their research skills. The increasing number of clinically based roles with a research component such as specialist or advanced practitioner, consultant nurse or consultant midwife or dedicated research posts have provided

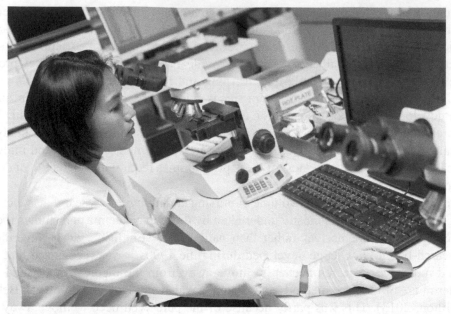

© Milkovasa / Shutterstock

Website
activity 1.4

Website
activity 1.5

Website
activity 1.6

nurses and midwives with further opportunities to gain research experience and in some instances to lead research (Evans et al., 2014). There is also now a wealth of research related resources available to nurses and midwives. These include peer reviewed journals, electronic databases and the evidence-based resources generated by organisations such as the Midwives Information and Resource Service (MIDIRS) and the National Institute for Health Care Excellence (NICE) (Allotey et al., 2012).

As a consequence of these developments, both nursing and midwifery have moved towards being regarded as a profession that is grounded in its own body of knowledge and scientific enquiry. However, the nurses and midwives should not become complacent. As we will see in later chapters, reluctance to implement research findings sometimes persists and there are many aspects of nursing and midwifery practice for which there is currently no research evidence. In addition, whilst there are probably more funding opportunities for nursing and midwifery research now than there were 20 years ago, this is still under-resourced, particularly in comparison to medical research. There is also a need to ensure that skilled researchers retain clinically focused roles, rather than move into academic or management roles. To ensure this is facilitated, dedicated research posts with appropriate scope and financial reward in a supportive environment are required to foster the next generation of nursing and midwifery researchers.

SUMMARY

In this chapter we have established what research is, why it is needed and why nurses and midwives need to be 'research-aware'. We have given an overview of the factors and pressures that have influenced the development of nursing and midwifery research over the last century. We have also introduced the concept of evidence-based practice, which will be explored in more detail in the following chapter.

FURTHER READING

Bohman, D.M., Ericsson, T. and Borglin, G. (2013) Swedish nurses' perception of nursing research and its implementation in clinical practice: a focus group study. *Scandinavian Journal of Caring Sciences*, 27(3): 525–533.

This Swedish paper focuses on many of the issues that we have raised in this chapter. As you read the paper, consider the extent to which the findings apply to your practice and the setting in which you work.

Borsay, A. and Hunter, B. (2012) *Nursing and Midwifery in Britain since 1700*. Basingstoke: Palgrave Macmillan.

This text provides a useful history of the development of the nursing and midwifery professions (particularly Chapters 4, 7 and 9).

> Don't forget to visit https://study.sagepub.com/harveyandland to watch videos, take quizzes and to follow specially designed web activities.

2

EVIDENCE-BASED PRACTICE

Within this chapter the concept of evidence-based practice is explored and compared with traditional methods of building research knowledge. In this chapter we will:

- explore why there has been a move toward evidence-based practice
- define evidence-based practice
- identify the levels of the hierarchy of evidence
- describe the process of evidence-based practice.

WHAT IS EVIDENCE-BASED PRACTICE?

Evidence-based practice is often perceived as a new way of working despite the fact that the origins of the evidence-based medicine movement can be traced back to Archie Cochrane, whose name is now given to the Cochrane Collaboration. In 1971 he was the first to suggest the idea that research should be grouped into summaries of evidence to make medicine more effective and efficient. The wider concept of evidence-based practice was a term developed in the 1990s to embrace elements of patient involvement, resources and clinical judgement (see Box 2.1). EBP has now become an accepted method of working.

As health care practitioners we are faced with the challenge of dispelling medical myths and supporting people in making realistic health care decisions. This can only be done if we understand what good evidence is, how rigorously it is produced and how applicable it is to the person we are caring for. This doesn't mean that each practitioner needs to research individual problems as they arise; on the contrary, this is not efficient or effective unless there really is no available evidence. Instead we need to understand the process of producing good clinical evidence and where it can be found. Developing skills in evidence-based practice is invaluable in a world where there is a wealth of printed information and of course the World Wide Web, which is usually the first port of call for the public when looking up symptoms or treatment for their ailments.

BOX 2.1   DEFINITION OF EVIDENCE-BASED PRACTICE

Evidence-based practice:

> is the integration of best research evidence with clinical expertise and patient values. (Sackett et al., 2001: 1)

Magazines rarely miss an opportunity to offer tips and tricks to achieve the perfect body. Slimming clubs compete by making promises about the new life that can be experienced if only we lost that weight, but what do we *know* about weight reducing diets? The only thing we know for sure is that to lose weight we must use more energy than we consume, but *how* we do this most efficiently and effectively is a subject of much debate. Diets in magazine articles are not usually aimed at the medically obese, but more generally at those who might have a goal of fitting into a wedding outfit or bathing costume, so they can range from the radical to the downright bizarre without too much fear of damaging health because the more radical the diet, the less likely we are to stick to it and reap any potential long term harm. Information contained in newspaper articles can be much more problematic. Reports claiming cures for cancer and other life changing illnesses are a daily phenomenon in the press, but surely it cannot be true that coffee can both cause and cure cancer as one high circulation UK newspaper alternatively claims on a regular basis. Take the news report in Box 2.2. The research study (Cullum et al., 2010) actually reports that compression bandaging is superior to ultrasound therapy to aid venous return, but the 'headline grabber' makes it appear that laughing might be just as important, even though this is not included in the research. Imbalanced reporting like this can be very persuasive and lead people to cling to unrealistic hopes when mixed with the ultimate desire to be thin or cured of an incurable disease.

BOX 2.2   A NEWS REPORT OF A RANDOMISED CONTROLLED TRIAL OF LEG ULCER CARE

LAUGHING 'BETTER THAN LATEST TECHNOLOGY FOR LEG ULCERS' (BBC, 2011)

Hospitals and health clinics are increasingly using low-dose ultrasound for leg ulcers. But the five-year study of 337 patients found it did nothing to speed up recovery, the *British Medical Journal* reported.

(Continued)

(Continued)

'HEARTY CHUCKLE'

Instead, the lead researcher said: 'They key to care with this group of patients is to stimulate blood flow back up the legs to the heart. The best way to do that is with compression bandages and support stocking coupled with advice on diet and exercise.

'Believe it or not, having a really hearty chuckle can help too. This is because laughing gets the diaphragm moving and this plays a vital part in moving blood around the body'.

WHAT CAME BEFORE EVIDENCE-BASED PRACTICE?

A traditional approach to health care practised by professions including medicine, nursing and midwifery over the years held that experience was the key to superior thinking and that this, together with training and common sense were sufficient to make decisions about how patients should be treated. It could be said that common sense is rarely common to all, and from hospital to hospital, in delivery suites, medical wards and operating theatres, variation in practice can occur, quite often dependent upon the opinion of the person in charge. It was also thought that a basic knowledge of the mechanisms of disease and principles of care would be a sufficiently good guide for practice but in fact it has led to some live saving therapies being withheld for years whilst ineffective or dangerous interventions continued long after there was good evidence to abandon them.

Take anti-thrombolytic therapy – 'clot busting' drugs. In 1992, an analysis of several randomised controlled trials established that a reduction in death by approximately 20% was achievable using anti-thrombolytics. A further 14 reviews of similar research did not mention the treatment or felt it was still experimental. This disagreement meant that it took a total of 25 years before anti-thrombolytic therapy was introduced as routine treatment and it doesn't take a great mathematician to work out how many lives might have been saved during this period if the therapy had been adopted earlier.

The problem with medicine it seems was that individual research studies of varying size and quality would demonstrate different findings and this ranged over a wide number of treatment areas. This made it possible that clinicians would pick their favourite treatments and justify them according to the particular paper that supported their belief, something that members of the public are minded to do when they bring newspaper clippings or website addresses to consultations. It became clear that something else was needed to improve care and to maximise the effect of research, and EBP takes a more objective approach. Whilst clinical experience and the development of clinical instincts are a crucial part of becoming a competent practitioner, information solely derived from experience and intuition may be misleading. Likewise the study and understanding of basic mechanisms of disease are necessary but on their own not a sufficient guide for clinical practice. Evidence-based practice uses certain 'rules' to interpret the literature to support treatment, and the EBP movement urges us to move from opinion-based decision making to evidence-based decision making.

The basis of evidence-based decision making comprises four elements shown in Figure 2.1. These elements need to be taken into consideration when we make care and treatment decisions.

There are many treatments that we take for granted, for example, pain relief interventions for childbirth, post-surgical pain or chronic pain arising from a long term condition. These interventions work for most of the people most of the time but using an evidence-based decision making model we can see how this intervention can be applied to each individual case (Figure 2.2).

In many routine cases the decision making process is relatively fast and one where there is no real need to investigate the evidence before treatment, but there still exists (and may well always exist) doubt about what constitutes effective treatment for a whole range of health care problems. This is why we need to have a structure to the process of finding the best evidence.

At the beginning of the chapter the traditional method of health care was described as based largely on expertise and opinion, which is viewed by evidence-based practitioners as unsatisfactory *unless there is no other available evidence.* Instead the

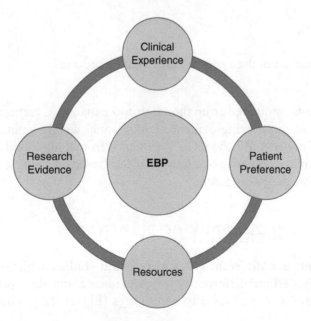

Figure 2.1   Elements of evidence-based practice

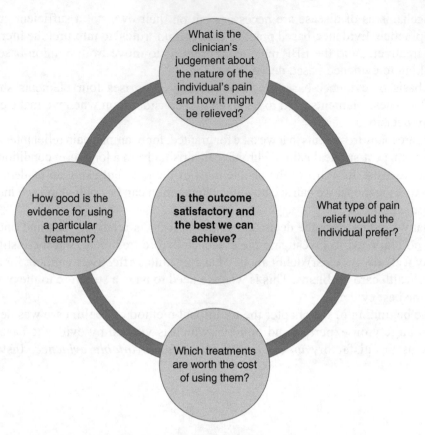

Figure 2.2   An example of the evidence-based decision process

evidence needs to be produced from thorough and exhaustive testing. One of the first lessons to be learnt about using evidence is that equal weight cannot be given to the different types of papers published. Good evidence from a high quality research study should not be dismissed because of a journal article based on a single author's opinion, however persuasive their arguments.

LEVELS OF THE HIERARCHY OF EVIDENCE

To distinguish between different types of research studies a hierarchy of evidence has evolved. This defines different types of evidence and then prioritises them in order of **rigour** and **generalisability** of findings (Figure 2.3). These are explained in turn below.

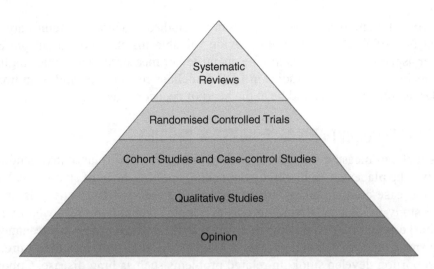

Figure 2.3 The hierarchy of evidence

LEVEL ONE: OPINION

At the base of the hierarchy of evidence is opinion. We all have opinions about the way the world works and perhaps solutions to its problems, and if we all agreed about this then it may be a better place. However, people seldom agree about the most basic ideas, so it is no wonder that health care practitioners fail to agree on aspects of care. This produces variation in practice and in the end we never get to find out whose opinion is the most useful. That said, there are many instances where the research evidence does not exist and while we wait for it to be produced we have no choice but to rely on opinion, but using an evidence-based approach that opinion needs to be formed by consensus from experts. Evidence-based guidelines will often include elements of expert opinion, but we need to acknowledge that guidelines are meant to be evolutionary and changed when new evidence is established. For example, the Scottish Intercollegiate Guidelines Network (2012) guideline for the management of perinatal mood disorders suggests that all pregnant women should be asked about family history of bipolar disorder in order to predict and reduce antenatal risk. Whilst there is no empirical research as yet to support the idea that the risk is increased if there is a family history, experts who developed the guideline are of the collective opinion that there may be a link.

LEVEL TWO: QUALITATIVE STUDIES

Qualitative studies form the next layer. Qualitative researchers may be unhappy at the thought that such studies are placed lower in the hierarchy than other types of studies, but the EBP model is oriented towards effective interventions, which are best determined by experimental and other types of quantitative studies. Qualitative studies are still an essential part of EBP as they often provide valuable insight into patient preferences and other aspects of care that cannot be quantified or measured in any meaningful way. The inclusion of qualitative studies in EBP guidelines reflects this and is an important reminder that the patient should be at the heart of decision making.

LEVEL THREE: COHORT AND CASE-CONTROL STUDIES

Studies that can measure the effectiveness of interventions (quantitative studies) can themselves be placed into a hierarchy depending upon the level of rigour involved and cohort and case-control studies are examples of these. A **cohort study** is an observational study in which a defined group of people (a cohort) is followed over time. The cohort can be followed prospectively, that is, the defined group, say teenagers who take up smoking, are followed up over a regular period of time into the future, to see what proportion develop smoking related problems such as lung disease. Cohorts can also be reviewed retrospectively so that adults who have lung disease can be assessed as to the proportion that might have developed it as a result of taking up smoking as a teenager. The rationale for this type of design is that it is not always appropriate or ethical to 'experiment' on people, for example, to make a particular group smoke in order to compare them to a similar group who do not to see which group develops a greater proportion of lung disease. In addition cohorts can reflect an element of time, which is a useful epidemiological resource (epidemiology is the study of populations rather than individuals). Examples of prospective and retrospective cohorts can be found in the further reading list.

Case-control studies are retrospective epidemiological studies where people (cases) who have contracted a particular disease are compared with a similar group who did not catch the disease. Case series studies are a description of more than one case, for example, a review of results of an HIV screening programme from which an overview of the spread of HIV/AIDS could be plotted.

LEVEL FOUR: RANDOMISED CONTROLLED TRIALS

As evidence-based models focus on the effectiveness of interventions, the gold standard for testing these is a randomised controlled trial (RCT). These evaluate interventions by comparing two or more treatments using a strict scientific process. When used to test treatments in the real world, the term **controlled clinical trial** (CCT) is often used. There are also terms used to define specific types of RCT, such as a double blind trial or prospective randomised trial, but all of these come under the umbrella of an experimental approach and are discussed in greater detail in Chapter 7. The principle of an RCT is to conduct a **fair test** of treatments to determine which is the most effective. This is done by controlling the research environment as much as possible to minimise the occurrence of **bias**, which might lead the researcher to make the wrong conclusions and to exclude the possibility of a 'chance' result, which again may lead to misleading results.

LEVEL FIVE: SYSTEMATIC REVIEWS

Single RCTs may not always provide a clear answer about the usefulness of an intervention, either because they are not large enough or may not represent high quality research. In this case it may be necessary to collate all the studies that address the same research question and analyse them *en masse* to see if they could provide a clearer answer. This approach is called a systematic review and involves following a very strict set of procedures to analyse existing research rather than collecting new (primary) data. The systematic review process is explained in Chapter 10 and is considered the best method of resolving therapeutic dilemmas. At the top of the hierarchy, systematic reviews can produce overwhelming evidence in favour of the use of a particular treatment or intervention that might resolve that dilemma; the review of anti-thrombolytics therapy described earlier is an example of this.

The hierarchy of evidence is a guide that classifies different types of research and indicates, for example, that if there is a high quality systematic review demonstrating that a particular treatment is effective, practitioners should not be tempted to adopt a different treatment found from results of a cohort study. Instead practitioners should always begin to look for effective treatments initially from systematic reviews, but if none is found then to follow the hierarchy down until appropriate evidence is found. This may seem an onerous task but in fact this is exactly how evidence-based guidelines are produced. This type of guideline is constructed by making a thorough investigation of all the evidence on a particular topic and placing it all together as a ready to go guide, but if practitioners are to trust the guidance that is given, then it is important to understand how rigorously it is produced.

THE PROCESS OF EVIDENCE-BASED PRACTICE: KEY STEPS TO FOLLOW

The process of identifying appropriate evidence has been developed into a structured process which always begins and ends with the patient (Figure 2.4).

It is essential that this process is detailed and transparent because:

- any flaws in the process can be identified that might lead to the wrong conclusions
- EBP is a continuous process and as new treatments are developed they will need testing against current ones. Having established a robust and transparent process for this means that evidence is produced incrementally and not on a trial and error basis.

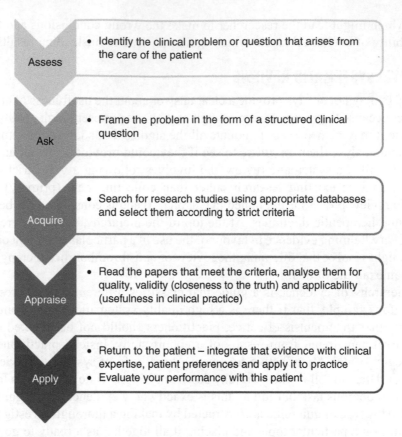

Figure 2.4   The evidence-based practice process

ASSESS

Assessment of the individual is fundamental in designing appropriate care. Experienced health care professionals are adept at identifying and managing routine problems, for example, if someone is dehydrated additional fluids will be introduced, or if their blood pressure is high, they can be given medication. Most of the time this diagnosis and treatment are something that can be done without the need to consult research evidence, but on occasion there is no clear indication of what the best treatment might be so assessment is equally important in the search for research evidence. Taking the earlier example of appropriate pain relief, imagine a clinical scenario where a pregnant woman who has opted for a home birth is considering her options for pain relief during labour. She has some literature on Transcutaneous Electronic Nerve Stimulation (TENS) and would like to try it. We know TENS is already used for pain control in labour, but does it provide effective pain relief? Does it affect the length of labour, interventions

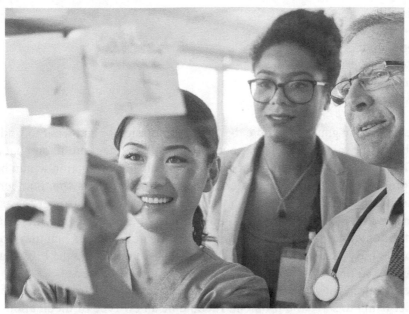

© sturti / iStock

in labour or the wellbeing of mothers and babies? Some colleagues may swear by it, others are indifferent, but personal professional opinion is, as indicated by the hierarchy of evidence, not ideal. It is a trial and error approach, which is poor for so many reasons, particularly where pain relief is concerned. Using the EBP process a full assessment and discussion with the woman will prompt a search for research that will, hopefully, provide an answer to her question.

ASK

Finding the best solution to the problem is impossible if the wrong question is asked, or if that question is 'fuzzy'. So once it is identified, a question needs to be framed in such a way that maximises the chance of finding a good solution. This means that the question needs to be clearly focused and clinically relevant, therefore we need to turn the problem into a simple research question. For example:

> Is transcutaneous electrical nerve stimulation (TENS) effective in providing pain relief during labour?

From this question we need to pick out the elements that are central to finding the answer and configured in a way that we can use it to search databases effectively. This is done by structuring the question in a particular way using the acronym PICO.

That is:

- Population
- Intervention
- Counter Intervention
- Outcome.

A **population** is the group of people that we are interested in and want to find research studies about. The more narrowly defined the population, the more likely that any solution we find will suit our patient group. In our example the population would be women who are pregnant. Others parameters could be identified such as age, number of pregnancies or home births, but we have to bear in mind that the narrower the population definition the less likely we are to find appropriate studies, whilst on the other hand a broad definition of the population may lead us to research findings that may not entirely suit our patient. By using a set of **inclusion** and **exclusion criteria** the PICO can also be refined further so that only the most relevant literature is retrieved.

The term **intervention** is used to mean any treatment or care option that we want to consider using to solve the problem. It could be a new type of medication, a wound dressing or a psychological intervention such as cognitive behavioural therapy (CBT). In this example it would be TENS. Having decided to look at the use of TENS, we then need to identify an intervention to compare it against (a **counter intervention**) and find studies that involve the use of TENS and the specified counter intervention. The comparison needs to be a fair one – an intervention which we might reasonably use instead. On occasion there is no comparable intervention so we might use 'standard care' or that which is established as current practice as a comparison. For our example we could use natural childbirth; that is, the process of labour and delivery not assisted by any pharmaceutical intervention.

Finally we need to identify an **outcome**; this should be aligned to the solution we hope to find and as close to the woman's wishes as possible. A good outcome for her would be that during labour she would be not need any form of pharmacological pain relief, but she would also like a safe delivery without mechanical intervention and not to have a longer labour than she might without TENS. It is important that we identify a single, primary outcome, one which is the main purpose of our quest for a solution. In this example it might be that not using gas and air, pethidine (Demerol) or having an epidural is the woman's main aim. It is essential that the primary outcome is measurable, otherwise there is no way to establish which intervention is best. The way to measure the outcome in our example is to count how many women resort to pharmacological pain relief in the TENS group of the research study and compare this with how many women resort to similar measures in the natural childbirth group. Determining a numerical difference between the two groups will tell us whether TENS is a good alternative. Research papers often include more than one outcome and we know that the woman in our example is also interested in whether TENS will affect the length of her labour and whether she might need a forceps delivery, so whilst searching for the evidence on TENS we will bear this in mind.

The PICO acronym is used to locate systematic reviews and RCTs but by altering it slightly it can be used to find different types of research questions. A PICOD for example includes an extra parameter – design – which would be used when we are certain that there are no systematic reviews or RCTs and therefore a search for cohort or case studies or surveys may be necessary. Only one type of design at a time should be used in a PICOD, it is impossible to compare the findings of a cohort study with a questionnaire survey. Equally, for a search of qualitative studies the inclusion of a comparison may not be relevant, so the acronym becomes PIO. PIOD may also be used; the addition of the 'D' denotes the *type* of qualitative design, for example, phenomenological or ethnographic studies (see Chapter 5),

---

THINK POINT ACTIVITY   2.1

Turn the following research question into a PICO:

In patients with opioid induced nausea and vomiting, which is the most effective anti-emetic: metoclopramide or haloperidol?

ACQUIRE

PICOs are a useful framework for locating papers that might answer the question posed by providing key search terms. Searching databases can be frustrating at the best of times so the use of explicit terms together with a well-defined search strategy helps filter out a huge amount of irrelevant material and increases the likelihood of finding the best evidence. A full explanation of the process of literature searching can be found in Chapter 13.

ASSESS

The papers that are found as a result of the search then need to be read and critically evaluated. This is a structured process which involves two elements:

1 An evaluation of the quality of the study.
2 The clinical significance of the findings.

The quality of a study is measured by assessing how closely the **research design** explained in the paper matches the standard convention for reporting that type of study.

This is to reassure ourselves that if the design is explicit and robust, we can then be more confident in the findings. The findings then need to be evaluated as to their clinical significance, in other words whether the paper gives an indication of whether or not the treatment is useful. Single studies may not provide an unequivocal answer on their own, so on occasion a third element is needed, an integration of the findings from several high quality studies, which would involve a process called a **meta-analysis**. The skill of **critical appraisal** and meta-analysis is explained in Chapter 10.

APPLY

Through this exhaustive process we hope to uncover a relevant solution to the problem posed and then return to our clinical scenario to determine whether it can be applied. Drawing together all parts of the EBP decision making process, the evidence has been retrieved, a clinical judgement can be made as to whether it can be applied and appropriately resourced and whether the patient (in our example the pregnant woman) finds the solution acceptable.

THINK POINT ACTIVITY   2.2

To find the answer to question of whether TENS is useful for the management of pain in labour visit the Cochrane library and read the following systematic review:

Dowsell, T., Bedwell, C., Lavender, T. and Neilson, J.P (2009) Transcutaneous electrical nerve stimulation (TENS) for pain management in labour. *Cochrane Database of Systematic Reviews*, Issue 2, Art. No.: CD007214. DOI: 10.1002/14651858. CD007214.pub2.

The process of retrieving evidence may seem daunting, but it has to be emphasised that in practice, the clinical health care professional should not be expected to undertake this themselves. It is estimated that over 2 million biomedical articles are published each year in 2,000 biomedical journals and 400 nursing and midwifery journals. A practitioner would need to read around 19 articles a day, 365 days a year to keep up with their specialist topic alone. Most of these articles are based on opinion or are of dubious scientific quality, but by adopting an evidenced-based approach a practitioner can acquire relevant, clinical information by using the many resources freely available on the Internet.

Website activity 2.1

SUMMARY

Using an evidence base for making decisions has now filtered through many areas of everyday life, for example, we have become familiar with evidence-based social work and evidence-based architecture. Evidence-based nursing and midwifery has taken some time to be adopted but it is clear that this model is here to stay. Effective, compassionate care that meets patient needs requires sound research evidence which tells us what does and does not work, where it works best and with whom. In summary, nurses and midwives must embrace scientific, quantitative evidence, acquire the skills to evaluate it and design quantitative studies that could assist in improving many aspects of care.

FURTHER READING

Barker, J. (2013) *Evidence-Based Practice for Nurses*. London: Sage Publications.

Providing both the theoretical background and practical applications of evidence-based practice, this book guides you through the process of identifying, appraising and applying evidence in nursing practice and prepares students for applying EBP skills in the classroom and on clinical placements.

McCow, J., Yevchak, A. and Lewis, P. (2014) A prospective cohort study examining the preferred learning styles of acute care registered nurses. *Nurse Education in Practice*, 14: 170–175.

This paper provides an example of a prospective cohort study on the preferred learning styles of registered nurses.

Evidence Based Nursing is a quarterly published journal from the BMJ that selects health related literature research studies and reviews that report important advances relevant to best nursing practice.

For a guide to EBP for nurses by nurses see the Academy of Medical-Surgical Nurses (AMSN) website: www.amsn.org/practice-resources/evidence-based-practice.

Schreuders, L.W., Bremner, A.P., Geelhoed, E. and Finn, J. (2014) Using linked hospitalisation data to detect nursing sensitive outcomes: a retrospective cohort study. *International Journal of Nursing Studies*, 51(3): 470–478.

This research explores the effect of using linked hospitalisation data on estimated incidence rates of several nursing sensitive outcomes by retrospectively evaluating relevant patient disease information.

Don't forget to visit https://study.sagepub.com/harveyandland to watch videos, take quizzes and to follow specially designed web activities.

3

THE DEVELOPMENT OF NURSING AND MIDWIFERY KNOWLEDGE

Within this chapter we will consider where nursing and midwifery knowledge comes from and what shapes this knowledge. In this chapter we will:

- identify the sources of nursing and midwifery knowledge
- establish the important role that research plays in the development of nursing and midwifery knowledge
- explore the three main research paradigms of positivism, interpretivism and pragmatism; this exploration will include the development of the paradigms over time, their assumptions, their values and the research approaches with which they are associated
- consider alternative, less common research paradigms such as post-positivism and feminism
- review the influence that research paradigms have on nursing and midwifery research
- examine the tensions between the paradigms of positivism, interpretivism and pragmatism.

SOURCES OF KNOWLEDGE FOR NURSING AND MIDWIFERY

Although this is a book about research and evidence-based practice, it is important to place this source of knowledge in the context of other types of nursing and midwifery knowledge. We will review these other sources and in doing this we will see that there is some overlap between the different types of knowledge (see Figure 3.1). However, when reviewing the sources of knowledge separately it is clear that they vary in their reliability and appropriateness. These are important factors to consider when using knowledge to support the decisions we make about the provision of care for patients, clients and their families.

Think about a time when, as a student, you went to work on a new placement. You almost certainly at some point asked your mentor or a member of staff, 'why do you do that this way here?' This could have been a question about the type of dressings used, routes and frequencies for taking temperatures or perhaps the visiting policy for family and friends. You may have asked the question because this was the first time you had encountered that particular aspect of care or you may have been told to use a different care strategy on a previous placement. Alternatively if you are a qualified nurse or midwife you may have been on the receiving end and have been challenged by students, patients, clients or relatives about your practice. These questions can reveal some uncomfortable truths when we examine the reasons why we do what we do, in other words the sources of the nursing and midwifery knowledge that underpins our practice.

THINK POINT ACTIVITY   3.1

Make a list of the different sources of nursing or midwifery knowledge. To help you do this, think about the types of knowledge that you have acquired that informs your practice. Where does this knowledge come from? Think also about the senior nurses and midwives that you have worked with. What informs their practice?

TRADITIONAL KNOWLEDGE

In the early decades of the twentieth century most nursing and midwifery practice was based on traditionally held beliefs about the best way to care for patients and clients. Over time, these beliefs became accepted truths and this knowledge was passed on to other nurses and midwives through word-of-mouth, custom and practice and socialisation. Once acquired, this knowledge became comfortable and familiar. Possessing that knowledge also created a sense of identity, empowerment and belonging amongst nurses and midwives.

However, practice based solely on tradition can lead to entrenched ways of working that perpetuate over time. There is little scope to question the knowledge base or change practice. As a consequence, this can lead to ritualistic ways of working that are not scrutinised, challenged or tested. This culture was able to persist at a time when nurses and midwives were not taught to challenge the knowledge base or those in positions of authority. Indeed if a practice was questioned the likely response would be 'because we've always done it this way'. Moving away from the comfortable security of practice based on traditional knowledge can be difficult for practitioners. Accepting that what you have been doing up to now has been ineffective, inappropriate and in some cases harmful, can lead to reluctance to acknowledge the need for change.

When we look back now, we can identify many examples of strange traditional or ritualistic practices from the past that were based on what we now realise is dubious evidence. Examples could include putting a handful of salt in bath water to promote healing, giving women an enema prior to childbirth, preventing parents from visiting their child in hospital or carrying out four-hourly observations of temperature, pulse and respirations on patients who were hospitalised solely because of mental health problems. We would like to think that practice is no longer based upon traditional knowledge that although accepted over time, is without any other foundation. However, it is unlikely that this is the case.

THINK POINT ACTIVITY   3.2

Identify examples of practice that are based solely on traditional knowledge. These might be examples from the past or from practice that you have personally encountered. How were the practices that you have identified able to perpetuate?

PERSONAL KNOWLEDGE

Personal knowledge is a source of knowledge developed by individual nurses and midwives through their experience and expertise over time and can therefore be enhanced through reflection on practice. Practitioners may also draw on knowledge, experience and expertise developed outside the health care system that they feel is relevant to their practice. Nurses and midwives may therefore believe that they have developed a knowledge base that has been acquired through the 'wisdom of experience'. These practitioners may also be regarded by their colleagues, patients, clients and relatives as being an 'expert'. The extent to which individuals are able to exert the wisdom of their experience will be determined by the position of power or authority that they hold. The stronger their position of power, the more senior their role or the higher their authority, the more likely that the knowledge they use to inform practice will go unchallenged. In the past, care was commonly delivered in accordance with the senior nurse or midwife's wishes: 'Sister likes it done that way'. Whilst we have hopefully moved away from such dominance, it may still be the case that some senior nurses and midwives are not challenged about the personal knowledge they use to make decisions about care.

As we have seen in Chapters 1 and 2, personal knowledge in the form of clinical experience and expertise is one of the four components required for evidence-based practice. However, it should not be used on its own as a source of knowledge. Using just personal knowledge to inform practice may lead to complacency and flawed judgements. In utilising personal knowledge practitioners may simply be drawing on traditional ways of working. In addition, having lengthy clinical experience and having a senior role does not necessarily mean that a practitioner is drawing on the most appropriate knowledge to inform their practice. This is because the knowledge that they have acquired through experience in one situation may not apply in another. Indeed, drawing exclusively on personal knowledge could lead to the perpetuation of poor, inappropriate or even harmful care. It may also mislead students, colleagues, patients, clients and relatives. For example, a nurse may believe through her years of experience that she has developed a dressing technique that promotes wound healing. However, any wound healing that has occurred using her technique may just be coincidental and there may be other tested methods available that lead to more effective wound healing.

THINK POINT ACTIVITY   3.3

Identify examples of practice that you have observed that appeared to be based on personal knowledge. Was the practice based solely on personal knowledge or were other sources of knowledge also used?

INTUITION AS A SOURCE OF KNOWLEDGE

Intuition is in many ways similar to personal knowledge. Intuition is used when practitioners believe that they instinctively know the best way to care for patients and clients. This innate form of knowledge is sometimes referred to as having a 'sixth sense', a 'gut feeling' or a 'hunch' about something. Practitioners may base their instinct about something on their previous experience of a similar situation. Alternatively they may encounter a new situation and feel they know instinctively how to deal with it. Either way, practitioners using intuition as a source of knowledge are usually unable to explain, rationalise or justify their actions to others. Nevertheless, we can probably all think of a situation where intuition played a part in informing the decisions that we or others made about care. However, the potential problem of using intuition and nothing else is that whilst you may be right, you may also be wrong. The latter scenario could have serious implications for the patient, client, relatives, the practitioner and the wider service.

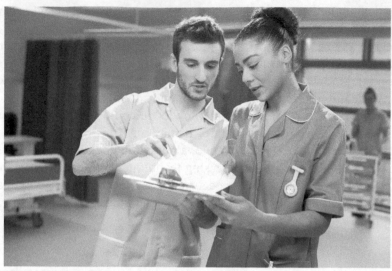

© sturti / iStock

THINK POINT ACTIVITY   3.4

Identify examples of practice that was based solely on intuition. These might be examples from your practice or that of others. Was the practice based solely on intuition or were other sources of knowledge also used?

KNOWLEDGE FROM OTHER DISCIPLINES

We have seen in Chapter 1 that in the early part of the twentieth century it was believed that the knowledge base required for nursing and midwifery practice was simplified medical knowledge (Jolley, 1987; Yuill, 2012). Although there has been a move away from medical dominance since then, knowledge from other disciplines quite rightly continues to inform nursing and midwifery practice. These other disciplines include psychology, human biology, sociology, medicine, pharmacology and physiology. The range of disciplines illustrates the diverse, complex and holistic nature of nursing and midwifery practice. However, if knowledge from other disciplines is used to inform nursing and midwifery practice it should not be directly lifted. It is imperative that it is *applied* to nursing and midwifery practice to ensure the problems and needs of individual patients, clients and families are met. It is also important that the professions of nursing and midwifery sustain their own identity by continuing to generate their own body of knowledge rather than relying solely on knowledge taken from a mix of other disciplines.

THINK POINT ACTIVITY   3.5

Identify examples of practice that was based on knowledge acquired from another discipline. These might be examples from your practice or that of others. Was the practice based solely on knowledge from another discipline or was it applied to nursing or midwifery practice?

RESEARCH

Well-conducted research studies provide the most reliable source of knowledge for nursing and midwifery practice. Whilst the other sources of knowledge that we have identified may on occasion have their place, these should always be underpinned by relevant research-based evidence. This will provide a solid foundation

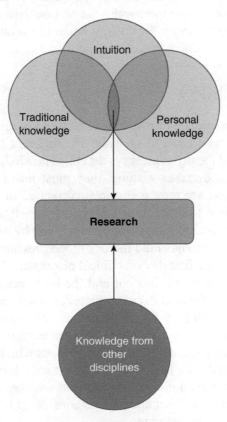

Figure 3.1   Sources of knowledge for nursing and midwifery

upon which care can be rationalised and justified. It will also ensure that practitioners are meeting their professional, ethical, legal and moral responsibilities. As we have seen in Chapter 2, the challenge for nurses and midwives is when it appears that there is no sound research relating to an aspect of care that they provide. In those cases, practitioners must use the 'next best' form of evidence that is available. Beyond that particular situation, the extent to which a practitioner uses research as a source of knowledge provides some insight into their beliefs about the value of research and the culture of the environment in which they work.

THINK POINT ACTIVITY   3.6

Identify examples of practice that was based on research. These might be examples from your practice or that of others.

Go back to the list of the sources of knowledge that you complied for Think point activity 3.1. How does your list compare with what we have described? Do you agree with our list? Is there anything from your list that you would add to ours?

RESEARCH PARADIGMS

Having identified the importance of research as a source of knowledge for nursing and midwifery practice, we now need to consider the different types of knowledge that research can generate and the different ways that this knowledge is produced.

Before a researcher undertakes a study, they must make a number of decisions. Firstly, which **phenomena** are they going to investigate? In the context of research, phenomena is the term used to describe what is being investigated and this can include any event, experience or attribute that can be perceived by the senses. In health care research, examples of phenomena could include blood pressure, wound healing, impact of bereavement or a student's first day on clinical placement. Next, the researcher must decide what exactly they want to find out and the best way of discovering that new knowledge. This will help them to decide which **research methodology** and method to use. The research methodology is the philosophy or principles of an approach to research which determines the way in which a research method is carried out. A research methodology incorporates a number of research methods which are the specific ways in which a study is conducted. The two most common methodologies are qualitative and quantitative. The methodology and method that the researcher chooses should be determined by what they want to find out and what is considered to be the most appropriate way of finding out that new knowledge.

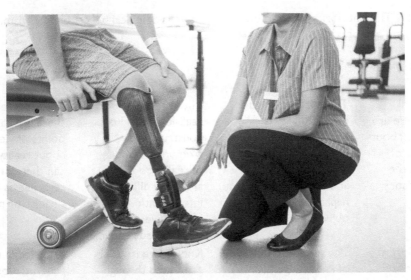

© Johnny Greig / iStock

The ways in which research may be conducted and new knowledge acquired are captured within different research paradigms. The word paradigm comes from the fifteenth-century Greek word *paradeigma* meaning 'show side by side' (Stevenson and Waite, 2011: 1038). In the context of research, a **research paradigm** can be described as being a school of thought, an over-arching view, a set of assumptions or a framework that consists of ideas, beliefs, opinions and values which guide the way researchers carry out a study. These ideas, opinions and values are sometimes referred to as the ontological, epistemological and methodological beliefs and these vary according to the different paradigms (**ontology, epistemology, methodology**) (see Table 3.1). The paradigm therefore provides a philosophical underpinning, a worldview or a general perspective about reality, the nature of knowledge and how it is created. The paradigm also shapes the way a research study is conducted and the way that new knowledge is developed. Each paradigm encapsulates a number of research methods in accordance with the paradigm's view of how knowledge is produced. The most commonly used research paradigms in health care are **positivism**, **interpretivism** (sometimes known as **naturalism** or constructivism) and **pragmatism**. Other less commonly used paradigms include **post-positivism** and **feminism**.

POSITIVISM

With its foundations in the sciences of physics, chemistry and mathematics, early proponents of positivism included philosophers and scientists such as Locke, Spencer, Comte and Newton (Crossan, 2003; Polit and Beck, 2014). Positivists believe that

Table 3.1   The ontological, epistemological and methodological beliefs of positivism, interpretivism and pragmatism

Ideas, opinions and values	Positivism	Interpretivism	Pragmatism
Ontological beliefs: these are the beliefs about the nature of being and the characteristics of reality.	There is one, singular reality. Reality is controlled by universal laws which apply irrespective of time and place. Reality is not haphazard. Reality is objective.	There are multiple realities. Individuals construct their own understanding of reality so there are many different interpretations. There is no universal truth. Reality is subjective.	It is accepted that there are varying points of view about reality. Reality can therefore be regarded as being singular or multiple.
Epistemological beliefs: these are the beliefs about the nature of knowledge and how it is generated.	The generation of knowledge is not influenced by the researcher. The researcher can therefore be independent, objective and value free. The researcher is 'outside' the research.	Knowledge is generated through shared understanding between individuals. The researcher's beliefs will influence the research. The researcher is 'inside' the research.	Knowledge can be generated both objectively and subjectively.
Methodological beliefs: these are the beliefs about the way research is conducted and knowledge is created.	The research involves fixed designs with emphasis on measured, quantifiable information. To establish cause and effect the researcher controls and manipulates events or people. Research methods include randomised controlled trials, cohort studies and case studies.	The research involves flexible designs with emphasis on detailed, narrative information. There is no attempt to control or manipulate events or people. Research methods used include phenomenology, ethnography and grounded theory.	The most practical approach is adopted. The researcher selects the most appropriate research method and design in order to address the study's aims and objectives. A variety of qualitative and quantitate research methods can be used.

facts and events do not occur haphazardly or randomly but instead have antecedent or underlying causes (Polit and Beck, 2014). Positivists therefore argue that an objective reality exists which is independent of human behaviour (Crossan, 2003). Advocates of positivism believe that measurable, objective and generalisable data are required in the generation and dissemination of new knowledge (Doyle et al., 2009). Positivists aim to be objective in their pursuit of knowledge and research undertaken within this paradigm uses quantitative approaches (Weaver and Olson, 2006). The key features of **quantitative research** include testing a theory, prediction, measurement and **objectivity** with the aim of explaining causal relationships using research methods involving structured, fixed designs (Ashworth, 2008). In order to achieve this, a reductionist approach is usually adopted. This means that the phenomena under investigation are reduced into manageable constituents so that they become objective, measurable components (Crossan, 2003). To facilitate objectivity the researcher adopts a position of neutrality or detachment during an investigation, 'outside' the research (Coyle, 2007). As a consequence of these features, positivism is often regarded as being the traditional 'scientific' research paradigm.

INTERPRETIVISM

Interpretivism developed as a counter movement to positivism and is based on the view that truth consists of multiple realities that are subjectively perceived by individuals (Denzin and Lincoln, 2011). Interpretivist researchers argue that reality is established and understood through the meanings that individuals generate from their world (Angen, 2000). Within interpretivism **subjectivity** is inevitable, indeed it is desirable. Humans are believed to have individual and often different interpretations about their experiences that are socially constructed (Robson, 2011; Polit and Beck, 2014). Interpretivism therefore places emphasis on understanding the meaning individuals give to their experiences, thoughts and feelings (Weaver and Olson, 2006; Denzin and Lincoln, 2011). As a consequence there is no single interpretation, truth or meaning. However, the notion of 'multiple realities' does not necessarily mean diverse realities. Interpretivists acknowledge that it is quite likely that there will be close similarities between the understanding and meanings of individuals who have encountered the same experience.

Interpretivists reject the view that truth can only be established by quantifiable methods (Robson, 2011). Interpretivists also argue that knowledge generated by obtaining an understanding of an individual's perspective and behaviours should occur in the settings in which they happen (Dykes, 2004; Denzin and Lincoln, 2011). Interpretivists use interactive and flexible qualitative methods, and the knowledge that the study produces may lead to the development of a theory (Weaver and Olson, 2006). Phenomena are explored through the eyes of individuals encountering the issue under investigation often through detailed descriptions of their experiences (Dykes, 2004; Weaver and Olson, 2006). Researchers work closely with participants and are therefore sometimes referred to as being 'inside' the research. By taking this approach, researchers endeavour to attain a relationship of mutual respect with research participants (Weaver and Olson, 2006; Birks et al., 2008). The research findings are the product of this interaction (Polit and Beck, 2014).

PRAGMATISM

Research undertaken within the paradigm of pragmatism aims to seek meaning and the context is also regarded as being important. Researchers who take this approach believe a person's experience is primarily determined by the situation rather than any antecedent causes (Greenwood and Levin, 2011; Creswell, 2014). The paradigm of pragmatism has been described as being the third or middle way between the opposing forces of positivism and interpretivism (Doyle et al., 2009). There are clear differences between the quantitative and qualitative methods that are allied to positivism and interpretivism (Bryman, 2012). Within the paradigm of pragmatism the researcher is able to use aspects of both qualitative and quantitative approaches in a **mixed methods study** because the outcome is more important than the process (Doyle et al., 2009; Creswell and Plano Clark, 2011). This paradigm has therefore been described as being eclectic, practical, logical, intuitive, dynamic and common sense (Doyle et al., 2009; Robson, 2011). Within this paradigm the researcher selects the most appropriate approach in order to address the aims and objectives rather than being constrained by the restrictions of the defined epistemological and ontological beliefs of a particular paradigm (Creswell, 2014; Polit and Beck, 2014). Pragmatism therefore overcomes the limitations of utilising an exclusively positivistic or interpretivist approach (Doyle et al., 2009) and it is argued that the mixed methods approach yields a more complete picture of the phenomena under investigation (Yardley and Bishop, 2008). This is achieved through the facility to collect both qualitative and quantitative data and the researcher's opportunity to adopt both structured and unstructured approaches (Bryman, 2012). Combining qualitative and quantitative methods in this way enables the researcher to draw on the strengths of interpretivism and positivism to measure the same or similar concepts. As a consequence the findings from these different approaches can be expanded, combined and compared. This combining of approaches, or **triangulation**, has the potential to strengthen the overall study if the findings are corroborated through the use of qualitative and quantitative methods (Teddlie and Tashakkori, 2009; Creswell and Plano Clark, 2011; Bryman, 2012).

OTHER RESEARCH PARADIGMS

Website activity 3.1

Although we have focused on positivism, interpretivism and pragmatism, there are other paradigms that influence nursing and midwifery research. We will explore two other paradigms here: post-positivism and feminism. Support for the paradigm post-positivism arose out of criticism of positivism. Whilst positivists maintain that the researcher is independent, objective and 'outside' the research, post-positivists believe that whilst every effort should be made to remain objective, the researcher will to some extent influence the findings. Post-positivistic research retains most of the features of positivism and usually takes a quantitative approach. However, proponents of post-positivism acknowledge that in research involving people it is not always possible to predict events and responses in the same way that a chemist can with chemicals in a test tube. Rather than establishing cause and effect, post-positivists aim to identify correlations or relationships. They endeavour to obtain **probabilistic knowledge,** in other words knowledge that 'probably' explains phenomena. In doing this, post-positivists acknowledge that there will always be some level of uncertainty about the findings.

Proponents of feminism regard the paradigms of positivism and post-positivism as being paternalistic and male-centred (androcentric) and reject them on this basis. To generate knowledge, researchers following the paradigm of feminism aim to work collaboratively with participants and create an atmosphere of cooperation, trust and mutual respect. Participants are encouraged to reflect on their experiences and feelings and this is usually, but not exclusively done using qualitative methods. Because of the collaborative nature of feminism it is particularly suited to exploring participants' experiences of domination, marginalisation, inequality, oppression, discrimination and exploitation. A key feature of this paradigm is to challenge conventional views and empower participants by giving a voice to those whose stories have not previously been heard and are under-represented in research. This paradigm is therefore particularly suited to research involving vulnerable groups and those who are 'invisible' to society. Gender is a central tenant of feminist research and researchers often aim to determine the ways in which perceptions of gender govern the lives of participants. Not surprisingly the majority of research using the paradigm of feminism has involved women and is particularly suited to midwifery and women's health research. However, the paradigm of feminism has also been successfully employed in studies involving other vulnerable groups such as children, immigrant populations and, in some situations, men.

THINK POINT ACTIVITY   3.7

In the context of health care, think of examples of individuals or groups of people who may feel dominated, marginalised, oppressed, discriminated or exploited. Consider whether using the paradigm of feminism would be likely to enable them to tell their stories.

Website
activity 3.2

USING RESEARCH PARADIGMS

You will recall that earlier in this chapter we said that the researcher's choice of method will reflect the underpinning research paradigm. But how are the decisions made about which paradigm and specific method to use? Trying to unravel this can be a bit like untangling the conundrum about the chicken and the egg, in other words, which came first? In deciding which research method to use, in some cases the purpose of the research will identify to the researcher which paradigm is the most appropriate and they will then select a method and design that follows that paradigm. However, in other cases a researcher's beliefs and values about the way in which research should be conducted will determine their preferred paradigm and thereby their preferred research methods. This preference will govern which phenomena they chose to investigate in the first place (see Figure 3.2).

It is likely that we all have a preferred research paradigm, one that we feel most comfortable with. This will be determined by our previous exposure to and experience of research and perhaps to some extent by the settings in which we work and the phenomena that we are interested in. We believe, however, that all research paradigms have something to offer and it is essential that the most appropriate paradigm is followed for each individual study. This means that sometimes researchers have to set aside their preferences if the study they are involved with is carried out following an alternative paradigm.

It is also the case that decisions about which paradigm to follow are not always made consciously by researchers when they embark on a study. This might be because the knowledge and experience that they have developed about research mean that they are able to make these decisions instinctively. However, it should always be possible to identify which paradigmatic stance that a study has followed.

We are aware that research paradigms can be difficult and challenging concepts to grasp. To some, grappling with research paradigms is akin to naval gazing. As you read this section, you may be thinking, do I really need to know this? It might be tempting to try to ignore research paradigms altogether or to focus solely on your preferred paradigm. However, it is important that we understand the paradigms commonly used in

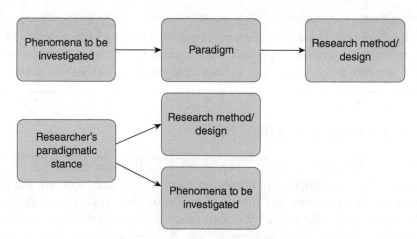

Figure 3.2 Using research paradigms

health care research. This is because any study we encounter will have been underpinned by a paradigm which we should be able to identify. This in turn will tell us about the beliefs, assumptions and values of the researcher.

Website
activity 3.3

RESEARCH PARADIGMS AND NURSING AND MIDWIFERY RESEARCH

In any era, one research paradigm usually dominates. Much health care research over the last century was dominated by the paradigm of positivism and involved medically orientated quantitative studies that were carried out to determine the underlying causes of disease and the most effective forms of treatment. As we identified in Chapter 1, those who led the drive for nursing and midwifery to be accepted as professions recognised the need for a unique body of knowledge that would be acknowledged by others, particularly within medicine and academia. In the pursuit of this knowledge, early nursing and midwifery research was almost exclusively undertaken within the then dominant paradigm of positivism using quantitative methods (Weaver and Olson, 2006).

In the latter half of the twentieth century the use of quantitative methods to investigate human phenomena, particularly in relation to nursing and midwifery practice, began to be questioned. The paradigm of positivism was felt to be inappropriate for studies that aimed to understand and interpret human behaviours and experiences in a detailed way (Crossan, 2003; Mapp, 2008). Consequently other paradigms began to be used and the most frequently adopted alternative was interpretivism. The paradigm of interpretivism was particularly suited to research endeavouring to gain insight into the experiences of patients, clients and their families in order to improve the quality of care (Foss and Ellefsen, 2002; Kingdon, 2004). Interpretivism is especially useful when little is known about a particular phenomenon (Richards, 2009) because it provides a way of exploring human behaviour in an in-depth way without the researcher superimposing their preconceived ideas or becoming entrenched in conventional ways of thinking (Broom and Willis, 2007). Interpretivism is also compatible with the holistic approach to nursing and midwifery care. As a result, **qualitative research** has played an increasingly important role in the evaluation and development of nursing and midwifery practice over the last few decades (Polit and Beck, 2014).

A further more recent paradigm shift has been made in the way that nursing and midwifery research is carried out. The move away from positivism to interpretivism in the latter half of the twentieth century has been followed by a shift towards the use of pragmatism in the past decade (see Figure 3.3). Pragmatism is now rapidly becoming the dominant, yet often understated, paradigm in health care research (Doyle et al., 2009). Pragmatism is particularly suited to nursing and midwifery research because it enables the researcher to investigate complex issues in the most appropriate way. Pragmatism therefore reflects and suits the problem-solving nature of nursing and midwifery practice.

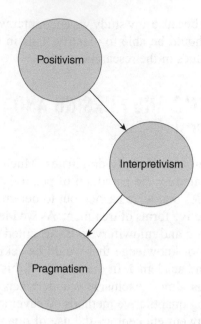

Figure 3.3   The paradigm shift in nursing and midwifery

TENSIONS BETWEEN THE RESEARCH PARADIGMS

We acknowledge that there are opposing views about the value of research paradigms. Some argue that the importance of paradigms has sometimes been over-emphasised (Crossan, 2003; Bryman, 2012; Yardley and Bishop, 2008) and that demarcations between different paradigms are not always clear cut (Foss and Ellefsen, 2002). It has also been argued that focusing on a particular paradigm constrains a person's understanding or acceptance of other perspectives (Dykes, 2004). However, an alternative view is that paradigms help researchers to select the most appropriate method for their research (Crossan, 2003).

There will always be tensions between the opposing paradigms of positivism and interpretivism. Positivists will continue to criticise interpretivism for its lack of objectivity. However, those advocating interpretivism see subjectivity as a key strength and not a weakness. Conversely, interpretivists advocate the holistic approach that interpretivism offers and regard the reductionist approach of positivism as a serious limitation.

Could it therefore be possible that the third or middle way of pragmatism is the perfect answer for nursing and midwifery research? It appears that the answer to this question is no, as pragmatism also has its critics (Morgan, 2007; Bryman, 2012). It has been suggested that the epistemological differences between quantitative and qualitative approaches are irreconcilable and any integration of the two approaches is often done in a superficial way (Mason, 1993; Yardley and Bishop, 2008). In addition, it is argued that

**Website
activity 3.4**

researchers often do not have the skills to use both approaches successfully (Bryman, 2012). The counter argument has been given that qualitative and quantitative approaches are compatible and that the fundamental goals of both approaches – the rigorous, scientific and context-sensitive generation of knowledge – are the same (Yardley and Bishop, 2008; Bryman, 2012). We reiterate our belief that all research paradigms have their place. It is essential that the most appropriate paradigm is followed for an individual study and the choice of paradigm should be determined by what the researcher wants to find out and the most appropriate way of finding out that new knowledge.

Website activity 3.5

SUMMARY

In this chapter we have identified the different sources of nursing and midwifery knowledge. In doing this, we have established the important role that research plays in the development of knowledge. We have also explored research paradigms, particularly positivism, interpretivism and pragmatism. Noting their philosophical differences has emphasised some of the on-going tensions between these research paradigms.

FURTHER READING

Dykes, F. (2004) What are the foundations of qualitative research? in Lavender, T. Edwards, G. Alfirevic, Z. (eds), *Demystifying Qualitative Research in Pregnancy and Childbirth*. Salisbury: MA Healthcare Ltd, pp. 17–34.

Morgan, D.L. (2007) Paradigms lost and pragmatism regained. *Journal of Mixed Methods Research*, 1(1): 48–76.

Weaver, K. and Olson, J.K. (2006) Understanding paradigms used for nursing research. *Journal of Advanced Nursing*, 53(4): 459–469.

These three sources explore the research paradigms and their use in nursing and midwifery research.

Jarvie, I. (2011) Philosophical problems in the social sciences: paradigms, methodology and ontology. In I. Jarvie and J. Zamora-Bonilla (eds), *The SAGE Handbook the Philosophy of Social Sciences*. London: Sage Publications, pp. 1–36.

This source explores some of the challenges and tensions associated with research paradigms.

Houghton, C., Hunter, A. and Meskell, P. (2012) Linking aims, paradigm and method in nursing research. *Nurse Researcher*, 20(2): 34–39.

This paper considers the application of paradigms to research practice.

Don't forget to visit https://study.sagepub.com/harveyandland to watch videos, take quizzes and to follow specially designed web activities.

4

QUANTITATIVE METHODOLOGIES: AN OVERVIEW

In this chapter we provide an overview of quantitative methodologies. We will:

- consider the quantitative methodology in the context of nursing and midwifery research
- explore the key features and the contrasting elements and principles of the quantitative methodology
- identify the research methods commonly allied to this methodology.

As we have seen in Chapter 3, the two main research methodologies are quantitative and qualitative. Over the next two chapters we will explore these approaches to research in more depth. This provides a good opportunity to remind ourselves what the term 'research methodology' means, because it is sometimes confused with 'research method'. However, the meanings of these two terms are inherently different and they should not be used interchangeably. The research methodology is the philosophy or principles of an approach to research which determines the way in which a research method is carried out. A research methodology incorporates a number of research methods, which are the specific ways in which a study is conducted. The research method therefore reflects the key principles of the methodology to which it is allied. Whilst the methods aligned to a particular research methodology have many core similarities in the way a study is conducted, they will also have some important differences that make each one unique. However, their commonalities align them to the same methodology.

In the following sections we will explore the characteristics and contrasting elements of the quantitative methodology. We will also outline the research methods that are allied to this approach. However, these will be explored again in greater depth in Chapters 7 and 9. As we explore the principles and key features of the quantitative methodology we will highlight the strengths and weaknesses of this approach. These have been hotly debated over time and as we shall see, supporters and opponents of this methodology hold strong and often contentious opinions about its merits.

THINK POINT ACTIVITY   4.1

Looking at the word 'quantitative' and make a list of the characteristics and key features that you think these this research methodology has. You may wish to refer to Chapter 3 to help you to complete this task.

The key characteristics of the quantitative research methodology are outlined in Table 4.1.

Table 4.1   Key characteristics of quantitative research methodology

Characteristics	Quantitative methodology
Underpinning paradigm	Positivism
Nature of evidence generated	Objective
Role of theory in relation to the research	Theory testing, deductive reasoning
Aim	Discovery of empirical (facts) evidence
Focus	Narrow, reductionist
Starts with	Hypothesis, null hypothesis or precisely worded research question
Purpose	Assessing cause and effect relationships or correlations
Design	Fixed, structured, pre-planned
Literature review	Supports development of the hypothesis or research question
Pilot study	Carried out with a small sample reflecting the sample for the larger study
Sample	Representative, usually large, size often determined by power calculation
Data collection	Extensive but with a narrow focus, usually under controlled conditions
Data collection tools	Structured, precise, devised before data collection begins
Setting	Controlled environment
Impact of variables	Impact of extraneous variables minimised through control of variables
Format of data	Numerical, quantifiable
Data analysis	Involves use of descriptive or inferential statistics

(Continued)

Table 4.1 (Continued)

Characteristics	Quantitative methodology
Position of the researcher	Outside the research
Presentation of results/findings	Usually referred to as results. Presented numerically using charts, tables and graphs
Specific ethical issues	Ensuring participants understand randomisation, monitoring the impact of the intervention
Criteria for assessing rigour	Validity, reliability
Outcome	Hypothesis is supported or refuted. Research question is answered. Findings generalised to the wider population
Examples of research methods	Experiments (RCTs), cohort studies, case-control studies

QUANTITATIVE METHODOLOGY

As we have seen in Chapters 1 and 3, much health care research during the twentieth century was dominated by the paradigm of positivism and so most research followed the quantitative methodology. Quantitative research measures cause and effect relationships, and **correlation**(s) (associations) between variables and enables researchers to determine the most effective form of intervention or treatment. It is therefore not surprising that health care research was predominantly quantitative particularly during the first half of the twentieth century because health care was progressing at a rapid rate at this time with the drive for better understanding about the causes of diseases, the development of new drugs and other therapies, advances in technologies and, indeed, the formation of the NHS itself. As the motivation to push forward the boundaries of health care continued, so the need for quantitative research was sustained.

In accordance with quantitative methodology the research following this approach begins with a **hypothesis** or a precisely worded research question. A hypothesis is a statement which predicts the relationship between the variables that are to be measured during the study. **Variable**(s) are the characteristics or entities that the researcher is interested in. They are called variables simply because they can vary. Examples of variables could include blood pressure, wound healing, patient satisfaction or birthweight. Within the hypothesis we should be able to identify two particular types of variable: the **independent variable**, the presumed cause, and the **dependent variable**, the presumed effect. The aim of a quantitative study is to test the hypothesis by measuring the predicted cause and effect relationship. In other words the study determines whether the independent variable has caused the dependent variable, the effect; or whether there appears to be a correlation between the cause and effect. For example, a hypothesis could predict that feeding a baby exclusively with mother's breast milk (the independent variable) rather than formula milk leads to a reduced incidence of newborn gastroenteritis (the dependent variable) (see Figure 4.1). The findings of the study will determine whether the hypothesis has been supported, i.e. it is correct, or refuted (rejected), i.e. it is incorrect.

Website activity 4.1

Note here that it is unwise to use the terms 'prove' or 'disprove' when making a statement about the hypothesis. To prove a hypothesis the researcher must have absolute certainty that the independent variable has caused the dependent variable. As we will see in Chapter 7, even when the findings of a study strongly indicate that the suggested cause and effect relationship is correct, there will always be an element of uncertainty, albeit that this may be very small. Therefore 'supported' and 'refuted' are the more appropriate terms to use. In some forms of quantitative research rather than testing cause and effect relationships, the findings identify whether or not there are correlations between variables. Probably the most famous of these is the work led by Richard Doll in the 1950s which showed the relationship between smoking and lung cancer (Doll and Hill, 1950).

The **literature review** has an important function in a quantitative study. Thorough examination of the literature at the outset of the study enables the researcher to review the current body of knowledge and identify any gaps in that knowledge. The literature review therefore helps the researcher to refine and justify the hypothesis or research question for their proposed study. In accordance with quantitative methodology research following this approach has fixed and structured designs. The research usually follows a linear process whereby participants are recruited, data are then collected and finally the data are analysed. The research therefore adopts an orderly and disciplined approach. The specific study design and conduct of the study is planned and finalised before the study begins. The researcher therefore knows exactly what will happen and when during the course of the study. These factors mean that obtaining the required approvals for quantitative research is relatively straightforward assuming

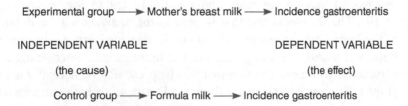

Figure 4.1   The cause and effect relationship between the independent and dependent variable

that those granting the approvals do not have any concerns about what is proposed (see Chapter 18). This is because they will be able to see exactly what the research will involve from start to finish.

Studies following quantitative methodology usually involve a large number of **participants** who are representative of the total population. **Probability sampling methods** are used, which means that potential participants have an equal or random chance of being invited to take part. The exact **sample** size is decided before the study begins and is often determined by a **power calculation**. This tells the researcher the minimum number of participants that are required to measure the impact of the independent variable (Bench et al., 2013). The power calculation therefore ensures that sufficient participants are recruited to reduce the likelihood that the findings are caused by chance (see Chapters 7 and 15). Large-scale quantitative studies may involve participants who are based in a number of different locations, including international settings. To ensure uniformity in the sample, the researcher must establish clear inclusion and exclusion criteria before participant recruitment begins.

Formal instruments are used for data collection. This means that they are structured and precise. The data collection tools are devised before the study begins and will probably be tested in a small-scale **pilot study**. If this indicates that the tools require further development, then they should be retested in a second pilot study before the main study begins. The most commonly used quantitative data collection methods are structured **questionnaires, Likert scales**, checklists and previously validated tools and standard instruments such as psychometric or biophysiological measures. If data collection methods such as **interviews, diaries** and **observation** are used they will be structured in a format to reflect the quantitative nature of the study. For example, closed questions will be used in an interview. Vast quantities of data will usually be generated because of the large number of participants. However, the data will generally be narrow in focus and will either be in numerical format or a format which can easily be converted to numbers; for example, a question in a questionnaire that asks participants how many times they have attended the out-patient department.

Quantitative data analysis involves the use of statistics. There are two types of statistics that might be used. **Descriptive statistics** are measures of central tendency and include the **mean, median** and **mode**. **Inferential statistics** are used when the researcher wishes to make inferences about the findings to the **wider population** (see Chapter 19). The statistical test that is used in the analysis will be determined by the nature of the hypothesis or research question. To assist the data analysis process, the numerical data will usually be computed and the findings calculated using a software package. In the research report, the findings will be presented numerically using charts, tables and graphs. Examples of these are shown in Figure 4.2, which includes a table and charts that present the same information about the number of admissions to a paediatric intensive care unit (PICU) over one year.

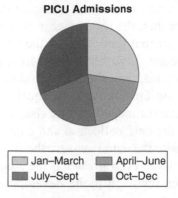

Months	Number of admissions to PICU
January–March	105
April–June	76
July–September	82
October–December	120

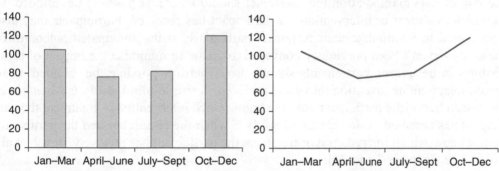

Figure 4.2 Examples of table and charts displaying the same information in different formats

---

THINK POINT ACTIVITY   4.2

Figure 4.2 shows a table and charts which present the same information about the number of admissions to a PICU over one year. Which format do you think presents the information most clearly?

As a consequence of the large, **representative, randomly selected** sample, the researcher should be able to **generalise** or apply the findings to the wider population. The findings will also determine whether the research question has been answered or if the hypothesis (or theory) has been supported or refuted. This is called **deductive reasoning**, which is theory testing.

A key characteristic of quantitative methodology is said to be objectivity. In order to facilitate this, the researcher must endeavour to reduce the risk of bias by minimising the impact that they have on the research. There are a number of ways in which this can be done. If within the research, participants are to receive different treatments or interventions, they should be randomised to determine which option they receive. This means participants have an equal chance of receiving the different options and the researcher (or indeed anyone else) cannot decide which option the participant receives. During the data collection and data analysis processes researchers may be tempted to manipulate the data to ensure the findings support the hypothesis. The temptation to do this could be even greater if the study has been funded by an organisation which has also been involved in the development of the intervention or treatment. To eliminate the risk of data manipulation the researcher should wherever possible be 'blinded' as to which treatment or intervention the participant has received. Participants may also be tempted to manipulate their responses particularly if the anticipated outcomes of the study haven't been previously conveyed to them. To minimise the impact of these changes in behaviour, participants should also, wherever possible, be 'blinded' as to which treatment or invention they have received. A **single-blind study** is when *either* the researcher *or* the participant does not know which intervention or treatment the participant has received. A **double-blind study** is when the researcher *and* the participant do not know which intervention or treatment the participant has received (Bench et al., 2013) (see Chapters 7 and 21).

Quantitative research can present a number of ethical challenges for the researcher. If the study involves randomisation of treatment or interventions it is essential that the researcher ensures that potential participants fully understand what the randomisation process means before they give consent. In other words, participants are aware that they have an equal chance of being allocated the different treatment or intervention options. In some situations, those giving consent may believe that the participant will receive a new treatment when in reality they have an equal chance of this not being the case.

Quantitative research has been very influential in determining the provision of health care. The findings of quantitative studies tell health care practitioners which treatments and interventions they should use. Quantitative studies can also tell health care managers and politicians how health care should be organised and funded. However, quantitative research is not without its critics. A common criticism is its fragmented and reductionist nature (Farrelly, 2013). In other words, quantitative research focuses only on an 'element' or 'part' of something, for example, a person's pain, diet or sleep pattern. Another concern is regarding the imbalance of power between the researcher and the participant because of the **control** that a researcher has over the conduct of the research. However, whilst strategies can be put in place to minimise potential bias from both the researcher and the participant, some would argue that it can be difficult to completely eradicate (Bench et al., 2013).

THINK POINT ACTIVITY   4.3

Summarise what you consider are the key strengths and weaknesses of the quantitative methodology.

EXAMPLES OF QUANTITATIVE RESEARCH METHODS

We will now explore the more commonly used quantitative research methods in nursing and midwifery research. These are:

- randomised controlled trials
- cohort studies
- case-control studies.

We will also consider **surveys** here, because although this method does not always follow quantitative methodology, it usually takes this approach. Whilst we provide an overview of these research methods here, they will be explored in more detail later in Chapters 7 and 9.

RANDOMISED CONTROLLED TRIALS

True experiments or randomised controlled trials are the highest level of quantitative studies. Indeed some regard RCTs as being the gold standard for all research (McCourt, 2005; Bench et al., 2013). The aim of an RCT is to test a hypothesis regarding a treatment or intervention. Half the participants recruited to the study will receive the new treatment or intervention and the remainder will receive the conventional treatment or a **placebo** (a mock or dummy treatment). Those receiving the new treatment or intervention are known as the **experimental group** and those receiving the conventional (usual) or placebo intervention are known as the **control group**. The outcomes for the two groups are compared and the findings will determine whether the hypothesis about the new treatment or intervention has been supported (see Box 4.1).

BOX 4.1   EXAMPLE OF AN RCT

Scientists have developed a new drug to control hypertension. The new drug is the independent variable (cause) and blood pressure is the dependent variable (effect). Participants

(Continued)

(Continued)

meeting predetermined inclusion criteria are recruited to the study. Whilst there are a number of possible RCT designs (Chapter 11) in its most basic format, half the group receive the new drug whilst the remainder receive the conventional treatment. Participant blood pressure levels are monitored over a predetermined period of time and this will reveal whether the new drug is more, less or equally effective as the usual treatment (see Figure 4.3).

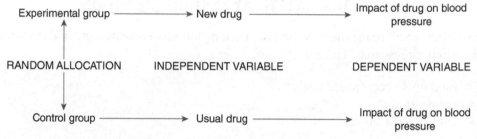

Experimental group ⟶ New drug ⟶ Impact of drug on blood pressure

RANDOM ALLOCATION   INDEPENDENT VARIABLE   DEPENDENT VARIABLE

Control group ⟶ Usual drug ⟶ Impact of drug on blood pressure

Figure 4.3   Illustration of the most basic RCT format

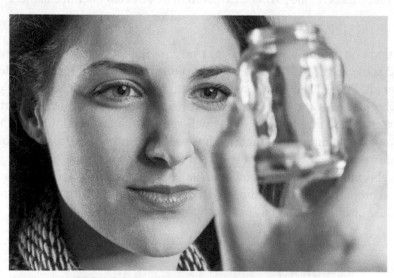

© InnerVisionPRO / iStock

The three essential characteristics of a true experiment (RCT) are:

Website activity 4.2

- randomisation
- manipulation
- control.

Participants are randomised to receive either the experimental or conventional treatment. The independent variable, in our example the drug used to manage hypertension, is manipulated. In an RCT 'control' can be identified in two ways. Firstly, this is the control group against which the findings of the experimental group are compared. It is also the control that the researcher exerts over the study to minimise the impact of other variables (factors) which may influence the findings. This is done by ensuring the conditions under which the study is conducted are as close as possible for both the experimental and control group. There are a number of different RCT designs (see Chapter 11) but the principle, to test the hypothesis using randomisation, **manipulation** and control, remains the same.

CASE-CONTROL STUDIES

Case-control studies and cohort studies are sometimes referred to as **observational studies** or **quasi experiments** (Connelly and Platt, 2014). Quasi means 'as if, almost' (Stevenson and Waite, 2011: 1176) so these two research methods are 'almost' true experiments. However, one of the essential characteristics of a true experiment, either randomisation or control, is missing. These elements are usually missing because of ethical or practical concerns. Consequently these studies are weaker than RCTs but they can reveal correlations between variables.

  Case-control studies compare cases, whereby the researcher compares people with a condition or problem, with people without that condition or problem. This is done retrospectively, in other words, the condition or problem has already occurred. The researcher recruits participants with the problem or condition and then recruits participants to the control group. These participants are as similar to the cases as possible, the difference being that the control group do not have the condition or problem. The differences between the two groups give the researcher an indication of the likely causes of the condition or problem (see Box 4.2).

BOX 4.2   EXAMPLE OF A CASE-CONTROL STUDY

Samina plans to compare mothers whose baby has been born with gastroschisis with mothers whose baby does not have the condition. Samina's research will explore aspects of the mother's pregnancy, rates of exposure and the mother's health with the aim that factors can be identified which explain why some women had a baby with gastroschisis and others did not.

COHORT STUDIES

Cohort studies are conducted prospectively. For this type of study, the researcher has an idea about a possible cause and effect relationship. Participants who are exposed to the presumed cause are recruited and followed up over a period of time to see if they experience or develop the presumed effect. The researcher also recruits and follows up participants who are as similar to the other group as possible, the difference being that the second group are not exposed to the presumed cause. The researcher assumes that the second group will not experience or develop the presumed effect. The findings will confirm whether the researcher's presumption about the cause and effect relationship is correct. Cohort studies generate a stronger form of evidence than case-control studies; however, they are more costly both in terms of time and financially (see Box 4.3).

BOX 4.3   EXAMPLE OF A COHORT STUDY

Samina may believe that smoking during pregnancy increases the likelihood of a mother having a baby with gastroschisis. Pregnant women who smoke will be recruited. The incidence of gastroschisis will be compared with that of a group of pregnant women who are as similar as possible to the first group except for the fact that they do not smoke.

SURVEYS

Survey research usually starts with a research question. It is the most commonly used research method and it usually takes a quantitative approach. Surveys enable researchers to gather information about attitudes, beliefs, behaviours and the prevalence, distribution and incidence of a variable. For example, a researcher may conduct survey research to find out people's opinions about smoking.

BOX 4.4   EXAMPLE ILLUSTRATING THE VALUE OF CONDUCTING A PILOT STUDY

A researcher, having carried out a pilot study, may discover that the instructions on how to complete the questionnaire are unclear and that the questions are ambiguous. The researcher may also discover that they have left insufficient space for participant responses and that the questionnaire does not in fact measure what was intended. So whilst carrying out a pilot study may seem time consuming and costly, it can save the researcher time, money and effort in the long run.

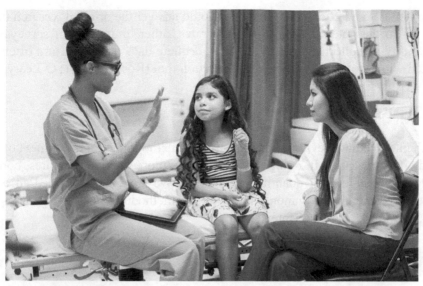

© Steve Debenport / iStock

Surveys can be used to collect data from large samples, often spread over a wide geographical area in a relatively straightforward and inexpensive way. The most commonly used method of data collection is questionnaires, and these should be tested in a small-scale pilot study before being used in the main study. This will provide the researcher with important information about the effectiveness of the questionnaire (see Box 4.4).

The format of the questionnaire will usually reflect a quantitative approach with the use of closed questions, Likert scales and multiple choice type answer options. However, questions adopting a more qualitative format may also be included. Key advantages of questionnaires are that they can protect participant **anonymity** and the participant can take time to think about their responses without intrusion from a researcher. It is important to note here that questionnaires and surveys are not the same thing. A questionnaire is a method of data collection and is a tool that can be used in a number of different research methods. A survey may also involve other methods of data collection such as interviews, diaries and observation.

Defining the **total population** and the sample inclusion and exclusion criteria is crucial when conducting a survey. Probability sampling methods are usually used, which means that the findings can be generalised to the wider population. However, the **response rates** to surveys, particularly postal surveys, can be low. In these cases, it is important to consider why participants did not respond and the possibility that the findings might be different if more participants had responded. Data from surveys will be analysed in accordance with the data type, i.e. quantitatively or qualitatively

Website
activity 4.3

(see Chapters 19 and 20) and the findings should answer the original research question. In addition to the potentially low response rates, other limitations of surveys include the possibility of collecting superficial or inadequate data. This is in turn often closely associated with poor design of the data collection tool (Robson, 2011; O'Leary, 2014).

SUMMARY

In this chapter we have reviewed the quantitative methodology in the context of nursing and midwifery research. In doing this, we have explored the key features, contrasting elements and principles of quantitative research. We have also provided an overview of the research methods commonly allied to this methodology. These methods will be explored in more detail in Chapters 7 and 9.

FURTHER READING

The following sources provide further discussion regarding quantitative approaches to research and their strengths and limitations:

Gray, D.E. (2014) *Doing Research in the Real World* (3rd edn). London: Sage Publications.

A practical guide to the basic theory you need to have considered before you can do anything else. Don't skip this stage, it is very important later on when you are looking at practical methods. See especially Chapter 2, 'Theoretical perspectives and research methodologies', pp. 15–39.

Ingham-Broomfield, R. (2015) A nurse's guide to quantitative research. *Australian Journal of Advanced Nursing*, 32(2): 32–36.

A quick breakdown of quantitative methodologies in nursing research.

Don't forget to visit https://study.sagepub.com/harveyandland to watch videos, take quizzes and to follow specially designed web activities.

5

QUALITATIVE METHODOLOGIES: AN OVERVIEW

In this chapter we provide an overview of qualitative methodologies. We will:

- consider the qualitative methodology in the context of nursing and midwifery research
- explore the key features and the contrasting elements and principles of the qualitative methodology
- identify the research methods commonly allied to this methodology
- explore the notion of 'scientific' research and the implications of the varying views of this on nursing and midwifery research.

As we have seen in Chapter 3, the two main research methodologies are quantitative and qualitative. In the previous chapter we explored quantitative methodologies in detail. It is now the turn of qualitative methodologies. In the following sections we will explore the characteristics and contrasting elements of the qualitative methodology. We will also outline the research methods that are allied to this approach. However, these will be explored again in greater depth in Chapter 8. As we explore the principles and key features of the qualitative methodology we will highlight the strengths and weaknesses of this approach. These have been hotly debated over time and as we shall see, supporters and opponents of this methodology hold strong and often contentious opinions about its merits. We will conclude the chapter by exploring the notion of 'scientific' research and the implications of the varying views of this on nursing and midwifery research.

THINK POINT ACTIVITY   5.1

Look at the word 'qualitative' and make a list of the characteristics and key features that you think this research methodology has. You may wish to refer to Chapter 3 to help you to complete this task.

The key characteristics of the qualitative research methodology are outlined in Table 5.1.

Table 5.1   Key characteristics of the qualitative methodology

Characteristics	Qualitative methodology
Underpinning paradigm	Interpretivism
Nature of evidence generated	Subjective
Role of theory in relation to the research	Theory generated, inductive reasoning
Aim	Discovery of meanings
Focus	Broad, holistic
Starts with	A broad research question, idea, problem or issue to be explored
Purpose	Understanding the meaning of behaviour, social phenomena and their relationships
Design	Flexible, evolving designs
Literature review	Provides a broad overview of the subject
Pilot study	Not carried out. However, experienced researchers may be consulted about aspects of the study
Sample	Small, relevant sample, size usually determined by data saturation
Data collection	Intensive but with a wide focus
Data collection tools	Semi or unstructured, may be devised as the study evolves
Setting	Natural setting
Impact of variables	No attempt to control variables, aim is to understand all factors that may influence the findings
Format of data	Rich, detailed, narrative descriptions
Data analysis	Involves looking for patterns in the data
Position of the researcher	Inside the research
Presentation of results/findings	Usually referred to as findings. Presented as detailed description illustrated with direct quotes or excerpts from field notes
Specific ethical issues	Potential impact of the research on participants and the researcher
Criteria for assessing rigour	Trustworthiness: credibility, dependability, confirmability, transferability, authenticity
Outcome	Research question is answered, issue is explored. Findings are specific to the sample. Theory generated
Examples of research methods	Phenomenology, ethnography, grounded theory

QUALITATIVE METHODOLOGY

Qualitative methodology has become increasingly popular in health research over the last 50 years (Walsh and Downe, 2006; Daly et al., 2007). Qualitative research enables us to gain an understanding of the behaviours, interactions, attitudes, beliefs, experiences and opinions of individuals or groups of people and in so doing we obtain a window into their world. These insights resonate with the fundamental elements and core principles of nursing and midwifery practice: an interest in people, empathy and the notion of holism. In order to achieve insights into the lives of patients, clients, their relatives and our colleagues, research following qualitative methodology usually takes place in the environment where the phenomena under investigation normally occur. For example, if we wanted to find out about the ways in which nurses or midwives interact with each other in a particular clinical setting, our research would be carried out in that location.

Qualitative research generally starts with a broad research question, a problem or an issue that the researcher wants to explore. Consequently, studies following this methodology are particularly suited to exploring phenomena about which little is previously known or reported. A literature review of the subject may be conducted at the start of the study to provide a broad overview of the subject, but the researcher must be careful to ensure that the findings of this review do not unduly influence the way in which they conduct their study. The researcher will return to the literature and use it in a more detailed way to provide a context for their findings (see Chapter 20).

Research methods adopting qualitative methodology have flexible, evolving research designs. This means that the researcher does not always know at the beginning of a qualitative study exactly how they will conduct the research. Participant recruitment, data collection and data analysis often occurs simultaneously. As a consequence, the initial data analysis may suggest to the researcher other, perhaps unexpected issues to explore. This may mean that the researcher recruits additional, more diverse participants and uses alternative methods of data collection. As a consequence of its emergent nature, it can sometimes be difficult for researchers to gain the required approvals to carry out research involving qualitative methods (Robson, 2011).

Studies following qualitative methodology usually involve small, relevant samples. **Non-probability sampling methods** are used (see Chapter 15) whereby participants are recruited because they have on-going or prior experience of the phenomena that the researcher is exploring (Mapp, 2008). Whilst the exact sample size is usually not determined at the start of the study, the researcher usually has a rough idea about the likely number of participants.

In determining the likely sample size, the researcher should consider the purpose of the study, the timeframe available and the need for **credibility**. To assist judgements about sample size, the researcher will decide upon the participant inclusion and exclusion criteria (Endacott and Botti, 2005). However, these may change if the initial data analysis suggests that the recruitment of different groups of participants would be beneficial. The simultaneous processes of participant recruitment, data collection and data analysis mean that the researcher is able to make their final decision about the sample size when **data saturation** is reached (see Box 5.1). This is when data collection and analysis does not reveal any new findings and so the recruitment of further participants is unnecessary.

BOX 5.1   EXAMPLE ILLUSTRATING DATA SATURATION

Sally plans to interview relatives about their experiences of witnessing the resuscitation of a family member. Sally thinks that 8–10 participants will provide her with sufficient data to obtain a comprehensive insight to relatives' experiences of witnessed resuscitation. However, as recruitment, data collection and data analysis progress it becomes apparent to Sally that there are aspects of the relatives' experiences that she still needs to explore and that she will need to recruit more than 10 participants. It is not until Sally has interviewed 20 participants that she feels she has reached data saturation.

The most commonly used qualitative data collection methods are interviews, diaries, **focus groups, participant** and **non-participant observation, case studies** and **life histories** (Endacott, 2005; Baker, 2006). These should reflect the qualitative nature of the study, so for example during observation, the researcher will document anything that appears of relevance. In many cases participants lead or influence the data collection process (Yardley, 2008). For instance, the participant's responses will drive the researcher's subsequent questions. The data collection process is intensive and vast quantities of detailed, rich data are generated, usually in the form of descriptive or narrative text. Most qualitative methods use strategies that involve data collection in a direct way in natural settings (Polit and Beck, 2014).

Whilst qualitative methods do not generally include a pilot phase (Richards, 2009), strategies are often used to enhance the development of data collection tools. This may include utilising evidence from other similar studies, consulting experienced researchers and peer review. Initial data analysis often informs subsequent data collection because the two processes usually occur concurrently (Jacelon and O'Dell, 2005; Polit and Beck, 2014). Data collection continues until data saturation is reached and this is facilitated by efficient sampling and management of data analysis (Richards, 2009).

Although qualitative methods generally involve small samples, large quantities of in-depth data are generated. Consequently, qualitative analysis software packages are often used to manage and organise the data in a way that can be difficult to replicate manually (Jacelon and O'Dell, 2005; Plummer-D'Amato, 2008). There are a number of different methods of qualitative data analysis, the most common of which is **thematic analysis** (Chapter 20). Whichever method is adopted, the purpose is to elicit meanings from the data and to provide an accurate portrayal of that meaning for others (Robson, 2011). The overall process of qualitative data analysis has been described as being **iterative** (Robson, 2011). This means that it is not a linear process with a clearly defined start and finish and it can be a time consuming and lengthy process. Qualitative research often involves repetition, whereby the data are constantly reviewed and revisited until the researcher feels that analysis of the data has been completed. In their interpretation of the data, the researcher will draw on their personal experiences whether intentionally or otherwise (Birks et al., 2008; Richards, 2009).

Qualitative methods can therefore be referred to as being subjective and dialectical, whereby the researcher is affected by the phenomena they seek to understand and in turn affects the phenomena themselves (Coyle, 2007; Birks et al., 2008). In accordance with qualitative methodology the researcher tries to set out with no or few preconceived ideas. In studies where the researcher has prior knowledge of the topic under investigation this can be a particular challenge. Consequently during the course of all qualitative studies the researcher should reflect on their preconceived ideas and the impact of these on their interpretation of the findings (Yardley, 2008). This is called **reflexivity**, it is an on-going process and it is done so that the researcher's preconceived ideas can be acknowledged through self-awareness (Richards, 2009; Darawsheh, 2014) (see Chapters 8 and 21) (see Box 5.2).

BOX 5.2   EXAMPLE ILLUSTRATING REFLEXIVITY

Adam is a mental health nurse and he is undertaking a qualitative study exploring clients' experiences of cognitive behavioural therapy. It is possible that as Adam carries out the study he will, albeit unwittingly, be influenced by his prior knowledge and preconceived ideas of CBT. Before the study begins Adam writes a reflective account of his thoughts about CBT. He also keeps a reflective journal as the study progresses. Adam shares his initial account and journal with his supervisor and they regularly discuss the possible impact of Adam's prior knowledge and ideas on the way he has carried out the data collection and data analysis processes. Adam acknowledges this possible impact in his thesis and in subsequent publications.

In the context of qualitative research, subjectivity is sometimes confused with bias. However, they are different issues and these terms should not be used interchangeably.

Subjectivity is a fundamental feature of qualitative research. Knowledge is generated through shared understanding between the researcher and participants. Consequently the researcher's beliefs and experiences influence the research. However, in the context of qualitative research, bias is when the researcher deliberately manipulates an aspect of the study such as the data collection process or analysis of the data in order to suit their desired outcomes or preconceived ideas. There may be a fine line between subjectivity and bias. Therefore the qualitative researcher should constantly monitor the impact of their preconceived ideas throughout the study by being reflexive.

The findings of a qualitative study are usually presented in a descriptive format with direct quotes from participants and excerpts from the researcher's **field notes** to illustrate the findings. The findings may also lead to the development of a theory; this is **inductive reasoning** (see Box 5.3), which could be tested in a larger-scale quantitative study.

BOX 5.3   EXAMPLE OF INDUCTIVE REASONING

A qualitative study involving a small number of women in one setting may culminate in the theory that mothers with postnatal depression feel let down by the health service. This theory could be tested in a quantitative study involving a large number of women from a diverse range of settings.

It is sometimes assumed that qualitative methods do not have the potential to cause harm (Baker, 2006). However, when feelings, behaviours and experiences are explored, sensitive or difficult issues may be encountered. The holistic nature of qualitative research also means that a wide range of sometimes unexpected issues may be revealed. In addition, the flexible nature of qualitative research means that researchers may not always be able to predict the way in which the study will evolve and thereby identify potential risks (Rogers, 2008). It can also be difficult for researchers to envisage how participants may respond (O'Leary, 2014). Therefore, during a qualitative study informed consent should be regarded as an on-going process rather than a single event and researchers should advise participants about sources of on-going support that they can access (Baker, 2006; Rogers, 2008) such as support groups and counselling services. Researchers should also think about the potential impact of a qualitative study on them and put strategies in place to ensure they are adequately supported should they find themselves exploring sensitive or emotionally challenging issues (Rager, 2005; Lalor et al., 2006) (see Box 5.4).

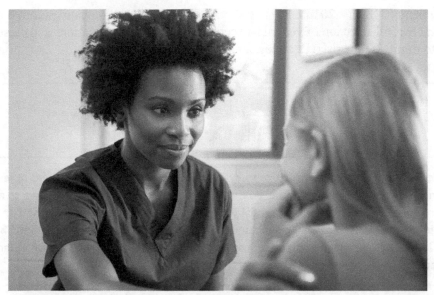

© Monkey Business Images / Shutterstock

BOX 5.4   EXAMPLE ILLUSTRATING THE POTENTIAL IMPACT OF A TOPIC ON THE RESEARCHER

Mandy is exploring parents' experiences of stillbirth. It is quite likely that the stories parents share with Mandy will be upsetting. The distressing nature of these accounts will be reiterated as Mandy transcribes the interviews and analyses the data. It is therefore essential that Mandy has regular meetings with her research supervisor to discuss the impact of these stories on her and to ensure adequate strategies are in place to support her.

As is the case in any research, participant **confidentiality** and protection of participant identity should be maintained (Mapp, 2008; O'Leary, 2014). However, this can be particularly problematic in research adopting qualitative methodology. Participants may be identifiable because of the small sample size, their biographical details or the use of only one study site. There is therefore a risk of inadvertent disclosure of participant identity (Baker, 2006), and avoiding breaches of confidentiality is a challenge for qualitative researchers (O'Leary, 2014). The use of participant codes, non-identification of the study site and careful selection of verbatim excerpts to be used in publications and presentations help to minimise the risk (Dearnley, 2005) (see Box 5.5).

BOX 5.5   EXAMPLE ILLUSTRATING THE PROTECTION OF PARTICIPANT IDENTITY

Rachel is carrying out a qualitative study involving parents with children who have a rare genetic disorder. Although Rachel does not identify the setting, it will be known to a number of people. It is therefore essential that Rachel does not use quotations in her thesis, publications or conference presentations that might identify a particular parent. The sort of identifiable information a parent may give in a piece of dialogue could for instance be that they have triplets or that they have recently moved to the UK.

Other situations where maintaining confidentially may be problematic occur when participants reveal issues of concern, or unsafe practice is observed or reported (Rogers, 2008). Researchers in the UK who are nurses or midwives are duty bound by their code of conduct (Nursing and Midwifery Council, 2015a) and the law. There may therefore be situations where the researcher has a moral, professional or legal obligation to disclose information to others, for example, the police or senior managers within the research setting (Manning, 2004; O'Leary, 2014). Discussion with the participant may enable individuals to self-disclose or seek appropriate help or support (Rogers, 2008).

Qualitative methodology has been criticised for being anecdotal and lacking 'scientific' rigour (Coyle, 2007; Plummer-D'Amato, 2008). The idiosyncratic nature of the research process has also been criticised. It is likely that two researchers conducting the same study, with the same participants, in the same setting, at the same time would describe the findings in different ways (Polit and Beck, 2014). However, rather than seeing this as a flaw, it can be argued that the potential for individual interpretation is the strength of qualitative methodology (Rolfe, 2006).

A further criticism of qualitative research is that the findings only apply to those who have participated in the study and the context in which the investigation took place. The intention of qualitative research is not to identify universal truths, generalise findings or establish causal relationships. Some regard this as one of the major limitations of qualitative research. However, the findings can provide insight into the experiences of participants and the context in which these experiences occur (Broom and Willis, 2007). The extent to which findings are applicable to different people in other settings can therefore be considered. Robson (2011: 160) describes this as being 'analytic or theoretical generalization'. In this way, the findings of a qualitative study can be substantiated by similar studies or corroborated by people who have had similar experiences (Angen, 2000; Yardley, 2008). Whilst the findings are time- and context-bound, they should appear plausible and may resonate with other similar populations or settings (Baker, 2006; Yardley, 2008). The written account of the research may therefore invoke in the reader a feeling of authenticity and realism (Angen, 2000).

EXAMPLES OF QUALITATIVE RESEARCH METHODS

We will now explore the more commonly used qualitative research methods in nursing and midwifery research. These are:

**Website
activity 5.1**

- phenomenology
- ethnography
- grounded theory.

We will also consider **action research** here, because although this method does not always follow qualitative methodology, it usually takes this approach. Whilst we provide an overview of these research methods here, they will be explored in more detail in Chapter 8.

PHENOMENOLOGY

Phenomenology is grounded in the ideology of Husserl and Heidegger (Johnson, 2000; Dykes, 2004; Mapp, 2008). Phenomenology aims to discover the meaning of a person's life and this is based on the premise that a person's reality is determined by their interpretations of their world. Whilst there are several different forms of phenomenology, the main purpose, to gain insight into the lives of the participants, is the same. The phrase that is often used in conjunction with a phenomenological study is the 'lived experience' of the participants (Walsh and Downe, 2006). For example, 'what is life like for young adults with insulin dependent diabetes?' or 'what is life like for pregnant women who self-harm?' Whilst nurses and midwives may feel they already know what life is like for the people they care for, phenomenological studies often reveal new, perhaps unexpected insights. This research method also enables researchers to focus on the whole person, in other words all aspects of their life, not just the condition, situation or problem that brings them into contact with health care professionals. Phenomenological studies involve small, **purposive samples** and the most commonly used method of data collection is semi-structured interviews or, as they are sometimes called, in-depth conversations (see Box 5.6). Diaries and case studies may also be used. A number of different methods of qualitative data analysis may be used. Analysis of the findings often culminates in the development of a theory.

BOX 5.6   EXAMPLE OF A PHENOMENOLOGICAL STUDY

Richard is carrying out a phenomenological study of the lived experience of men living with a partner who abuses alcohol. Richard recruits 12 men and he uses semi-structured interviews and diaries as methods of data collection.

ETHNOGRAPHY

The roots of **ethnography** are in social anthropology, and this research method is used when researchers wish to explore the behaviours and beliefs of groups of people (Walsh and Downe, 2006) (see Box 5.7). Ethnographers are interested in the cultures, customs, language, interactions and the actions of groups.

BOX 5.7   EXAMPLE OF AN ETHNOGRAPHIC STUDY

Kate wants to gain a greater understanding of children with life-limiting conditions. An ethnographic study carried out in a hospice setting would enable Kate to explore both individual's and group behaviours, the ways in which children interact with each other and the verbal and non-verbal ways in which they communicate with each other about their situation.

The most commonly used method of data collection in ethnography is observation, which is carried out in the setting where the group usually comes together. Observation may be supported by other data collection methods such as interviews, diaries and focus groups. The sample size for an ethnographic study will be determined by the setting in which the study takes place and the number of group members who are willing to take part in the study. The purpose of the data analysis is to explain group behaviours and, like other qualitative methods, may culminate in the development of a theory.

GROUNDED THEORY

Grounded theory has its origins in sociology and was first described by Glaser and Strauss in the 1960s (Punch, 2014). Grounded theory is used when the researcher aims to explore phenomena by developing a theory that explains an aspect of human behaviour. This method is used when little is known about the phenomena under investigation. A grounded theory study usually starts with the researcher's intention to find out more about a particular topic rather than a specific research question. The theory that is ultimately developed is said to be 'grounded' in reality, in other words the theory has its foundations in the data collected about the phenomena. Researchers include any data source that they feel will inform the development of the theory. Consequently a variety of data collection methods may be used and these could include in-depth interviews, diaries, focus groups, images such as photographs and pictures, observation and exploration of documentation. Whilst predominantly associated with qualitative data, grounded theory may also incorporate quantitative approaches (see Box 5.8).

BOX 5.8   EXAMPLE OF A GROUNDED THEORY STUDY

Peter wishes to find out about living with schizophrenia. For his grounded theory study Peter interviews people who have schizophrenia, carries out focus groups with people whose relative has schizophrenia and interviews health care professionals who work with clients and their families. Peter also observes clients attending out-patient clinics and examines literature about schizophrenia including material produced by user groups and charities.

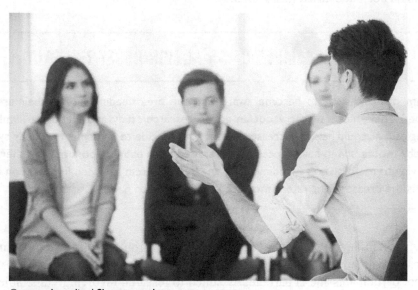

© g-stockstudio / Shutterstock

As with other qualitative methods recruitment of participants, data collection and data analysis occur simultaneously. This is an important feature of grounded theory as the initial data analysis will help the researcher to identify issues to explore with subsequent participants and other possible data sources. Data analysis usually involves the **constant comparison** method, whereby data are compared and contrasted in order to refine the theory. Multiple approaches to grounded theory have evolved over the last 50 years and it is important to note that Glaser and Strauss subsequently had different views about the way in which grounded theory should be conducted.

ACTION RESEARCH

Action research, sometimes known as collaborative, emancipatory or **participatory research**, usually follows qualitative methodology. Kurt Lewin's work on change theory and group dynamics in the 1940s provides the foundation for this research method (O'Leary, 2014). Action research takes a cyclical approach to solving problems. Whilst there are a number of different models of action research, they usually involve flexible designs. The research starts with a problem which is recognised and acknowledged by a group of people. The aim of the research is to assess the problem, implement an intervention or change that the group feels will address the problem and then evaluate the impact of the intervention or change. The evaluation will identify if further strategies are required to address the initial problem. The effect of these additional interventions or changes should subsequently be evaluated. The research is concluded when the initial problem has been addressed (see Box 5.9).

BOX 5.9   EXAMPLE OF AN ACTION RESEARCH STUDY

A team of health visitors become aware that the breastfeeding rate in their area has dropped. They decide to carry out an action research study and identify a number of strategies that could help to increase the rate. They decide to implement a 'buddy system', whereby mothers who have successfully breastfed their baby support new mothers who are trying to establish breastfeeding. After the buddy system has been in operation for six months the breastfeeding rate is measured and is found to have increased.

Website activity 5.2

A theory is often developed relating to addressing the problem. For action research to be effective, the collaboration and commitment of all those involved is required. The research empowers participants and is particularly suited to research involving vulnerable groups, such as children and people with mental health problems or learning disabilities.

In the consideration of quantitative and qualitative methodologies we have acknowledged some of the strengths and weaknesses. In many cases, the strengths of one methodology address the considered weaknesses of the other. However, some researchers are firmly positioned in one camp and consider the opposing methodology too flawed to be used.

Website
activity 5.3

> ## THINK POINT ACTIVITY   5.2
>
> Summarise what you consider are the key strengths and weaknesses of the qualitative methodology.

Website
activity 5.4

WHAT IS 'SCIENTIFIC RESEARCH'?

The terms 'science' and 'scientific' have featured in our exploration of quantitative and quantitative methodologies in Chapters 4 and 5. This is therefore an appropriate point to consider what these terms mean in the context of research and whether they can be applied to both qualitative and quantitative methodologies.

> ## THINK POINT ACTIVITY   5.3
>
> In the context of research, what do the terms 'science' and 'scientific' mean to you? Do you think these terms can be applied to both qualitative and quantitative research?

With its foundations in the sciences of physics, chemistry and mathematics, the paradigm of positivism and thereby quantitative research has traditionally been acknowledged as being science-based and therefore scientific (Broussard, 2006; Patton, 2015) (see Chapter 3). As a consequence of this view and the conventional hierarchies of evidence, the conclusion that is often drawn is that if quantitative research is scientific, then qualitative research is not (McCourt, 2005; Grubs and Piantanida, 2010). This in turn leads to the view that quantitative research is valuable and therefore qualitative research is not. But what do we mean by 'scientific'? In the context of research, scientific means systematic study that is undertaken in a rigorous, ethical and robust way in accordance with the key principles of the method used. We argue that these features can be evident in both quantitative and qualitative research (McCourt, 2005; Yardley and Bishop, 2008; Bryman, 2012). Whilst qualitative research may seem haphazard and disorganised to some, the methodological strength of this approach is its responsiveness and flexibility. It is imperative, however, that the researcher using a qualitative method does so in accordance with the principles of that particular method and is able to justify methodologically what they have done and why.

Website
activity 5.5

As we will see in later chapters (7, 8, 9, 21), there are strategies that researchers should use to ensure that their research, whether quantitative or qualitative, is sound. If these strategies are adopted both quantitative and qualitative research can be systematic, rigorous and a genuine form of science (Giorgi and Giorgi, 2008). Both can be of great value to nursing and midwifery practice. We suggest that those who argue that qualitative research is not scientific are usually strongly allied to the paradigm of positivism and therefore believe the only way to conduct research is using quantitative methods. However, traditional hierarchies of evidence are being challenged (Daly et al., 2007). We support this recent reconsideration and propose the hierarchy of evidence for qualitative research outlined in Chapter 10 in order to recognise the rightful place of scientific qualitative studies.

SUMMARY

In this chapter we have reviewed the qualitative methodology in the context of nursing and midwifery research. In doing this, we have explored the key features, contrasting elements and principles of this approach to research. We have also provided an overview of the research methods commonly allied to this methodology. These methods will be explored in more detail in Chapter 8.

Finally we have explored the notion of scientific research and considered the extent to which this label can be applied to quantitative and qualitative research.

FURTHER READING

The following sources provide further discussion regarding qualitative approaches to research and their strengths and limitations:

Green, J. and Thorogood, N. (2014) Qualitative methodology and health research. In J. Green and N. Thorogood, *Qualitative Methods for Health Research* (3rd edn). London: Sage Publications, pp. 3–34.

A good overview which helps to orientate qualitative research and the role of theory in real health contexts.

Mills, J. and Birks, M. (eds) (2014) *Qualitative Methodology: A Practical Guide*. London: Sage Publications.

Both authors are based in the Centre for Nursing and Midwifery Research at James Cook University. They are expert researchers who trace the history and philosophical underpinnings of different methodologies. Featured methodologies include action research, discourse analysis, ethnography, grounded theory, case studies and narrative inquiry.

Don't forget to visit https://study.sagepub.com/harveyandland to watch videos, take quizzes and to follow specially designed web activities.

6

MIXED METHODOLOGIES: AN OVERVIEW

This chapter will build upon the issues and concepts explored in Chapters 3, 4 and 5 to provide an overview of mixed methodologies. In this chapter we will:

- discuss the development of mixed methods research
- explore the key features of mixed methods research
- review different models of mixed methods research
- examine the value of mixed methodologies to nursing and midwifery research
- consider the reasons why mixed methodologies are being increasingly used in health care research.

As we have seen in Chapter 3, the paradigm of pragmatism is increasingly being used in health care research and has been described as being the 'middle way' between the opposing paradigms of positivism and interpretivism (Doyle et al., 2009; Farrelly, 2013) (see Figure 6.1).

In Chapters 4 and 5 we identified the inherent differences between quantitative and qualitative research methods, which are allied to the paradigms of positivism and interpretivism, respectively (Bryman, 2012). In accordance with the paradigm of pragmatism,

Interpretivism	Pragmatism	Positivism
Qualitative methods	Mixed methods	Quantitative methods
Phenomenology		Randomised controlled trials
Ethnography		Cohort studies
Grounded theory		Case-control studies

Figure 6.1   The research continuum

the researcher is able to use both qualitative and quantitative methods in one mixed methods study (Bishop and Homes, 2013), for example, a randomised controlled trial and grounded theory within one study. A study that involves two (or more) methods from the same paradigm is not generally regarded as being a mixed methods study (Bryman, 2012). For example, a study involving ethnography and phenomenology would be regarded as being a qualitative study. A mixed methods study is therefore defined as being a study that involves both qualitative and quantitative methods in one study (see Box 6.1).

In accordance with the definition above, this means that within one study there will be elements that are quantitative in approach by being structured and pre-planned, whilst other parts of the study will be more qualitative in nature by being flexible and evolving. As a consequence during the course of one study, both quantitative and qualitative data can be collected (see Figure 6.2). The mixed methods approach therefore enables the researcher to use different approaches to measure the same or similar concepts (Farrelly, 2013). This in turn provides a more comprehensive insight into the phenomena under investigation (Yardley and Bishop, 2008).

BOX 6.1   AN EXAMPLE OF A MIXED METHODS STUDY

A study may be conducted to examine a new investigative procedure (see Figure 6.2). The research could include a randomised controlled trial to measure how effective the new procedure is in comparison with conventional investigative procedures. The research could also include a qualitative study to explore participants' experiences of the new procedure.

There have been varying reports of the extent to which mixed methods are used in health care research (Alise and Teddlie, 2010; Bishop and Homes, 2013). Use of this approach should be determined by the research question, aims and objectives. Combining qualitative and quantitative methods in one study is of particular relevance to nursing and midwifery research where studies tend to focus on complex issues that involve human beings. Investigating multifaceted concepts and issues using exclusively qualitative or quantitative approaches runs the risk that the issue under investigation will be inadequately understood or explained. In other words, it may only reveal one side or part of the story. Combining approaches in one study strengthens the research by drawing on the positive aspects of both interpretivism and positivism and through corroboration of the findings (Teddlie and Tashakkori, 2009; Creswell and Plano Clark, 2011). This combining of methods and corroboration of findings is sometimes referred to as triangulation and this has the potential to strengthen the overall study through validation of the findings (Bryman, 2012; Loke et al., 2014) (see Chapter 21).

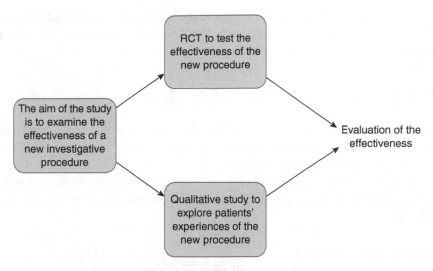

Figure 6.2   Illustration of a mixed methods study

The researcher's decisions about which particular approach to use and when should be determined by the study's aims and objectives. Pragmatism does not support any particular view of epistemology, ontology or methodology; these are determined by the context of a specific study (Houghton et al., 2012). This is made possible within the paradigm of pragmatism because achieving the aims and objectives of the research is more important than the process (Creswell, 2014; Patton, 2015). This practical, problem-solving approach is something that nurses and midwives should be familiar with and it is therefore particularly suited to nursing and midwifery research (Houghton et al., 2012; Farrelly, 2013).

As is the case with other research terminology a mixed method study may be referred to by other terms. Rather than mixed methods this type of research is sometimes called **multiple**, **combined or blended methods research** or **mixed strategy** or **multi-strategy research** (Robson, 2011; Bryman, 2012). Whilst all of these labels indicate the distinctive feature of this research method, it is most commonly referred to as mixed methods research and so we will continue to use this term throughout the book.

Creswell and Plano Clark (2011) suggest that mixed methods research was first mooted in the 1950s. After an initial period of resistance this approach began to be more widely accepted, particularly during the 1980s. A review of the literature published in English between 1999 and 2009 found that most mixed methods studies originated in the United Kingdom and North America (Östlund et al., 2011). Whilst some may remain firmly allied to either qualitative or quantitative research (Farrelly, 2013), the mixed methods approach is becoming more commonly used in research, particularly in health care (Doyle et al., 2009; Bryman, 2012). There are now journals and conferences specifically dedicated to mixed methods research. Funding bodies and other journals are also becoming increasingly receptive to this approach to research.

MODELS OF MIXED METHODS RESEARCH

Website
activity 6.2

There are a number of different models (sometimes called typologies) of mixed methods research and they are often labelled in different ways (Yardley and Bishop, 2008; Teddlie and Tashakkori, 2009; Creswell and Plano Clark, 2011; Robson, 2011). These place varying emphasis on the sequence, timing and weight to be given to the qualitative and quantitative elements within a study. When selecting which model to use, the researcher must consider:

- the purpose of the study
- the priority to be given to the qualitative and quantitative approaches
- theoretical perspective to be taken
- resources available
- researcher expertise
- whether the different elements could or should be undertaken simultaneously or concurrently (Teddlie and Tashakkori, 2009; Creswell and Plano Clark, 2011).

In making these decisions the researcher must also consider if the initial data could or should inform subsequent data collection and at which point the data become 'mixed'. This 'mixing' could occur during data collection, data analysis or when the findings are interpreted. The practical nature of the paradigm of pragmatism provides the facility for the researcher to make all of these choices.

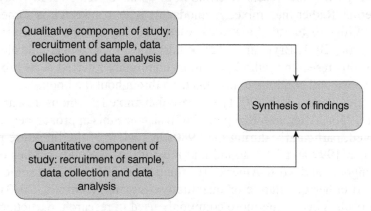

Figure 6.3   Parallel model of mixed methods research

Whilst a number of different models have been described, they can be described as being of three main types: **parallel, sequential** and **embedded**.

The parallel model (sometimes referred to as the **triangulation model**) is when the qualitative and quantitative components are carried out at the same time but the findings are not synthesised until both sets of data have been analysed separately (see Figure 6.3 and Box 6.2). A recent systematic review of mixed methods research identified that this model was most commonly used (Bishop and Homes, 2013).

BOX 6.2   EXAMPLE OF A PARALLEL MIXED METHODS STUDY

A large-scale study is carried out to examine the effectiveness of simulation as a teaching and learning strategy for student nurses. Some members of the research team conduct an RCT to test the effectiveness of simulation in comparison to traditional teaching and learning methods on the students' acquisition of clinical skills. At the same time other members of the research team undertake a qualitative study exploring the students' perception and experiences of simulation. Once all data are collected and analysed the findings are synthesised into the final summary of the study findings.

The sequential model of mixed methods research is when the qualitative and quantitative elements are undertaken separately and one leads to and informs the other (see Figure 6.4 and Box 6.3). Therefore preliminary data analysis is undertaken after the first phase so that the findings can inform the second phase. The order in which the elements are undertaken, i.e. qualitative followed by quantitative or quantitative

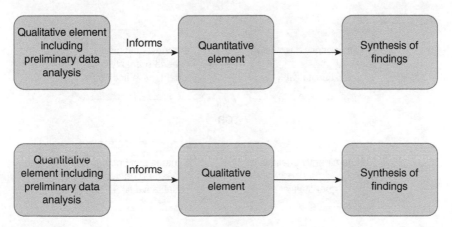

Figure 6.4 Sequential model of mixed methods research

followed by qualitative, will be determined by the aims and objectives of the particular study. For example, a grounded theory study may lead to the development of a theory or hypothesis which is tested in a large-scale quantitative study. Conversely, a large-scale quantitative survey may highlight issues that the researcher subsequently explores in a phenomenological study. Teddlie and Tashakkori (2009) suggest that the sequential model is more manageable for the solo researcher.

BOX 6.3   EXAMPLE OF A SEQUENTIAL MIXED METHODS STUDY

Gloria is exploring fathers' experiences of being present during complicated childbirth. For the first phase of her study, Gloria observes complicated deliveries where the baby's father is present. She uses a structured data collection tool to collect quantitative data. Having analysed the data, Gloria identifies a number of issues that she explores further during the second phase of the study when she carries out qualitative, semi-structured interviews with the fathers about their experiences.

The embedded mixed methods model is when one component (qualitative or quantitative) is embedded or 'nested' within the other component (see Figure 6.5 and Box 6.4). The embedded component is intentionally secondary to the component into which it is nested. Researchers use this model when quantitative or qualitative data will facilitate achievement of the study's aims and objectives within a study which predominantly takes the opposite approach.

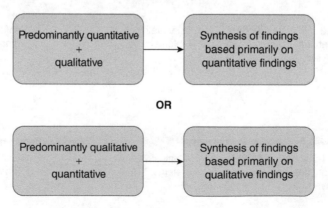

Figure 6.5   Embedded model of mixed methods research

BOX 6.4   EXAMPLE OF AN EMBEDDED MIXED METHODS STUDY

A national quantitative survey is undertaken to investigate midwives' experiences of case-load midwifery. The researchers take the opportunity to carry out qualitative interviews with 10 midwives to provide further insight into their experiences. Whilst the findings of the interviews are referred to, the report focuses mainly on the findings of the quantitative survey.

Whichever model of mixed methods research is used, the researcher will at some point synthesise the qualitative and quantitative findings. The processes for doing this will be explored in Chapters 19 and 20.

ADVANTAGES OF MIXED METHODS RESEARCH

THINK POINT ACTIVITY   6.1

Make a list of the reasons why you think mixed methods research is becoming increasingly popular in health care research. What do you think are the advantages or benefits of using this research method?

There are a number of advantages and benefits of using the mixed methods approach in health care research. A mixed methods study:

- enables researchers to explore different perspectives in one study
- enables researchers to explore different aspects of complex phenomena in one study
- facilitates a holistic approach to investigating phenomena
- avoids the researcher being forced to take either a qualitative or quantitative approach
- draws on the strengths of both qualitative and quantitative research
- reduces the impact of any weaknesses associated with either qualitative or quantitative approaches
- is particularly suited to interdisciplinary research especially if the different disciplines involved in the study have a stronger affinity with one paradigm
- facilitates collaborative working

- offers a more practical approach to research
- may reveal new knowledge in one part of the study which can be further explored in subsequent parts of the same study
- provides a greater depth and breadth of understanding and insight about phenomena and thereby enhances the evidence base
- is cost-effective by including a range of approaches in one study rather than each element being undertaken as a separate piece of research
- increasingly meets the needs of policy makers, service providers and funding bodies through the provision of comprehensive findings within one study.

Mixed methods research could also be regarded as being 'fashionable,' 'trendy' or 'of the moment'. In other words, it is rapidly becoming the dominant approach to health care research (Doyle et al., 2009) and the situation may soon arise when researchers will have to justify why they are *not* doing a mixed methods study.

DISADVANTAGES OF MIXED METHODS RESEARCH

THINK POINT ACTIVITY   6.2

Make a list of potential disadvantages or drawbacks of using mixed methods.

It must be acknowledged that there is a negative view of mixed methods research (Bryman, 2012). A number of drawbacks and disadvantages of using this approach have been suggested:

- the inherent differences between quantitative and qualitative research are such that they cannot be mixed
- there is the risk that one philosophical standpoint dominates the other
- it may lead to power struggles within the research team
- the qualitative elements may be valued more highly than the quantitative elements or vice versa
- the researcher or research team may not be sufficiently experienced to ensure both the quantitative and qualitative elements are carried out appropriately
- a mixed methods study could be more time consuming and therefore also more costly
- it may lead to fragmented research which lacks a clear focus
- synthesising qualitative and quantitative findings can be complex and may involve large amounts of data; it is essential that the essence of all data is not lost.

A further potential drawback of the mixed methods approach is that because its popularity is currently on the increase, it may at some point diminish in popularity. In other words, 'the bubble may burst'. The well-documented paradigm war between positivism and interpretivism that we discussed in Chapter 3 may in time be replicated with a standpoint taken against pragmatism and the mixed methods approach.

FACTORS TO CONSIDER WHEN UNDERTAKING A MIXED METHODS STUDY

Having decided to use a mixed methods approach as determined by the research questions, aims and objectives there are other factors the researcher should consider. We have identified some of the drawbacks and limitations of mixed methods research and these should be deliberated and addressed by the researcher or research team before they embark upon such a study. Research skills training may be required before the study begins to ensure that both the qualitative and quantitative elements can be adequately addressed. This may be costly both in terms of time and resources (Farrelly, 2013). This may be less problematic if the study involves a team of researchers as it is more likely that the skill requirements will be met by the team as a whole. Team members could be specifically recruited in accordance with the skills required to meet the study's aims and objectives. This may be more challenging for the lone researcher, who will need to ensure they can undertake all aspects of the study.

Website activity 6.3

In addition to skills training, the lone researcher should also consider arranging support and guidance from appropriate experts or supervisors. However, some of the concern that a researcher will not be sufficiently knowledgeable about both qualitative and quantitative research probably dates from an era when students were taught about only one approach as determined by the particular discipline that they were from. Students from all health care disciplines, particularly nurses and midwives, are now exposed to both quantitative and qualitative research (see Chapters 1 and 3) and as such, concerns about the attainment of adequate research skills should diminish over time.

There should be a clear rationale for the inclusion of both qualitative and quantitative elements in one study. This should not appear to be 'window dressing' or a way to appease critics or to increase the chances of securing funding. Within the rationale, consideration should be given to the model to be used, the emphasis that will be placed on the qualitative and quantitative elements, at which point the 'mixing' of data will occur and how the findings will be synthesised (Yardley, 2008). Consideration should also be given to the length of time that each element will require. For example, the qualitative component may take longer than the quantitative part and so equal lengths of time should not be allocated to each phase. Being clear about these factors before the study begins will reduce the risk of the study becoming disjointed and lacking focus. It should also minimise power struggles between members of the research team when the study gets underway.

SUMMARY

In this chapter we have described the development of mixed methods research. We have explored the key features of this research approach and have reviewed the different models or typologies that the researcher could use. We have also established the reasons why this methodology is being increasingly used in health care research and have identified the particular value of this approach to nursing and midwifery research.

FURTHER READING

Creswell, J.W. and Plano Clark, V.L. (2011) *Designing and Conducting Mixed Methods Research* (2nd edn). London: Sage Publications.

This is a clear guide for anyone hoping to design a mixed methods study.

Doyle, L., Brady, A.-M. and Byrne, G. (2009) An overview of mixed methods research. *Journal of Research in Nursing*, 14(2): 175–185.

Östlund, U., Kidd, L., Wengström, Y. and Rowa-Dewar, N. (2011) Combining qualitative and quantitative research within mixed method research designs: a methodological review. *International Journal of Nursing Studies*, 48(3): 369–383.

These two sources provide further discussion regarding the strengths and limitations of mixed methods research and the application of specific models.

See also the interdisciplinary *Journal of Mixed Methods Research* – http://mmr.sagepub.com/.

Don't forget to visit https://study.sagepub.com/harveyandland to watch videos, take quizzes and to follow specially designed web activities.

PART II

UNDERSTANDING RESEARCH METHODS AND DESIGNS: THE THEORY

7

RANDOMISED CONTROLLED TRIALS

This chapter explores the experimental method in health care, in particular the randomised controlled trial. In this chapter we will:

- determine the appropriate use of randomised controlled trials in health care research
- discuss the features of a randomised controlled trial design
- using an example construct a simple experiment randomised controlled trial.

EXPERIMENTAL METHODS

Experimental methods adopt the underlying theory of positivism (see Chapter 3), that is, that knowledge can be absolute or certain. Experimental research involves the active manipulation of variables under the control of the researcher (Clamp et al., 2004) and attempts to study how participants will react to the manipulated conditions through monitoring one or more outcome measures. Experimental methods attempt to establish laws and principles by developing hypotheses that can be accepted or rejected through the use of structured tests under controlled conditions. The data collected from these tests are often 'counted', that is, they are numerical in form, which can be analysed using a range of statistics to make sense of data. This is a very simplified explanation of what is involved in the design of an experiment in a clinical setting study but as we progress through the chapter we will see how the randomised controlled trial has become more sophisticated over time to overcome inadvertent errors in a study's conclusion but more positively to make sure that the results provide the most transparent conclusions.

EXPERIMENTS AS FAIR TESTS

Without fair tests of treatments and interventions we risk, as health care practitioners, concluding that useless or harmful treatments are helpful, or dismissing as useless treatments that are actually useful (The James Lind Library, www.jameslindlibrary.org/). The material in The James Lind Library illustrates the evolution of fair tests of medical treatments over the centuries and explains some of the key historical research since the time of Daniel in the Old Testament who is attributed as conducting the first experiment. The key concepts here are the need to make a comparison of two or more treatments, or of one treatment with no treatment, which are fair, because steps have been taken to minimise the effects of bias and chance (these concepts are explained more fully later in the chapter).

BOX 7.1   DEFINITION OF EXPERIMENTAL DESIGN

Experimental design is:

a formal, objective, systematic process in which numerical data are utilised to obtain information about the world ... to describe, test relationships and examine cause-and-effect relationships. (Grove et al., 2014: 28)

Experimental designs in health care are often boasted as the most 'rigorous' of all research designs or, as the 'gold standard' against which all other designs are judged (see Box 7.1). If we can demonstrate with some certainty that one drug is better than another or that in a high proportion of cases, patients and clients would benefit more from a certain treatment, then experimental research designs probably are the most rigorous because they can demonstrate these things with some certainty. That said they are *only* the most rigorous for certain types of research questions where the effects of treatments or interventions are being studied. See Figure 7.1 for an illustration of the experimental process. For example, we might set up an experiment to test two different types of wound dressings. Participants with leg ulcers would be divided at random into two groups. One group would have their ulcers dressed with one type of dressing and the other with the second type. All aspects of the experiment would be tightly controlled and at the end of the experiment, the researcher would measure which group had the best ulcer healing rates.

RANDOMISED CONTROLLED TRIALS

Randomised controlled trials are used in several types of experimental research, such as laboratory experiments, but they can also be called randomised clinical trials or controlled clinical trials, which indicate that they are used in health care to test treatments or interventions on people or patients. They follow very strict procedures or protocols and all steps of the process must be transparent.

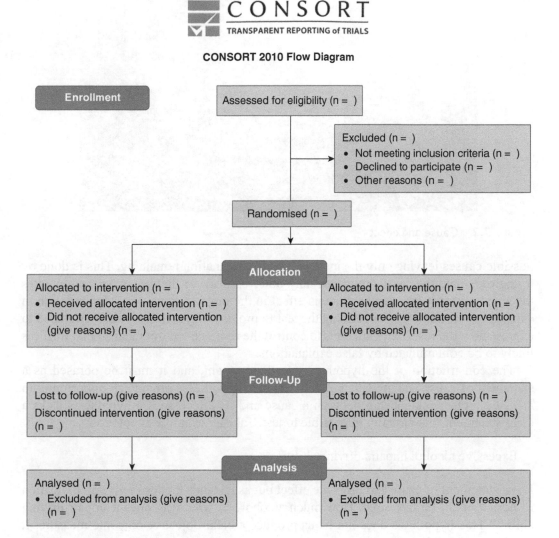

Figure 7.1   Flow diagram illustrating the process of conducting an experiment

ESTABLISHING A HYPOTHESIS

The researcher begins by making a statement (a hypothesis) that predicts a direct relationship between a cause and its effect. Take a look at Figure 7.2. What has caused that ripple? The most probable answer is that a drop of water from above has caused it, but that is not the only explanation.

A fish may have taken an insect from under the surface or indeed the ripple may be a result of the effect of a whirlpool. In an experiment it is the researcher's job to rule out

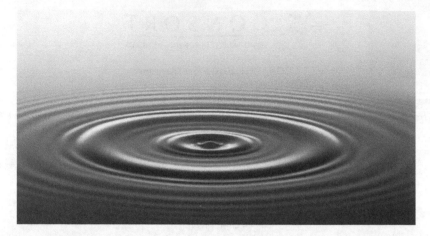

Figure 7.2   Cause and effect

possible causes leaving only the most *plausible* explanation remaining. This is done by trying to isolate the cause (ruling out any other causes), so the researcher manipulates the situation to try and demonstrate its effect in the most obvious way. Manipulation in experiments is *not* a way of bending the test to prove the hypothesis, it is a term used to express how the researcher attempts to control the research environment so that it is less likely to be contaminated by false explanations.

The construction of the hypothesis is all important, and it must be phrased as a statement of cause and predicted effect. The best hypotheses provide an opportunity to *measure* a clear relationship between a cause and its effect, so if a hypothesis lacks a clear statement it is virtually impossible to test. Take an example hypothesis:

Excessive alcohol impairs driving ability.

It *is* a statement of cause and probable effect but as it stands it doesn't give an indication of how it could be measured. How much alcohol? In what way does it impair driving ability? This hypothesis does not let us produce a clear objective outcome measure. It would be better phrased as:

Blood alcohol levels in excess of 80 mg/100 ml reduce driving reaction times for braking by one third.

This way an experiment can be designed to demonstrate this cause and effect using an objective measure. In experimental design, the cause is termed the independent variable and the effect, the dependent variable, so for the above example, a blood alcohol level in excess of 80 mg/100 ml is the independent variable and reduction in reaction time is the dependent variable. In practical terms what we might do to test this is to give people increasing amounts of alcohol and then test their reaction times on a driving simulator.

By increasing the amounts of alcohol we are manipulating the independent variable which we hypothesise is the cause of the reduction in reaction times. The reduction in the reaction times is hypothesised to be the effect of alcohol and is dependent on the amount of alcohol given. This cause and effect relationship can then be measured by recording the reaction times at the beginning of the experiment and again at the end to see how many more seconds it takes for people to brake.

We often hear people say 'research proves ...', which is in fact incorrect. Hypotheses don't provide absolute proof about a situation; they just attempt to confirm that the information from an experiment is the best explanation we have at present. It is usual to propose a further hypothesis at the same time, one which states the opposite position to the original. For example:

Blood alcohol levels in excess of 80 mg/100 ml *do not* reduce driving reaction times for braking by one third.

The first hypothesis is labelled H_1 whilst the second is called the null hypothesis and is labelled H_0. Providing both statements in experimental research is called a two tailed hypothesis.

The statistical analysis of the data gathered during the experiment is designed to establish whether or not there is a cause and effect but statisticians actually do this by attempting to *reject* the null hypothesis (H_0), which means the researcher may then *accept* the original hypothesis (H_1). In our example, if we gather data in our alcohol and reaction times study, appropriate statistics are used to reject the statement:

Blood alcohol levels in excess of 80 mg/100 ml *do not* reduce driving reaction times for braking by one third.

Therefore we have to accept the hypothesis:

Blood alcohol levels in excess of 80 mg/100 ml reduce driving reaction times for braking by one third.

THINK POINT ACTIVITY   7.1

Generate a hypothesis and null hypothesis from the following question:

Does sleep have an effect on concentration?

Remember that your hypothesis must be formed in such a way that it has an objective measurable outcome.

POPULATION AND SAMPLING

Having established the hypothesis, the researcher needs to design an experiment that will test it as rigorously as possible to make sure that no errors creep in that will unwittingly provide an inaccurate answer. The first step towards this is to find participants who are eligible for our experiment, that is, they represent the type of people who could support the acceptance or rejection of the hypothesis. We also need these people to exhibit the same characteristics, in other words to be as similar as possible to each other in respect of what we are trying to achieve; these people are called the study population.

Experimental researchers would like the world to be populated by genetically identical twins because if they are going to test the efficacy of a new drug they would like to give one twin that drug and another a placebo. Since identical twins are physically similar in every way there is a greater opportunity of demonstrating a difference in the effect of a drug and a placebo, but experimentation would be severely limited if researchers were to restrict their study population to twins so they need to find a way of producing a study population that is as similar as possible by other means. They do this in two ways by:

- specifying eligibility criteria for inclusion in the study
- randomly sampling from the study population.

ELIGIBILITY CRITERIA

Eligibility refers to the potential inclusion of all those people who might exhibit the characteristics we are looking for and who could constitute the study population. It is often easier to state who we would *exclude* rather than begin with who we should include. With reference to our hypothesis, for example, we should exclude people who don't drive as they won't be able to operate the driving simulator, but we might consider excluding other people such as those who are alcohol dependent as we might assume that they have higher tolerance levels. There may be a range of other characteristics that we might want to include such as limiting the age range of participants to between 18 and 25, or indeed placing an age limit of over 50. There is no right or wrong in this example as long as the inclusion and exclusion criteria are explicit and there is a clear explanation of why the particular criteria have been selected.

In health care this criteria is often more complex. Take an example where people with diabetes would constitute the study sample. The experiment might rely on that population being type 1 or type 2 and then we might consider whether they need to be a certain age and free from complications such as peripheral neuropathy. When designing their experiments researchers should have used the strictest inclusion and exclusion criteria to make sure the target population is clearly defined. When the researcher is clear about the population they can recruit people to the study who meet the criteria and are willing to participate. Recruitment should be conducted using the principles of informed consent; this is explained in more detail in Chapter 18.

RANDOM SAMPLING

Random sampling is a method of picking a sample from the study population where everyone has an equal chance of being chosen; see Chapter 15 for a more detailed explanation of this process.

SAMPLE SIZE

A well-designed trial should include an optimum number of participants: too many and the study becomes unwieldy, its cost becomes too high and, most importantly, the participants are burdened unnecessarily. If there are not enough participants there may be a chance that even with the appropriate statistics the study will fail to reach appropriate conclusions and again that participants have been recruited unnecessarily.

Students learning about research for the first time, when asked 'what is an appropriate sample size?' will often respond with a round number, usually 100. This is because they think that this figure will produce a neat sample for analysis, but it is less straightforward than that. Rather than pluck a number from the air, a sample size calculation needs to be made based on the individual features of the study. For a more detailed explanation of calculating the sample size see the suggested reading and browse the Internet for a sample size calculator.

RANDOM ASSIGNMENT

The key to the success of an experiment is the random assignment of the participants to receive either the new treatment we want to test or perhaps a placebo. It is possible in our alcohol experiment that we could use just one group and measure the increasing effect on braking times, but the researcher may decide to use two groups, the first (called the experimental arm) where the participants begin with zero blood alcohol levels and then are tested at several points afterwards when they have ingested alcohol. The second group (the control arm) would also have a zero alcohol level to begin with and throughout the experiment. Their reaction times would be tested at each point at **Website** the same time as the experimental group and in theory the control group should have **activity 7.1** similar reaction times all the way through the experiment.

The purpose of random assignment is to create two groups that are characteristically equal at the baseline (before the start of the study). In fact, even with random assignment we never expect that the groups we create will be exactly the same. How could they be, when they are made up of different people? We rely on the idea of probability and assume that the two groups are probabilistically equivalent. So, if we randomly assign people to two groups, and we have enough people in our study, we have a good chance of assessing whether the cause has the effect we anticipate. It is usual to measure the important characteristics of each group before the start of the experiment. For example, if our inclusion criteria states that the participants should be a mixture of males and females, the numbers of each would be counted in both groups. Similarly if the stipulated age range is 18–25 years old then an average age would be calculated for each group, and so on. In our example we may test all of the participants' braking times and calculate an average reaction time for each group, just in case the random assignment has placed drivers with more extraordinary reaction times in one group as this may skew the final result and we falsely accept or reject our hypotheses. Whilst there may be minor differences, the two groups should be balanced or in other words, 'look the same'. This is what is called baseline equivalence and is illustrated in Figure 7.3.

The purpose of baseline equivalence is to establish that both groups are indeed similar, but when the experiment is completed we would expect the 'balance' to shift in that the reaction times within the experimental (alcohol) group would be markedly slower than the control (non-alcohol) group (see Figure 7.4).

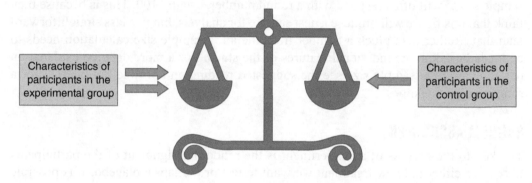

Characteristics of participants in the experimental group

Characteristics of participants in the control group

Figure 7.3   Before the experiment: baseline equivalence

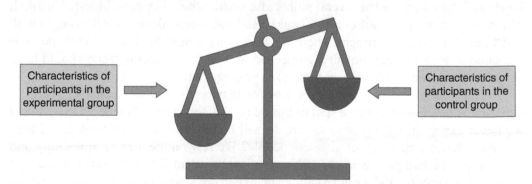

Characteristics of participants in the experimental group

Characteristics of participants in the control group

Figure 7.4   After the experiment: the difference in the effect of the interventions

CONCEALMENT

We have already discussed that a good experiment relies on minimising bias and chance, and one of the most important ways of minimising bias is to hide or conceal which treatments each group is receiving. So although the researcher will know that the experimental arm will receive the experimental treatment and the control arm will receive an alternative treatment or placebo, it is very important that the researchers should not be aware of which group is which in the administration of either treatment as it might influence how they measure the effects. Similarly participants should be unaware of which group they are in as it might influence the way they report their reaction. For example, imagine we have invented a new headache tablet that we have named 'Headaway' and we would like to test it against a placebo. If we told the participants in the experimental arm that they were receiving Headaway then they might report that their pain was relieved more effectively.

There is some controversy about the placebo effect – the idea that people who have been given a placebo believing it to be a real treatment have been known to demonstrate relief of symptoms.

THE PLACEBO EFFECT EXPLAINED

There are three types of concealment, also called masking or blinding, and the most common is called double blinding. Double blinding is where two parties are unaware of the treatment allocated to the participants, most often it is the participant and carer (nurse, doctor) or the participant and researcher, and if the experiment involves a medicine, this is usually done by packaging the medicine in identical forms so that both the placebo and the experimental drug appear exactly alike. Of course this becomes more complex with different types of treatment so different methods would be used. For example, in some trials of acupuncture, attempts have been made to provide sham acupuncture treatments, that is, those that mimic acupuncture, but which do not have a therapeutic effect.

In our example it is not possible to conceal the fact that the experimental arm are drinking alcohol and it is difficult to persuade the control arm that they might be, so the only option here is to make sure the researchers analysing the data do not know which participants are in which group, this is called a single blind trial.

Triple blind trials mean that participants, carers and researchers are all unaware of which treatments are allocated to whom.

It is important to remember when reading a paper that reports a randomised controlled trial that the process of concealment is clearly articulated, but we must also bear in mind that where it is not possible to conceal treatments we make an objective assessment as to whether this results in significant bias to the study.

DATA COLLECTION

Different forms of data collection are described in Chapters 16 and 17 but the most often used in randomised controlled trials is termed structured observation. This can take many forms including the collection of blood samples where the structured observation involves analysing the samples. In our reaction time study it may be by measuring blood alcohol levels and the time it takes to brake from a certain point to coming to a halt. This could be measured in metres or feet and inches *or* by recording the *time* this takes, but all of these measurements can be classed as structured observation.

Data collection in the form of questionnaires or other instruments that measure an effect such as depression scales may also be used in a randomised controlled trial to measure the effect of a treatment, but they *must* be valid and reliable; that is, they must demonstrate the ability to measure the variable under investigation and must be able to do this consistently across different participants and situations. For more information on **validity** and **reliability** see Chapter 21.

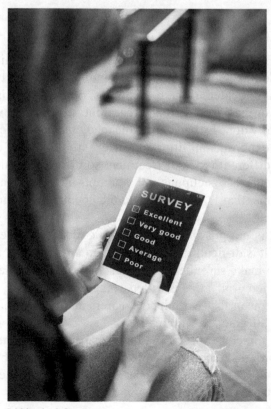

© Warchi / iStock

INTENTION TO TREAT ANALYSIS

Intention to treat analysis (ITT analysis) is usually described as 'once randomized, always analyzed' (Gupta, 2011: 109). It is a process by which the researcher makes sure that data from *all* the participants are analysed according to the trial protocol and according to the groups to which they were randomly assigned, regardless of their adherence to the entry criteria, regardless of the treatment they actually received, and regardless of subsequent withdrawal from treatment or deviation from the protocol.

ITT analysis avoids over-optimistic estimates of the effect of an intervention as a result of participants dropping out of the study perhaps because they don't like the side effects of the treatment or because they've died.

Take an example of a comparison of weight loss diets. Using the process described above we could compare the 'superfast weight loss diet' against a traditional reduced calorie diet. Using ITT analysis, the results actually demonstrate that the superfast diet is not effective whereas the reduced calorie diet is effective, but not using the principles of ITT analysis, we could get very different results. Why? Because of certain events that actually happened in the study:

- People on the effective low calorie diet lose weight and stay in the study.
- On the ineffective superfast weight loss diet some will lose weight regardless and will stay in the study, but those who fail to lose weight in this group are more likely to drop out, if only to try something else.

See how the results of this may be calculated in Table 7.1 (The sample of 100 has been chosen for simplicity!). With the superfast weight loss diet only 20 people complete the study and only 15 of those lose weight, so by ignoring the 80 people who didn't complete the study we can say that 15/20 lost weight, which produces the final result of 75%. With the traditional reduced calorie weight loss no one drops out and 50/100 (50%) lose weight. This gives the impression that 25% more people lose weight on the ineffective diet.

Table 7.1 Analysing results without using ITT analysis

	Sample	Number of people who drop out	Number of people remaining who lose weight	% of people in the study who lose weight
Superfast weight loss diet	100	80	15/20	75
Traditional reduced calorie diet	100	0	50/100	50

In Table 7.2 we analyse all the data, regardless of drop outs, so that in the superfast weight loss diet 15/100 lose weight, which means that 15% of the people on this diet lose weight compared to the 50/100 or 50% who were on the traditional reduced calorie diet.

Table 7.2 Analysing results using ITT analysis

	Sample	Number of people who drop out	Number of people who lose weight	Proportion of all people who lost weight	% of people in the study who lose weight
Superfast weight loss diet	100	80	15	15/100	15
Traditional reduced calorie diet	100	0	50	50/100	50

MINIMISING BIAS AND THE PLAY OF CHANCE

The findings from a study where the participants in the sample represent a wider group are often extrapolated to a larger population. That is, if a new medicine is shown to be more effective than an older one in a specific sample following a randomised controlled trial, we assume that it would be effective in most or all of the population that have similar characteristics. Occasionally, the sample may not reflect the wider population and these deviations from the true population may be due to chance – also called variation – which is called **random error**. Chance can never be eliminated entirely, but it can be minimised by repeating the measurements, and by increasing the size of the study.

Bias is a preference or disposition to favour a particular conclusion, see Table 7.3 for types of bias that can occur in randomised controlled trials. Bias results from poor study design and cannot be corrected for at the analysis stage.

Table 7.3 Types of bias

Type of bias	Meaning
Selection bias	A systematic difference between those selected into the sample and those not selected. The sample is therefore not representative of the population
Allocation bias	A systematic distortion of the data as a result of the way in which participants were allocated to the experimental or control group
Detection bias	Systematic differences in the assessment of the outcome between the experimental and control group

Type of bias	Meaning
Observational bias	Suggests that the observations are informed or contaminated by the observer's beliefs, prejudices or background assumptions
Performance bias	Systematic differences in the care provided to participants in the experimental group compared to the control group
Attrition bias	Systematic differences in the loss of participants from the experimental and control group
Confounding bias	Occurs when a spurious association is made at the analysis stage between the intervention and the measurement, which, in reality, results from a different or secondary measurement
Recall bias	Differences in reporting experiences between those who have and those who do not have the outcome of interest; occurs particularly in retrospective studies
Publication bias	Occurs when only the available literature is reviewed concerning a trial rather than all the literature pertaining to the trial

ISSUES IN EVALUATING RANDOMISED CONTROLLED TRIALS

The structure of randomised controlled trials has become more precise as researchers try to eliminate the occurrence of bias or chance that will produce inaccurate conclusions. Experiments conducted in a laboratory setting can be controlled very tightly to avoid this (although even here bias and chance are a possibility) but randomised controlled trials are conducted in the real world with all the potential pitfalls that introduces, so when evaluating a study for its use in practice we need to assess the *clinical* importance of its findings. For example, we might find that in a trial that compares two treatments for high blood pressure we conclude that its findings are robust because the researchers have followed all the rules of experimental design. The study shows that the experimental treatment lowers diastolic blood pressure *on average* by 1 mmHg more than the control treatment. The researchers correctly claim this is a statistically significant finding, yet clinically how much difference would this make? If we take into account the potential side effect of each of the treatments, is the new treatment still attractive? This brings in a second issue, which is the similarity of the trial participants to your patients. This requires a degree of professional judgement and objectivity as on occasion we may have personal preferences that over-ride the evidence.

A third issue is the choice of outcome measure. This is important as we might choose a treatment based upon results that are actually irrelevant or of lesser importance. In studies of wound care it is often easier (and cheaper) to report how easy a dressing is to apply or how comfortable it is for the patient, but what we really need to know is whether it is effective in accelerating wound healing or reducing infection.

Length of follow up after the trial has been completed is also a consideration. We know now, for example, that the drug Vioxx whilst relieving arthritic pain also increased the incidence of heart attacks and strokes, whilst the so called 'new' or atypical antipsychotics cause weight gain and heart disease in the long term.

SUMMARY

Randomised controlled trials are a well-established means by which doctors and other health scientists determine the efficacy of medicinal products and interventions. Historically, the research priorities of nurses, midwives and allied health professionals addressed different areas of care, which did not lend them to experimental research of this type. This situation has changed in recent times and as health professionals take responsibility for interventions it is necessary that they understanding how good experimental evidence is produced. There are also several areas of health care, for example, wound care in the UK, where nurses conduct their own trials and have become extremely proficient in their conduct.

FURTHER READING

Akobeng, A.K. (2005) Understanding randomised controlled trials. *Archives of Disease in Childhood,* 90: 840–844.

A clear guide and a good starting point.

Greenhalgh, T. (2010) *How to Read a Paper: The Basics of Evidence Based Medicine* (4th edn). Chichester: Wiley-Blackwell.

This sets out the key themes and questions needed to understand other people's research.

Jadad, A.R. (2007) *Randomized Controlled Trials: Questions, Answers, and Musings* (2nd edn). Oxford: Blackwell.

This book is a convenient and accessible description of the underlying principles and practice of randomised controlled trials and their role in clinical decision making.

McRum-Gardner, S. (2010) Sample size and power calculations made simple. *International Journal of Therapy and Rehabilitation,* 17(1): 10–14.

A good, accessible discussion of quantitative research within health.

Don't forget to visit https://study.sagepub.com/harveyandland to watch videos, take quizzes and to follow specially designed web activities.

8

QUALITATIVE METHODS

This chapter builds on Chapters 3 and 5. In this chapter we will review qualitative methods in detail and we will:

- explore the qualitative methods of phenomenology, ethnography and grounded theory and their theoretical underpinnings
- review the practical, logistical and research governance issues to be considered when using these three methods in nursing and midwifery research
- appraise the strengths and limitations of phenomenology, ethnography and grounded theory.

As we have seen in Chapters 3 and 5 the underlying principles of interpretivism determine the ways in which qualitative research is carried out. These principles influence the sampling strategies, choice of methods of data collection and the way in which they are conducted, the type of data collected and the way that the data are analysed. In Chapter 5 we gave an overview of phenomenology, ethnography and grounded theory. In this chapter we will explore these methods more closely. This exploration will include the practical and logistical factors including research governance issues that the would-be researcher should take into consideration as they plan and then carry out their study.

The detailed exploration of phenomenology, ethnography and grounded theory will enable us to review their strengths and limitations. This will support the critical appraisal of these methods (see Chapter 22) and help would-be researchers decide the most appropriate method to use for their study. Strategies that the researcher may use to enhance the **trustworthiness** of studies using these methods will be considered in more detail in Chapter 21.

PHENOMENOLOGY

The foundations of phenomenology can be found in the ideologies of Husserl and Heidegger (Johnson, 2000; Dykes, 2004; Mapp, 2008). Phenomenology is used when researchers wish to gain insight into the experiences of individuals and is based on the notion that a person's reality is determined by their interpretations of their world. Phenomenology facilitates this process by enabling participants to describe and explain their lived experiences (Brinkmann and Kvale, 2015). A person's account therefore helps others to understand what life is like for them. The phrase that is synonymous with phenomenology is the 'lived experience' of the participants (Walsh and Downe, 2006). For example, 'what is the lived experience of pregnant women with gestational diabetes?' or 'what is the lived experience of people who are fulltime carers for a partner with Alzheimer's disease?' Whilst some findings from a phenomenological study may be unsurprising, new, often unexpected insights may also be revealed (Hunter, 2007).

THE UNDERPINNING PHILOSOPHIES OF PHENOMENOLOGY

The underpinning philosophies of nursing and midwifery are congruent with that of phenomenology (Van der Zalm and Bergum, 2000; Weaver and Olson, 2006). Like nursing and midwifery, phenomenology is person-centred and holistic and requires skills of communication, observation and interpersonal interaction (Koch, 1995; Murtagh and Folan, 2014). Nurses and midwives need to understand the perspective of patients, clients and their families so that they can care for them effectively (O'Leary, 2014). The phenomenological approach provides a way of gaining this insight by enabling the researcher to focus on the 'whole' person; in other words all aspects of the participant's lives, not just the condition, situation or problem that brings them into contact with health care professionals in the first place.

Phenomenology is derived from philosophy and its epistemological position is based on the belief that knowledge is revealed when meaning and understanding are established (Van der Zalm and Bergum, 2000). Phenomenology is based on the assumption that individuals encounter their experiences with and through others and that they play an active role in shaping their experience (Polit and Beck, 2014). A person's experiences and perceptions are therefore influenced by the context in which they occur. They are also embedded in and cannot be separated from their culture and personal history (Johnson, 2000; Robson, 2011).

DESCRIPTIVE AND INTERPRETIVE PHENOMENOLOGY

There are two main approaches to phenomenology: **descriptive** and **interpretive**. The differences between these approaches are determined by their theoretical underpinnings

(Dykes, 2004). However, it has been suggested that over-emphasis has been placed on these philosophical differences and the literature on phenomenology can be contradictory (Silverman, 2015). Descriptive phenomenology is grounded in the ideology of Husserl (Johnson, 2000; Dykes, 2004), which focuses on the concept of the 'life world' or 'lived experience' (Koch, 1995). The aim is to describe an individual's perception or account of their experiences (Smith, 1996). Descriptive phenomenology does not require the researcher to have prior knowledge or experience of the phenomena under investigation. To many proponents this lack of prior knowledge is desirable (Mapp, 2008). It enables the researcher to explore issues unhampered by any preconceived ideas that they might have about the topic under investigation and they can explore issues with an open mind (see Box 8.1).

BOX 8.1   AN EXAMPLE OF A DESCRIPTIVE PHENOMENOLOGICAL STUDY UNDERTAKEN BY A RESEARCHER WITH NO PRIOR KNOWLEDGE OR EXPERIENCE OF THE TOPIC

A team of health visitors have decided that a descriptive phenomenological study of mothers' experiences of postnatal depression would provide them with better insight into families encountering this condition and this in turn will help them to provide more effective care in the future. Funding is obtained and a researcher, Sally, is recruited. Sally is not a health care professional and she has no prior personal or professional experience of postnatal depression.

In situations where the researcher is familiar with the phenomena under investigation Husserl advocated that they set aside, suspend or 'bracket' prior knowledge, assumptions, beliefs and prejudices (Johnson, 2000; Giorgi and Giorgi, 2008). This is sometimes referred to as **bracketing**. The researcher usually does this before the study begins, by reflecting (usually in the form of a written account) on what they know, believe and assume about the topic. Bracketing assists data collection and analysis by increasing the likelihood that the reported findings describe the participants' experiences and perceptions (Johnson, 2000). This is because the researcher can refer back to their reflective account and check that they are not superimposing their own prior knowledge, experiences and beliefs on the study. Bracketing therefore enables the researcher to be receptive to participants' accounts (Brinkmann and Kvale, 2015). It is not a way of eradicating the researcher's prior knowledge, but it enables the researcher to look anew at phenomena and if necessary question their prior assumptions (see Box 8.2).

Website activity 8.1

BOX 8.2   AN EXAMPLE OF A DESCRIPTIVE PHENOMENOLOGICAL STUDY UNDERTAKEN BY A RESEARCHER WHO HAS PRIOR KNOWLEDGE OF THE TOPIC

Using the example of the phenomenological study of postnatal depression, rather than appointing Sally, the team appoint Gloria to undertake the study. Although Gloria has no personal experience of postnatal depression, she is a registered nurse and midwife and most recently has been working as a practice nurse in a primary care setting. Prior to undertaking this descriptive phenomenological study, Gloria writes a detailed reflective account which explores her knowledge, professional experiences and assumptions about postnatal depression. Gloria constantly refers to this account during data collection and data analysis to ensure the participants' accounts are the focus of the study.

THINK POINT ACTIVITY   8.1

What challenges might Gloria face as she writes her reflective account? How long do you think the account would be and how long do you think it would take her to write it?

Heidegger developed an alternative phenomenological approach known as interpretive phenomenology or hermeneutics (Johnson, 2000; Mapp, 2008). This approach to phenomenology attempts to interpret, analyse or explain the participants' experiences (Walker, 2014) (see Box 8.3). In doing this, interpretive phenomenology rejects the notion of bracketing (Dykes, 2004). Heideggerians argue that a researcher's understanding of participants' accounts is grounded in their own personal experiences. Researchers cannot therefore bracket their prior knowledge, assumptions and beliefs (Koch, 1995; Johnson, 2000). Within interpretive phenomenology the researcher's preconceptions are therefore an essential factor in the interpretation process. Interpretive phenomenology consequently requires the researcher to have prior knowledge of the phenomena (Mapp, 2008). The key difference therefore between descriptive and interpretive phenomenology is an ontological difference regarding the nature of reality (Koch, 1995).

BOX 8.3   AN EXAMPLE OF AN INTERPRETATIVE PHENOMENOLOGICAL STUDY

Continuing the example of the phenomenological study of postnatal depression, Gloria decides to take an interpretative phenomenological approach to the study. This means that she uses her prior knowledge and professional experiences to explore the mothers' experiences of postnatal depression.

PHENOMENOLOGICAL RESEARCH: SAMPLING

Whichever approach is adopted, phenomenological research follows the underlying principles of qualitative research whereby participant recruitment, data collection and data analysis occur concurrently. Phenomenology requires participants who have encountered the events or experiences that the researcher is investigating (Walker, 2014). Therefore non-probability, purposive sampling strategies are used (see Chapter 15). This means that the researcher decides on the required inclusion criteria for participants (e.g., this might include: age range, sex, geographical location, ethnicity) and then specifically invites people who meet the criteria to take part. In accordance with qualitative methodology, the exact sample size of a phenomenological study is not usually known before the study begins. However, the researcher should have a rough idea of the number of participants that they are likely to recruit and Brinkmann and Kvale (2015) suggest a sample of between five and 25 participants is usually sufficient. When deciding the likely sample size, the researcher should consider:

- the aim(s) and objective(s) of the study
- the accessibility and availability of potential participants
- the timeframe available
- the need to ensure trustworthiness (see Chapter 21).

The sample should include sufficient variation to ensure that a comprehensive range of experiences can be described. This means that participant inclusion criteria may change during the study if the initial data analysis suggests that the recruitment of different groups of participants would be beneficial. Another factor that will determine the final sample size is data saturation. This is when data collection and data analysis do not reveal any new findings and so the recruitment of further participants is deemed unnecessary (see Chapter 15).

PHENOMENOLOGICAL RESEARCH: DATA COLLECTION AND DATA ANALYSIS

The most commonly used method of data collection in phenomenology is semi-structured interviews during which participants are encouraged to reflect upon their experiences and feelings. The phenomenological interview is often regarded as being an engaged, in-depth conversation. Narrative accounts are generated which provide as accurate a portrayal as possible of the participant's lived experience (Johnson, 2000; Van der Zalm and Bergum, 2000; Giorgi and Giorgi, 2008). Questions posed within a phenomenological interview should therefore enable participants to describe their feelings, experiences and actions regarding the phenomena under investigation (Brinkmann and Kvale, 2015). It is essential that participants tell their story without interruption. Consequently the researcher and participant can be said to be co-authors of the data (Robson, 2011). Other methods of data collection may also be used such as diaries and case studies (see Chapter 17).

Phenomenological interviews are usually audio-recorded to facilitate transcription and data analysis. The recording should then be transcribed verbatim (word for word) into a word-processing document. A 30-minute interview will probably yield six to eight pages of dialogue (data). To manage the transcripts and organise the data analysis process researchers often use qualitative data analysis software packages such as NVivo because this can be difficult to do manually (Jacelon and O'Dell, 2005; Plummer-D'Amato, 2008). Whilst there are a number of different methods of qualitative data analysis, the most commonly used method in phenomenology is thematic analysis. This is where sections

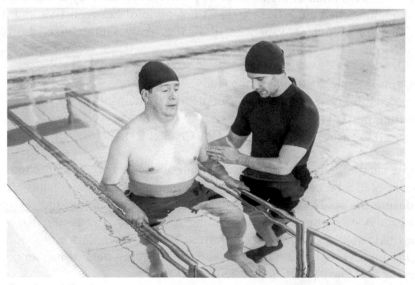

© andresr / iStock

of the data are coded into broad themes each of which usually contain a number of sub-themes (see Chapter 20). The themes identified in a phenomenological study may culminate in the development of a theory (see Box 8.4).

Website
activity 8.2

BOX 8.4   AN EXAMPLE OF THEORY DEVELOPMENT IN PHENOMENOLOGICAL RESEARCH

A phenomenological study of carers' experiences of looking after an adult relative with a learning disability could lead to the development of the theory that they feel abandoned by the health and social care services.

PHENOMENOLOGICAL RESEARCH: ETHICAL ISSUES

General research governance issues such as informed consent, participant confidentiality and the approvals processes are discussed in Chapter 18. However, in addition to these core issues that apply to all research methods, there are a number of other specific research governance issues that the would-be researcher should consider before embarking on a phenomenological study. The holistic nature of phenomenology may mean that the study encroaches on aspects of participants' lives that neither they nor the researcher had originally anticipated and sometimes unexpected sensitive, ethical and moral issues may be revealed (see Box 8.5).

BOX 8.5   ILLUSTRATION OF THE HOLISTIC NATURE OF PHENOMENOLOGICAL RESEARCH

The holistic nature of phenomenology means that during interviews with women about their postnatal depression, all aspects of their life may be discussed. For some women this might include topics such as financial difficulties, feelings of ambivalence towards their baby or domestic abuse.

It is therefore imperative that potential participants fully understand the purpose and possible scope of the study when they give consent. They should also be reassured that they can withdraw from the study at any time if they wish without adversely affecting their on-going care. The researcher should also have strategies in place before the study begins to deal with any sensitive issues and this includes the provision of on-going support for both the participant and themselves (Murtagh and Folan, 2014). If the participant discloses information during the interview that the researcher feels should be reported, he/she should be mindful of their professional responsibilities (Nursing and Midwifery Council, 2015a; 2015b) and follow the guidance in Chapter 18.

There is the possibility that participants will find discussing their feelings and experiences distressing (Corbin and Morse, 2003; Rogers, 2008). However, researchers should ensure that the phenomenological interview does not become a counselling session as this could place both researcher and participant in a vulnerable situation and jeopardise the whole study. The researcher should therefore constantly evaluate the apparent impact on participants throughout the interview (Rogers, 2008) and have strategies in place to provide participants with support if this is required. Most commonly the researcher arranges direct access to a counselling service or participants are given a debriefing sheet at the end of the interview identifying possible support that they can access if they wish (Baker, 2006).

Another situation that the researcher should constantly monitor is the potential impact of an imbalance of power (Brinkmann and Kvale, 2015). The phenomenological approach provides participants with a level of control over what they disclose. The potential for an imbalance of power is therefore reduced in comparison with other research methods (Corbin and Morse, 2003). However, there is always a risk that participants reveal more than they intend (Corbin and Morse, 2003; Brinkmann and Kvale, 2015). This in turn may raise ethical dilemmas for the researcher with regard to confidentiality and participant anonymity (see Chapter 18). The researcher should not unduly coerce participants during phenomenological interviews and when probing questions reveal no further information the researcher should assume the participant has disclosed all that he or she intends.

Whilst research participants are generally well protected during a study, researchers may be vulnerable during phenomenological studies particularly in relation to the exploration of sensitive or emotionally challenging topics (Rager, 2005; Lalor et al., 2006). Strategies should therefore be put in place to support the researcher. These can include keeping a reflective diary, periodically taking time out and regular discussion with their research supervisor (Johnson and Macleod Clarke, 2003; Rager, 2005).

**Website
activity 8.3**

THINK POINT ACTIVITY   8.2

List the strengths and possible limitations of phenomenology. It may help you to look at the examples of this type of study that we have used in this chapter.

ETHNOGRAPHY

A simple way of distinguishing between phenomenology and ethnography is that phenomenology focuses on individuals whilst ethnography usually focuses on groups of people. In contrast to phenomenology, ethnography also explores the setting or world in which individuals or groups of people come together whereby researchers explore the behaviours and beliefs of groups of people or of individuals within a group (Walsh and Downe, 2006; Dove and Muir-Cochrane, 2014). The roots of ethnography are in social anthropology when during the nineteenth century predominantly white, middle- and upper-class anthropologists such as Boas, Mead and Malinowski discovered, lived with and studied previously unknown or unreported communities (Denscombe, 2010; Patton, 2015). If we were to read some of these studies now, we would probably feel uncomfortable about the paternalistic ways in which they were written (Cruz and Higginbottom, 2013). However, whilst we cannot condone this approach, we should take into account the era in which these studies were written and the attitudes and wider political agenda at the time.

In the twentieth century, ethnographic researchers such as Whyte and Powdermaker began to turn their attention closer to home and focused on Western cultures and communities (Denscombe, 2010; Patton, 2015). Ethnographers use this research method when they wish to find out about the culture, customs, language, interactions, values, beliefs and actions of a group. In doing this, the researcher endeavours to gain insight into the social, psychological, political and economic factors that impact upon the group and the way in which it functions (Ploeg, 2008). In the context of ethnography it is argued that the culture brings individuals together and then binds them as a group. An ethnographic study therefore attempts to unravel the different aspects of the culture and the ways in which these influence group behaviour. In order to do this, ethnographers explore the key features and characteristics of the culture. This might include:

- accepted behaviours
- expectations about behaviours that are conveyed either overtly or covertly to those who join the group
- the group's social traditions, values, beliefs, opinions and ideas
- the system of communication, which may include signs, gestures, slang, abbreviations, terminology and language
- the group's artefacts or symbols that represents the group.

MACROETHNOGRAPHY AND MICROETHNOGRAPHY

An ethnographic study may focus on a group of any size. Studies that involve large groups such as a whole community are sometimes referred to as **macroethnography** whilst studies involving smaller, more focused groups such as people working in a particular

Website
activity 8.4

place of work may be referred to as **microethnography** (Cruz and Higginbottom, 2013). Ethnographic researchers believe that a person's behaviours and experiences are shaped by the culture of the group to which they belong (O'Leary, 2014). The researcher therefore endeavours to explore the behaviours, values and practices of groups through **thick description** of these factors (Geertez, 1993). This requires detailed description and interpretation of both the context and group activity (see Box 8.6).

BOX 8.6   AN EXAMPLE OF AN ETHNOGRAPHIC STUDY

Joe wants to understand the issues that affect health care professionals working in an inner city emergency care department. An ethnographic study will enable him to explore individual practitioner and group behaviours, the ways in which they interact with each other, their verbal and non-verbal communication, and factors that appear to facilitate and disrupt the group.

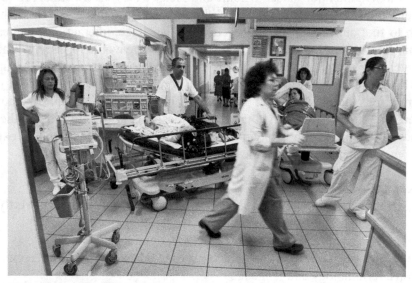

© ChameleonsEye / Shutterstock

ETHNOGRAPHIC RESEARCH: THE SETTING AND THE SAMPLE

The setting for an ethnographic study will be determined by the purpose of the research and the environment in which the group comes together (see Box 8.7). The researcher must therefore successfully negotiate access to the proposed study site with the gate-keepers. The sample size for an ethnographic study will be determined by the setting in which the study takes place and the number of group members who are willing to take part in the study. In accordance with the principles of qualitative research, non-probability sampling is adopted and the specific strategy of **convenience sampling** is usually used (see Chapter 15).

BOX 8.7   AN EXAMPLE ILLUSTRATING THE NEGOTIATION OF ACCESS FOR AN ETHNOGRAPHIC STUDY

Continuing the example of Joe's ethnographic study, to achieve the aims of his study this has to take place in an inner city emergency care setting. There are three such departments in the area where Joe lives. He approached the gate-keepers to all three sites and was able to successfully negotiate access to two of them. He was then able to recruit participants in both care settings.

ETHNOGRAPHIC RESEARCH: DATA COLLECTION AND DATA ANALYSIS

In ethnographic studies data collection and data analysis usually occur concurrently, and data collection will continue until data saturation is reached (see Chapters 15, 17 and 20). In order into gain insight into the group's behaviours, the most commonly used method of data collection is observation, which is carried out in the setting where the group comes together (Patton, 2015). This is sometimes referred to as collecting data 'in the field'. The terms that are often used in relation to ethnography are that the researcher 'immerses' themselves in the group and becomes 'intimate' with them. This means that the researcher spends time with and becomes part of the group. The rationale for taking this approach is that this strengthens the likelihood that the researcher will observe normal rather than contrived patterns of behaviour. Immersion and intimacy also enable the researcher to attain an '**emic**' or 'insider's' perspective of the group's behaviours. There are several different approaches to observation which may be used in ethnographic research. This may be done overtly or covertly whereby participants do or do not know that they are being observed. The researcher may also adopt a participant or non-participant approach to the observation. In participant observation, the researcher functions within the group whilst recording their observations. In non-participant observation, the researcher is not involved in group activities (see Chapter 17).

One of the potential limitations of observation is the possibility that participants change their behaviour because they are aware that they are being observed (Walsh and Baker, 2004; Patton, 2015). This was one of the reasons researchers gave in the past for undertaking covert observation. However, ethical concerns about observing participants without them being aware mean that this strategy is now rarely adopted. Consequently the researcher needs to consider other ways of ensuring that they observe normal patterns of behaviour (O'Leary, 2014). Strategies may include spending time with the group before the observations begin or discounting the initial period of data collection.

The researcher may document their observations as events occur or immediately afterwards, using pen and paper or by describing their observations on a digital voice-recorder. Alternatively they may use video cameras to record group activity. Whatever approach is used, the observations must be transcribed into a word-processing document. These observations when in documentary format are usually referred to as field notes and these can be extensive (Walsh and Baker, 2004). In ethnography, observation may be supported by other data collection methods such as interviews, diaries, focus groups, and media such as photographs, drawings and pictures (see Chapter 17).

Even short periods of observation can yield several pages of field notes. Ethnographic researchers therefore often use qualitative data analysis software packages to manage the field notes and organise the data analysis process. As is the case in phenomenological studies, the most commonly used method of data analysis in ethnographic research is thematic analysis (see above and Chapter 20). Whatever method of data analysis the ethnographic researcher uses, it is essential that they try not to impose any preconceived ideas that they might have on data collection and data analysis (Cruz and Higginbottom, 2013). A number of strategies can be used to minimise the risk of this occurring, probably the most common is reflexivity (Richards, 2009; Darawsheh, 2014). This is where the researcher considers the impact that they have had on the way in which the research has been conducted and the data analysed (see Chapter 5) (Cruz and Higginbottom, 2013).

The aim of data analysis is to explain group behaviours. In so doing, **tacit knowledge** is often revealed. In other words, activities and behaviours are identified which the group have not previously discussed or openly acknowledged. However, they recognise these activities and behaviours when the researcher reports their findings to them. As is the case for other qualitative methods, ethnographic research may culminate in the development of a theory (see Box 8.8).

BOX 8.8   AN EXAMPLE OF THEORY DEVELOPMENT IN ETHNOGRAPHIC RESEARCH

Joe's ethnographic study may lead to his development of the theory that hierarchical patterns of working inhibit the professional development of junior team members.

ETHNOGRAPHIC RESEARCH: ETHICAL ISSUES

In addition to the core research governance issues that will be discussed in Chapter 18, ethnographic research presents other research governance issues that the would-be researcher should consider before embarking on a study. The researcher may have difficulty obtaining permission for access from gate-keepers and this can be particularly problematic in health care settings (Walsh and Baker, 2004). Senior personnel may be concerned about the researcher's 'hidden agenda' even if there is none. Likewise health care professionals who are potential participants may be concerned about the real purpose of the research even if the aims and objectives of the study are fully explained (Gelling, 2014). This scepticism may arise from the increasing use of observation (albeit via covert video-recordings) to expose poor standards of health care over recent years.

Website activity 8.5

One of the challenges of endeavouring to recruit a group of people is that whilst the majority of the group may be willing to participate, some individuals may not. Potential participants should not be made to feel obliged to take part simply because other group members have agreed. However, this can present the researcher with practical and logistical challenges when arranging periods of data collection as they will need to ensure that those who have not consented to the study will not be present or can easily be excluded during the process. Similarly, problems arise when a participant in an ethnographic study wishes to withdraw part-way through the study. In most other types of research when this happens, all data involving that person can be destroyed at the participant's request. However, this may not be possible if, for example, observation of a group involving that participant has already taken place. Potential participants should be made aware of this when their consent is taken and if they subsequently decide to withdraw.

The researcher should have strategies in place before the study begins to deal with any difficult issues that may arise during an ethnographic study and this includes the provision of on-going support for both the participants and themselves. If the researcher observes activities or behaviours during a period of observation that he or she feels should be reported, their professional responsibilities should be fulfilled (Nursing and Midwifery Council, 2015a; 2015b) and the guidance in Chapter 18 followed.

As we have seen, central to ethnographic research, and the use of observation in particular, is the researcher immersing themselves in the group and becoming intimate with them. However, there is a very fine line between this enabling the researcher to achieve thick description and the researcher becoming so immersed in the group that they become over-familiar with the participants and either anticipate or begin to filter out behaviours and activities (Denscombe, 2010). This is sometimes referred to as the researcher 'going native'. This may be done deliberately or unintentionally, as researchers lose their perspective on the nuances of group behaviour. A number of strategies can be implemented to reduce the risk of the researcher going native. This could include maintaining a reflective diary, periodically taking time out and regular discussion with their research supervisor.

Website
activity 8.6

> ## THINK POINT ACTIVITY   8.3
>
> List the strengths and possible limitations of ethnography. It may help you to look at the examples of this type of study that we have used in this chapter.

GROUNDED THEORY

As we identified in Chapter 5, grounded theory has its origins in sociology and symbolic interactionism. It was first described by Glaser and Strauss in the 1960s and was used in their studies of people dying in hospital (Grubs and Piantanida, 2010; Punch, 2014). Glaser, Strauss, Corbin and Charmaz have subsequently become the authorities on grounded theory research (Markey et al., 2014). To some extent, grounded theory is something of a misnomer because it is not a theory in itself. It is instead a research method which enables the researcher to develop a theory inductively that describes and explains phenomena in order to provide a better understanding of people's lives, their attitudes and their behaviours (Brunstad and Hjälmhult, 2014). The theory that is developed is said to be 'grounded' in reality, in other words the theory has its roots in the data that have been collected about the phenomena.

Grounded theory is an ideal method to use when no prior theory about the phenomena under investigation exists (Maz, 2013). It is therefore a particularly useful research method for the professions of nursing and midwifery, which are still establishing their body of knowledge. Grounded theory is also an appropriate method to use if the aim of a study is to gain a more detailed understanding of factors affecting the health of patients and clients. Theories developed from grounded theory studies therefore inform nursing and midwifery practice and can be used to develop models, frameworks, policies and standards of care.

A grounded theory study begins with the recognition that greater insight to a phenomenon is required. This recognition can be generated into a general idea, problem or concern rather than a specific research question. During the course of the study it is essential that the researcher has an open mind about the topic under investigation. For this reason, it is advocated that the researcher should not undertake a detailed literature search and review at this stage (Holloway and Galvin, 2015). Whilst the researcher may have a level of knowledge and beliefs about the phenomena, they should not be unduly influenced by their preconceived ideas. This can be difficult because researchers are inevitably drawn to subjects that they are interested in and for clinical nurses and midwives the topic may be an aspect of their work. Being reflexive by keeping a reflective journal is probably the most effective way that a researcher can consider the impact that they have on the way in which the research is conducted (Richards, 2009; Darawsheh, 2014) (see Chapters 5 and 21).

GROUNDED THEORY RESEARCH: THE SETTING AND THE SAMPLE

In grounded theory participants are sometimes referred to as **data sources**. As is the case with phenomenology, the researcher using grounded theory does not know at the beginning of the study where the study will be conducted or how many participants will be involved because participants are recruited as the study progresses. Non-probability sampling strategies will be used throughout the study. Initially purposive or convenience sampling will be used whereby participants who the researcher feels will be able to inform the study will be recruited. During the initial period of data collection and data analysis the researcher looks for factors that may possibly explain the phenomena under investigation (Maz, 2013). Having identified these factors, the researcher identifies further participants or data sources who may be able to provide insight into these issues (Patton, 2015). Further participants will be then recruited using **theoretical sampling** (see Chapter 15). The means that the researcher specifically recruits participants who they think will help them to refine or challenge the theory that is being developed (Grubs and Piantanida, 2010). The evolving theory therefore determines the researcher's recruitment of subsequent participants (Bryman, 2012). Theoretical sampling continues until the theory has been finalised.

GROUNDED THEORY RESEARCH: DATA COLLECTION AND DATA ANALYSIS

In grounded theory the researcher will use whichever data collection method they think is appropriate. Likely data collection methods include in-depth interviews, focus groups, diaries, observation, semi-structured questionnaires, images such as photographs and pictures and exploration of documentation. Initially the data collection will be predominantly qualitative. However, as the theory becomes more refined, quantitative data may also be collected. Indeed, Glaser came from a predominantly quantitative philosophical stance (Maz, 2013).

An essential feature of grounded theory is that recruitment of participants, data collection and data analysis occur simultaneously (Brunstad and Hjälmhult, 2014). This enables the researcher to identify the required characteristics of further participants, issues to explore with them and the type of data collection methods to use. This is described as being an iterative or cyclical process.

A grounded theory study is likely to generate large quantities of data in the form of transcripts and field notes. Researchers therefore often use qualitative data analysis software packages to manage the data and organise the data analysis process. Data analysis involves the constant comparison method using open, axial and theoretical coding (Grubs and Piantanida, 2010; Corbin and Strauss, 2015). The researcher compares the data that they have collected from different sources and looks for confirmations and contradictions, similarities and differences. This therefore means that if new issues are found in data collected subsequently, the researcher should go back to the initial data to see if those issues can be identified there. This process of constant comparison also enables the researcher to identify other potential data sources that will inform the theory. This constant comparison helps the researcher to cultivate, refine and challenge the theory and triangulation of data, in other words using different types of data from a range of sources and participants strengthens the theory that is ultimately developed. It is often mistakenly suggested that the theory emerges from the data. This implies that the theory appears spontaneously, as if by magic. This perception of theory development seriously undervalues the role of the researcher, who must, through the recruitment of appropriate participants, rigorous data collection and data analysis, develop and refine the theory. The researcher is therefore integral to the development of the theory (Grubs and Piantanida, 2010) and one of the challenges they face is knowing when the theory is sufficiently refined (see Box 8.9).

BOX 8.9   AN EXAMPLE OF A GROUNDED THEORY STUDY

Rosie wants to find out about parenting a child with Down's Syndrome. For her grounded theory study Rosie begins by carrying out interviews with five parents who have a child with Down's Syndrome. To further explore some of the issues that Rosie identifies in the analysis of the interviews she carries out three focus groups with other parents who have a child with Down's Syndrome. As a consequence of some of the issues that these family raise, Rosie observes families attending out-patient clinics and support group meetings over a period of four weeks. She also examines literature about Down's Syndrome including material produced by health care professionals, user groups and charities. The theory that Rosie finally develops focuses on the feelings of failure and isolation that parents experience.

THINK POINT ACTIVITY   8.4

What other possible data sources and data collection methods do you think Rosie might involve in her study?

GROUNDED THEORY RESEARCH: ETHICAL ISSUES

In addition to the core research governance issues discussed in Chapter 18, grounded theory research presents other research governance issues that the would-be researcher should consider before embarking on a study. These issues often relate to factors associated with the data collection methods such as interviews and observation, which we have previously discussed in this chapter. The flexible and evolving

Website activity 8.7

nature of grounded theory means that researchers can rarely predict at the start of the study which data sources or methods of data collection will be involved. This means that when research governance approvals are applied for, researchers can usually only describe the initial or earlier phase of the study. Consequently further approvals may be required as the study evolves (see Chapter 18).

Multiple approaches to grounded theory have evolved over the last 50 years and it is important to note that Glaser and Strauss subsequently had different views about the way in which grounded theory should be conducted (Patton, 2015). Strauss began to work with Corbin in 1980s and Glaser became critical of Strauss and Corbin's techniques for data analysis and theory development (Denscombe, 2010; Markey et al., 2014).

Website
activity 8.8

THINK POINT ACTIVITY   8.5

List the strengths and possible limitations of grounded theory. It may help you to look at the examples of this type of study that we have used in this chapter.

SUMMARY

When reading qualitative studies you may have noticed that researchers do not always indicate which specific method they have used, for example, Gergett and Gillen (2014) and Lindgren et al. (2015). There may be a number of reasons for this and it does not necessarily mean that the studies presented in this way are flawed. However, we anticipate that this chapter has provided you with sufficient information for you to decide for yourself when reading such research papers.

Website
activity 8.9

In this chapter we have explored phenomenology, ethnography and grounded theory. In doing this we have considered some of the strengths and limitations of these three methods and in particular the practical, logistical and research governance issues that the would-be researcher should try to address. Some of the issues we have discussed in this chapter such as sampling strategies, methods of data collection and data analysis, and research governance issues are explored in greater detail in subsequent chapters.

Website
activity 8.10

FURTHER READING

Hunter, B. (2007) 'The art of teacup balancing': reflections on conducting qualitative research. *Evidence Based Midwifery*, 5(3): 76–79.

In this paper, the author reflects upon her experiences of carrying out qualitative studies and identifies a range of factors which exemplify the value of this approach to research.

Silverman, D. (2013) *A Very Short, Fairly Interesting and Reasonably Cheap Book about Qualitative Research* (2nd edn). London: Sage Publications.

This book gives a more detailed discussion regarding phenomenology, ethnography and grounded theory.

PHENOMENOLOGY IN ACTION

Murtagh, M. and Folan, M. (2014) Women's experiences of induction of labour for post-date pregnancy. *British Journal of Midwifery*, 22(2): 105–110.

Walker, W.M. (2014) Emergency care staff experiences of lay presence during adult cardiopulmonary resuscitation: a phenomenological study. *Emergency Medicine Journal*, 31(6): 453–458.

ETHNOGRAPHY IN ACTION

Batch, M. and Windsor, C. (2015) Nursing casualization and communication: a critical ethnography. *Journal of Advanced Nursing*, 71(4): 870–880.

Dove, S. and Muir-Cochrane, E. (2014) Being safe practitioners and safe mothers: a critical ethnography of continuity of care midwifery in Australia. *Midwifery*, 30(10): 1063–1072.

GROUNDED THEORY IN ACTION

Brunstad, A. and Hjälmhult, E. (2014) Midwifery students learning experiences in labor wards: a grounded theory study. *Nurse Education Today*, 34(12): 1474–1479.

McCarthy, B., Andrews, T. and Hegarty, J. (2015) Emotional resistance building: how family members of loved ones undergoing chemotherapy treatment process their fear of emotional collapse. *Journal of Advanced Nursing*, 71(4): 837–848.

Don't forget to visit https://study.sagepub.com/harveyandland to watch videos, take quizzes and to follow specially designed web activities.

9

SURVEYS, ACTION RESEARCH AND HISTORICAL RESEARCH

This is the third chapter in which we review specific research methods in detail. This chapter builds on Chapters 3, 4 and 5 and in it we will:

- explore the scope and purpose of surveys, action research and historical research and their theoretical underpinnings
- review the practical, logistical and research governance issues to be considered when using these three methods in nursing and midwifery research
- appraise the strengths and limitations of surveys, action research and historical research.

In Chapters 7 and 8 we have explored specific quantitative and qualitative research methods. However, as we identified in Chapters 4 and 5, there are some research methods that cannot be pigeon-holed so easily because they may adopt a quantitative *or* qualitative approach, or a mix of both. In this chapter we will review in detail three such methods: surveys, action research and **historical research**. This exploration will include the practical, logistical and research governance issues that the would-be researcher should take into consideration as they plan and then carry out their study.

The detailed review of surveys, action research and historical research will enable us to review their strengths and limitations. This will support the critical appraisal of these methods (see Chapter 22) and help would-be researchers decide the most appropriate method to use for their study. Strategies that the researcher may use to enhance the validity, reliability and trustworthiness of studies using these methods will be considered in more detail in Chapter 21.

SURVEYS

We recognise that no important decisions in life should be made until all the relevant information is gathered, scrutinised and digested. This is also true in our professional lives, where proposed changes in practice or procedures need to be prefaced by an analysis of the current situation. Survey research can be used as a tool by which a situation can be explored in a number of different ways to produce the most illuminating answers.

Most people will have participated in a survey at some time in their life, from being approached by people with clipboards outside a supermarket to those who telephone you asking you to rate your experience of a recent holiday. Surveys remain one of the most common methods used in research and originate from the commercial world, the examples above providing data for market research. The word 'survey' can also sometimes be used inappropriately when people are really referring to a specific method of data collection such as a questionnaire or interview. This is common in the business world, where researchers might ask you to complete a survey when they are actually asking you to complete a questionnaire. It is important to make the distinction that strictly speaking the term survey should be used to express the method of a particular type of research and questionnaires are the method of data collection often used in surveys. A survey is a research method which can be quantitative or qualitative in approach. Surveys gather information about attitudes, beliefs, behaviours and the prevalence, distribution and incidence of a variable, usually using questionnaires, diaries or observation.

The term 'survey' is all encompassing, and can include a variety of different research designs (see Chapter 11). Survey research can measure responses from individuals or groups and it is invaluable in the collection of demographic data. The survey method is preferred when a large volume of data is required and the most well-known survey is probably the US or UK population census, which utilise the whole population. However, under normal circumstances this is not practical, so a survey will engage a sample of the total population with the aim that the sample should be representative of the total population. If the sample is deemed to be representative, the findings can then be generalised, that is, assumed to reflect the responses that would have been given by all of the people had they been asked. In survey research the most common methods of sampling involve either random or convenience sampling strategies. The latter may lead to the generation of biased, non-representative findings. There also are surveys that aim to engage hard to reach populations, for example, asylum seekers or sex workers, and in this case a snowball sample may be used (for further discussion on sampling, see Chapter 15).

THE PURPOSE OF SURVEY RESEARCH

Surveys describe reality; they can provide data regarding prevalence, incidence, trends, attitudes, opinions, characteristics, experiences and behaviours. They often take a quantitative approach with the collection of quantifiable data from a large representative sample. However, it must be remembered that researchers may take a more qualitative approach, particularly if the aim of the survey is to collect information about people's thoughts, feelings and experiences. Therefore, the underpinning philosophy of a survey will be influenced by the approach taken (qualitative or quantitative, interpretivist or positivist) (see Chapter 3).

There are two distinct types of survey:

- The **descriptive survey**: this aims to describe as accurately as possible the situation as it is.
- The **explanatory survey** or **analytical survey**: this aims to establish cause and effect relationships or associations between variables without the use of experimental manipulation.

These two types of survey provide a framework and under this umbrella there are different approaches or designs that could be considered, such as the longitudinal survey design (may also be called cohort or trend surveys), cross-sectional surveys (sometimes known as the 'one-shot' or 'one-hit' survey design) or correlational survey design (see Chapter 11).

THINK POINT ACTIVITY   9.1

What do you think are the advantages and limitations of the survey method?

The method(s) of data collection used in surveys may take a qualitative or quantitative approach or a combination of both. The method used will be determined by: the population, sample, the nature of the data being sought and the resources available to the researcher. The most commonly used methods are illustrated in Box 9.1. A more detailed consideration of each of these is given in Chapters 16 and 17.

BOX 9.1   METHODS OF DATA COLLECTION USED IN SURVEYS

- Questionnaire: postal, email, electronic or distributed directly to participants.
- Interviews: face-to-face, Internet, video-link or telephone.
- Focus groups: face-to-face, Internet, video-link or conference telephone.
- Observation: overt or covert, participant or non-participant.
- Diaries.

The advantages of surveys include:

- Surveys can be used to research a wide range of topics.
- Surveys can be efficient, cost-effective and relatively economical to carry out.

- Surveys can be used to collect data from a wide geographical area, particularly if postal questionnaires or telephone interviews are used.
- An extensive amount of data can be generated.
- Surveys have in comparison to some other research methods fewer ethical implications; they do not involve invasive techniques or treatments.
- If the sample is representative of the population, survey findings can be generalised to the total population thus promoting internal and external validity (see Chapters 15 and 21).
- Multiple methods of data collection can be used in a survey to validate data.
- Surveys can be replicated.

The limitations of the survey method include:

- Internal and external validity is influenced by the sampling strategy used (see Chapters 15 and 21).
- Surveys tend to be used to collect exclusively quantitative data. Some would regard this as being a limitation.
- It is difficult to assess validity and reliability without access to the data collection tool (see Chapter 21).
- Surveys are often carried out without adequate planning/design.
- Surveys may yield low response rates.

In summary, surveys are an extremely practical and useful method for gathering large amounts of data, but they are sometimes employed by researchers who view them as a 'quick and dirty' way of gathering information. Surveys should be undertaken with the same rigour as any other design as only then will the information they contain be of any real value.

Website activity 9.1

ACTION RESEARCH

Action research is sometimes alternatively known as participatory, collaborative or emancipatory research, and Kurt Lewin's work on change theory and group dynamics in the 1940s is generally acknowledged as providing the foundation for this research method (O'Leary, 2014). Action research takes a cyclical, problem-solving approach (see Figure 9.1) and requires the collaboration of the team involved in the research through all stages of the study. This collaborative approach provides a useful mechanism for empowering or emancipating participants. It is therefore particularly suited to research involving vulnerable groups in health care settings such as children and people with mental health problems or learning disabilities. Action research can also be used as a means of engaging those who might otherwise

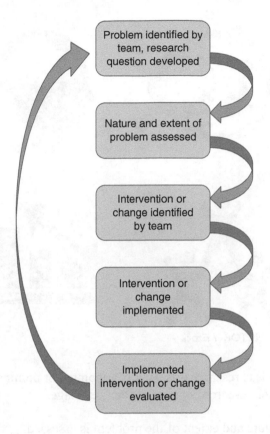

Figure 9.1   Cyclical research process of action research

be sceptical about research or feel threatened by it. Indeed, it has been suggested that engaging and empowering participants may be more important than solving the problem (Robson, 2011).

Action research is commonly used in educational and feminist research, and has also been used to facilitate organisational change (Robson, 2011). Action research was commonly used in nursing and midwifery research in the 1980s with proponents including Hunt, Chevasse and Webb. The particular strength of action research during this era was that it empowered nurses and midwives to be involved in research and supported the development of an evidence base. It is perhaps now less commonly used because of the practical and logistical challenges, which we will explore later in this section.

An action research study begins when a problem is identified and acknowledged by a group of people who agree to work together to try to solve the problem in the setting

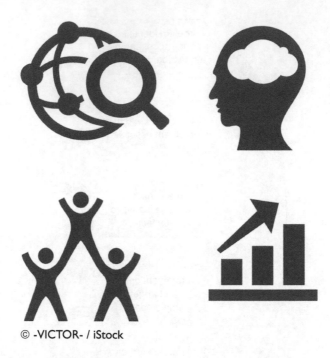

© -VICTOR- / iStock

in which it occurs. A lead researcher is usually appointed or nominated by the team. The first cycle of the action research consists of four key stages:

1 Assess: the nature and extent of the problem is assessed.
2 Plan: an intervention or change is identified which the group feels is likely to address the problem.
3 Implement: the intervention or change is implemented.
4 Evaluate: the impact of the intervention or change is evaluated.

Nurses will recognise these as being the four stages synonymous with those of the nursing process and all nurses and midwives should be familiar with the problem-solving approach to the provision of patient/client care.

Website activity 9.2

In an action research study, evaluation of the implementation of the intervention or change will identify if further interventions or changes are required to address the initial problem. Sometimes the evaluation identifies new or previously unrecognised problem(s) that the team feels should be solved. If either of these situations is the case, the cycle begins again, with the group proposing further interventions or changes. The effect of these additional interventions or changes should subsequently be evaluated. The research is concluded when the initial problem has been addressed and a theory is often developed which relates to addressing the problem (see Box 9.2).

BOX 9.2   EXAMPLE ILLUSTRATING ACTION RESEARCH

It has been noted that the job satisfaction of staff working in a practice area has deteriorated over the last year. The staff decide to carry out an action research study and identify a number of strategies that they feel could help improve staff morale. One of these strategies, a professional development programme, is implemented and subsequent evaluation shows that staff morale has improved slightly. However, staff feel there is scope for further improvement. On more detailed investigation it is identified that some staff felt excluded from the professional development programme, whilst others felt it did not meet their personal needs. The programme and access to it is therefore reviewed and changes made. Subsequent evaluation shows that morale had improved to a level the staff were happy with.

At the outset of a study using research action, beyond addressing the initial problem, the research team rarely knows how the study will evolve and how many cycles will be required. There are a number of different models of action research available which commonly adopt a flexible and evolving approach generally associated with qualitative research. However, action research designs can in some cases constrain the research process by implying a required order (Deery, 2011).

The data collection method(s) adopted in an action research study should be determined by the nature of the study. Traditional data collection methods such as interviews, questionnaires and focus groups may be used (see Chapters 16 and 17). However, these may not be appropriate for the participants that action research often endeavours to engage. Therefore, in these cases, less traditional methods such storytelling, photography, role play and artwork may be more appropriate.

For action research to be successful the collaboration and commitment of all those involved is required and should be evident throughout each stage of the research process including the design, conduct and dissemination. Team members therefore become active rather than passive participants of the research. However, maintaining collaboration and commitment and ensuring everyone has their say about the way in which the research is conducted can be a challenge. Some team members may become dominant, whilst others feel excluded if their views are not acknowledged or they may feel coerced into adopting the consensus view in order that the research can continue.

Participants who decide to opt out of the study may become disruptive and destructive and if too many participants drop out, it may not be possible to sustain the research. Equally the need for democracy may mean that the lead researcher feels they are losing control of the research. The blurring of roles between being a participant, a colleague and a co-researcher can also unsettle the status quo and this may in some cases jeopardise the research (Gelling and Munn-Giddings, 2011). Action research may also reveal previously unacknowledged problems or uncomfortable truths which the group or individual members may be reluctant to accept. The skills set of the lead researcher is therefore paramount and should include managing and avoiding conflict, facilitating collaboration and maintaining team motivation.

The flexible and evolving nature of action research can also present research governance challenges. Obtaining approvals and informed consent from participants can be problematic because the research team does not know at the outset how the research will evolve. Consequently approvals and informed consent may only be given for the first cycle and these will need to be obtained again for any second or subsequent cycles. Maintaining the anonymity and confidentiality of participants can also be a challenge as all participants will know who has been involved in the study.

One of the criticisms of action research commonly stated is that the implementation of change can be undertaken without the need to make it into a research study. Whilst that might be the case, action research formalises the change process and provides a motivation to ensure that change is implemented and the (anticipated) subsequent improvement is carried through to its conclusion. Knowing at which point to end the research can, however, be a problem. Whilst the research team may prefer to continue the cycles until the problem is completely solved or eradicated, a level of problem-solving may have to be accepted.

Despite its critics, action research has its strengths. It has been described as being democratic and egalitarian (Lingard et al., 2008). It can promote team working and enables all team members to take ownership of the research. It also provides an established mechanism for developing care and service provision.

Website activity 9.3

THINK POINT ACTIVITY   9.2

Summarise the advantages and limitations of action research.

HISTORICAL RESEARCH

Nursing and midwifery historical research has become increasingly popular over recent years for a number of reasons. The emergence of autobiographical accounts, television series and films focusing on health care in the past have whetted our appetite for an insight into the lives of health care professionals, the context in which they worked and the patients, clients and families they looked after (Holme, 2015). The anniversary of important events such as the outbreak of the First World War, the discovery of antibiotics and the establishment of the NHS have also motivated researchers to examine health care in the past with a fresh pair of eyes. The growing interest in historical research has also been promoted by the increasing number of professional organisations and university departments that focus on this type of research. It must also be acknowledged that in an era when the research governance and other logistical factors can seem to make nursing and midwifery research prohibitive, historical research can often be regarded as being more straightforward and therefore in some ways an easier option for MSc and PhD students.

Historical research involves the collection and analysis of data that relate to people, places and events in the past. In the context of nursing and midwifery, one of the main reasons for doing this is to obtain new insight and to develop our understanding about the foundations of the professions and health care practice more generally. Learning about the past in this way informs the present (Fealy et al., 2010). In some cases it can also tell us about the future by predicting trends and patterns. Therefore, in some instances, historical research can prevent us from 'reinventing the wheel'. The findings of historical research can also correct misunderstandings, romanticised views of the past and inaccurate information (Holme, 2015). For example, Toms and Shepherd's work identified the falsification of information by mill owners which enabled high levels of child labour to be maintained in the nineteenth century (Elton, 2014). Finally, historical research can provide a foundation for further studies.

The historical researcher needs to be organised and systematic in their approach to the research. The process begins with the identification of a topic or an area of interest and from this a research question should be developed. This in turn will identify the type of data needed in order to answer the question. The researcher must then establish the existence, location and accessibility of the data and if applicable find out whose permission is required in order to access them. Once any necessary agreements have been obtained, the researcher collects and then analyses the data. This may seem a relatively straightforward process. However, establishing the existence of data and negotiating access to them can be time consuming. A financial cost may also be involved because in some cases a fee may be charged to access data. Another challenge that a researcher may sometimes encounter is rather than having insufficient data, having to confine them (Rafferty and Wall, 2010). A clearly focused research question that, for example, relates to a specific geographical area or group of people will help resolve this problem.

An increasingly popular way of capturing data about service provision, care delivery, patients and clients is by accessing clinical databases. Whilst researchers must acquire the appropriate permissions and approvals to access these and in some cases may also be charged per data-set to do so, databases nevertheless provide a ready-made data source (Loke, 2014; Sinclair, 2015). Organisations such as universities and hospitals are also increasingly digitising their archives and those they have acquired through previous mergers and reorganisations. This means, for example, that universities often hold a wealth of material from former schools and colleges of nursing and midwifery.

Historical research generally takes a qualitative approach. This is because at the start of the study, the researcher often does not know where their investigation will take them. The evolving research design synonymous with historical research may lead the researcher to unexpected sources and types of data. Two broad sources of data are likely to be accessed. These are primary sources, which are first-hand accounts found for example in letters, diaries and autobiographies, or secondary sources, which report the second-hand accounts of others. These secondary sources can be found, for example, in newspaper articles, edited texts and biographies. Wherever possible, the researcher should try to access primary sources to check that nothing has been missed or that inter-pretations are correct. In some cases, the researcher's investigation may lead them to people who are willing to tell their story either in an interview or focus group.

Website activity 9.4

THINK POINT ACTIVITY   9.3

Make a list of the possible data sources, both primary and secondary, that a researcher might access. Compare your list with ours, which can be found on the companion website.

The amount of historical data available to researchers is increasing all the time as the archives of organisations, libraries, hospitals, universities and private collections are digitalised and can be accessed via the Internet. Having located the data, the researcher faces a number of challenges. Determining the reliability and authenticity of the data can be problematic, particularly given the increasing amount of erroneous information found on the Internet. Wherever possible, the researcher should determine if the author of the material is a reliable authority. They should also try to verify or corroborate information from a range of sources. The researcher should also consider if the infor-mation was written contemporaneously. If not, the impact of incomplete recollection, 'rose tinted spectacles' or the effect of other subsequent events or knowledge should be considered. The possibility of a hidden agenda at the time of data recording should also be considered. For example, the minutes of a meeting when infection rates on a particular ward were discussed may 'gloss over' uncomfortable truths. The researcher should also try to determine whether the material is complete or if it could have been altered. In some cases, 'translation' may be required to clarify jargon, terminology, accepted slang and abbreviations used at the time. Weights, measures and currencies may also need to be clarified. In some instances a word may have a different meaning now than in the past.

The method of data analysis required will be determined by the type of data collected: qualitative or quantitative (see Chapters 19 and 20). In analysing the data the researcher will face further challenges. Care should be taken not to generalise or oversimplify the findings. The nuances of individual stories should be captured. The researcher should therefore determine the extent to which an individual data source is representative of people more generally or of the wider situation. The data should also be analysed in the context of the social, cultural, religious, economic and political agenda at the time (see Box 9.3).

BOX 9.3   EXAMPLE ILLUSTRATING HISTORICAL RESEARCH

Beth wishes to investigate the role of nurses who worked at her local hospital around the time of the First World War. Beth has heard that nurses from the hospital were sent to work at the Western Front. Beth wants to find out if this rumour is true and, if it is, she wants to know if nurses volunteered for this work or were sent, where they worked, how long they worked there, the conditions in which they worked, and their roles and responsibilities. Beth obtains permission to access the hospital archives. This includes nurse records and reports, nurses' diaries and testimonies. Having explored the data Beth believes she has found evidence that indicates the impact the nurses' work during the First World War had on subsequent nurse training at the hospital.

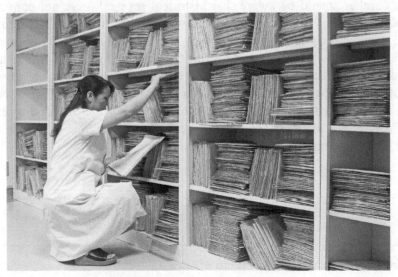

© Yuangeng Zhang / Shutterstock

THINK POINT ACTIVITY   9.4

What other data sources could Beth access? What factors might determine her being able to use these sources?

Website activity 9.5

One of the perceived attractions of historical research is that the requirements of informed consent from the person or people that the data relate to is generally not required. However, informed consent would of course be required if participants were recruited to take part in interviews or focus groups. Researchers should remember that they have a duty of care to data sources. Documents and artefacts should be handled and stored appropriately. Researchers should also be mindful that people mentioned in the research are usually unable to correct inaccuracies, or defend their words or actions. To protect individuals, wherever possible they should be anonymised.

Permission may also be required to access archived material. The person from whom permission is required will advise the researcher if further research governance issues need to be addressed. In the case of health related material, it is possible that the researcher may only be able to access anonymised data. The 30-year rule in relation to access to public records and the 100-year rule regarding access to medical records (Rafferty and Wall, 2010) should also be considered along with the requirements of the Data Protection Act (1998) and the Freedom of Information Act (2000) (see Chapter 18).

Website activity 9.6

The researcher should be aware that historical research may not conform to traditional perceptions of health care research, which tends to focus on improving care. Historical research may also be regarded by some as being nothing more that naval gazing. Indeed, many papers reporting the findings of historical research often do not provide sufficient information about the methodological approach taken in order to facilitate evaluation of the study's rigour (Fealy et al., 2013) (see Chapter 22). However, this research method enables us to learn about the past and to explain the present (Fealy et al., 2010). In some cases it can also reveal uncomfortable truths and challenge ideas, assumptions and stereotypes.

THINK POINT ACTIVITY   9.5

Summarise the advantages and limitations of historical research.

SUMMARY

In this chapter we have reviewed surveys, action research and historical research in detail. This exploration included the strengths and limitations of these three research methods. We have also considered the practical, logistical and research governance issues that the would-be researcher should take into consideration as they plan and then carry out their study.

Website activity 9.7

FURTHER READING

SURVEYS

Gerrish, K. and Lathlean, J. (2015) *The Research Process in Nursing* (7th edn), Chichester: Wiley-Blackwell.

This book illustrates the significant advances in nursing research and the importance of evidence-based practice. Chapter 19 provides a good resource for both the novice and the more experienced researcher.

Toepoel, V. (2015) *Doing Online Surveys*. London: Sage Publications.

This book provides a detailed exploration of the use of online surveys.

ACTION RESEARCH

Coghlan, D. and Brannick, T. (2014) *Doing Research in Your Own Organization* (4th edn). London: Sage Publications.

A general action research title that explores the specific challenges of conducting research in your own organisation and with colleagues.

McDonnell, P. and McNiff, J. (2015) *Action Research for Nurses*. London: Sage Publications.

Williamson, G.R., Bellman, L. and Webster, J. (2012) *Action Research in Nursing and Healthcare*. London: Sage Publications.

These two texts explore the use of action research in nursing and health care settings.

HISTORICAL RESEARCH

Chatteron, C. (2012) What is the 'best evidence' for researching nursing history? *The Bulletin*, 1 (2): 5–20.

A paper that considers conducting historical research. It can be accessed via the UK Association for the History of Nursing website: www.nursing.manchester.ac.uk/ukchnm/ukahn/ (last accessed 1 June 2016).

Lange, M. (2013) *Comparative-Historical Methods*. London: Sage Publications.

An easy-to-follow introduction which showcases classic analyses, offers clear methodological examples and describes major methodological debates. It is a comprehensive, grounded book which understands the learning and research needs of students and researchers.

Don't forget to visit https://study.sagepub.com/harveyandland to watch videos, take quizzes and to follow specially designed web activities.

10

SYSTEMATIC REVIEWS

> This chapter provides an overview of systematic reviews and the process of producing one. In this chapter we will:
>
> - establish the difference between narrative literature reviews and systematic reviews
> - discuss the need for systematic reviews
> - describe the process of systematic reviews.

From the very beginning of student life and our continuing professional development we learn to write assignments in an academic manner. This involves using critical analysis, and to support this analysis we use relevant literature. If we are honest what we probably do is to search the literature for papers that agree with the statement we are making and reference them whilst ignoring the papers that disagree with our view. As our learning continues to mature, we may add the odd reference that presents an opposing view, but the balance of the argument will always favour our own opinions. This bias is not limited to student assignments, but has been a feature of medical reporting and found in the allied health literature for many years. Take the example in Chapter 2 on evidence-based practice: although there was good evidence from a systematic review to suggest that anti-thrombolytics reduced the risk of death from a heart attack, several other concurrent publications on the subject ignored the review altogether. This bias resulted in the delay in the routine use of this medication by almost 25 years.

One of the most wide ranging types of paper published is a literature review, which involves a scholarly analysis and summary of several papers relating to a particular topic. Sometimes called traditional or narrative reviews, they are also called critical summaries or commentaries and they have been useful in the past because the reader can learn about a topic, its underpinning theories and current issues without having to read all the individual papers themselves. Whilst narrative reviews have largely been replaced by systematic reviews in academic journals, examples can still be found (see McDougall et al., 2014). Health care education programmes often employ an assessment that requires the student to conduct a literature review on a chosen topic and it is a useful way of allowing them to demonstrate knowledge of current research literature. The problem with this type of review in terms of retrieving reliable research evidence is that like an academic assignment, the author may not have begun with an open mind. Apart from subjectivity and potential bias, a narrative review does not provide information about which papers were included or which were left out and why. Without this **audit trail** the reader cannot assess if author bias has been introduced. A further problem is that a range of papers containing different study designs may be included in the review together with opinion pieces, which the author treats equally and this we know from the chapter on evidence-based practice may lead to misleading conclusions.

THE ADVANTAGES OF A SYSTEMATIC REVIEW

The overall aim of a systematic review is similar to a narrative review, which is to locate, evaluate and summarise papers on a particular topic, but systematic reviews do this in a much more open and structured way. It has a similar purpose to a narrative review, that is, it saves practitioners an enormous amount of time in conducting their own search of papers and it also helps them make informed decisions about the treatments they offer to patients. Narrative reviews are a good way for health care professionals to keep up to date with their general area of practice, whilst systematic reviews aim to produce unequivocal evidence on a specific intervention. It would be misleading to suggest that systematic reviews always provide the answer to a clinical problem: the collection of papers may fail to reveal a definitive answer or do not meet the quality criteria required to provide reliable evidence. The failure to produce good evidence is not a failure of a systematic review, it merely highlights the need for more research on a particular topic and cautions practitioners against using that treatment until a definite benefit is found. For an example of this see Foster et al. (2015).

USES OF A SYSTEMATIC REVIEW

There are several reasons why systematic reviews should be done:

- to keep up to date with the latest research
- to determine whether new treatments are more effective that old ones
- to determine whether existing treatments are harmful or not worth the cost of using them
- to underpin clinical guideline development
- to inform treatment and care decisions
- to avoid wasting research resources on topics where the evidence is already clear
- to support a bid for research funding to produce new evidence.

Systematic reviews are transparent in their construction and content so that they are open to external scrutiny and this also means that it can be repeated by the same authors or others to take into account new studies at a later date. In this way evidence is built and consolidated without having to start from scratch each time. A major advantage of a systematic review is the effort to remove all possible bias from the process providing more plausible and robust results.

QUANTITATIVE SYSTEMATIC AND QUALITATIVE SYSTEMATIC REVIEWS

A quantitative systematic review is the product of a specific type of research called secondary research. Primary research of any design will involve participants, human or animal, or involve cells, molecules or chemicals, for example. Quantitative systematic reviews focus on the results of primary research found in research papers to find out which treatment is the best. Following an evidence-based practice model, quantitative systematic reviews of clinical evidence only report on the results of randomised controlled trials or cohort studies, for example, a comparison of the effectiveness of a new drug treatment against an existing one or the best method for treating wounds.

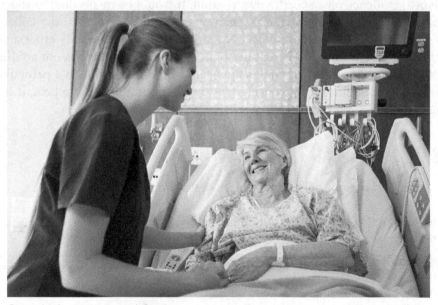

© monkeybusinessimages / iStock

Systematic reviews may also involve an assessment of psychosocial interventions such as cognitive behavioural therapy for obsessive compulsive disorder and epidemiological questions such as the incidence of obesity amongst teenagers. By incorporating an economic evaluation, systematic reviews can also discover whether more expensive treatments are actually more beneficial than cheaper alternatives.

Qualitative systematic reviews adopt the same philosophy and process, but draw on primary research that employs a qualitative design. The results from qualitative research can take the form of an analysis of interviews, focus group discussions or observational analysis to name a few, so there is an additional challenge in the qualitative systematic review process to make sure that the results can be combined in a meaningful way. In a quantitative review combining data involves integrating the statistical data from each study in the form of a meta-analysis, whereas in a qualitative review, the results are combined using meta-synthesis.

THE SYSTEMATIC REVIEW PROCESS

The process of producing a systematic review is similar to the evidence-based practice process, which is to assess, ask, acquire, appraise and apply. The difference is that the EBP process is used to find existing best evidence that can be applied to practice, whereas the systematic review process tries to uncover 'new' evidence. The need for a systematic review usually arises when there is a therapeutic dilemma that is a disagreement about the best treatment for a particular problem. Imagine there are 12 research studies on the topic of using saline to flush intravenous lines rather than heparin to maintain their patency. Four studies show that heparin is better, another four studies are not conclusive and a final four demonstrate that saline is better (it is surprising how often this occurs regarding a number of different topics). Without looking at all 12 papers the practitioner may find one of the papers and decide to go by its findings, which means there is a two in three chance that it could be misleading and the 'evidence' suggested may even be harmful to their patient. Using the systematic review process, all 12 papers would be read and each assessed for the quality of the research – validity, reliability and lack of bias – then the data would be pooled together and treated as one study (aggregated) to see if there is a clearer picture of whether or not the treatment works. The process should be very rigorous and completely transparent, which makes it time consuming, so systematic reviews are usually produced by a team of authors. Busy practitioners should not feel obliged to undertake this process but do need to understand how systematic reviews are produced, to trust that the integrity of the review will provide safe and effective advice. The process of systematic review is illustrated in Figure 10.1.

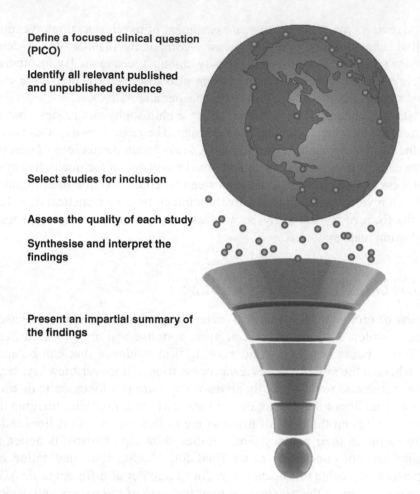

Define a focused clinical question (PICO)

Identify all relevant published and unpublished evidence

Select studies for inclusion

Assess the quality of each study

Synthesise and interpret the findings

Present an impartial summary of the findings

Figure 10.1   The systematic review process

STAGES IN THE SYSTEMATIC REVIEW PROCESS

CONSTRUCT A FOCUSED CLINICAL QUESTION

As with the beginning of the EBP process, a question usually arises from a practical problem, which might be to find out whether one treatment is better than another, using a clearly focused question. The aim of a systematic review is to find all the papers that address a specific question and they need to be located by a number of means, mostly by using electronic databases although this is not the only method that can be used. A focused question provides a means by which each potential sources of literature can be searched consistently. The elements of the PICO are illustrated in Figure 10.2.

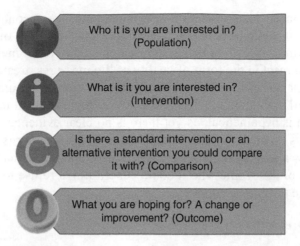

Figure 10.2 The structure of a PICO

A further advantage of a clearly focused question is the specification of an outcome measure – this is in effect what we want to achieve for our patient. The practitioner's aim may be to 'help the patient to feel better' but there is a need to discover what it is exactly that will help them to do this and then to make an objective judgement whether or not it was successful. Without measurement the effect of any intervention cannot be evaluated. Physical treatments such as anti-hypertensive medicines are an example of a treatment that is easily measured by recording blood pressure before and after medication, but with treatments such as anti-depressants, it is not quite so straightforward. Outcome measures need to be objective so whilst it is important that someone taking anti-depressants 'feels better', it cannot be used as the main measure to evaluate a treatment's effectiveness. The reason for this is that some people might feel a great improvement in their situation using a particular anti-depressant whilst others taking the same medication may only acknowledge a slight improvement. A subjective approach does not provide practitioners with sufficient evidence to be confident that 100% of the people (or as close to that number as possible) who take the medication will benefit. The most important measure, called the primary outcome measure, should where at all possible be measurable in an objective way, so the benefits of a given intervention can be assured.

THINK POINT ACTIVITY 10.1

The outcome measure in a PICO must be measurable. In this chapter the example of anti-depressants has been used as an example of how just asking the patient whether they feel better is not enough. Identify the ways in which a researcher could measure an improvement in depressive symptoms.

External verification that an intervention or treatment manages a condition effectively is essential otherwise it would be pointless using it, but it is, of course, of equal importance that the person taking it *does* feel better so research studies often include patients' perceptions of the treatment in the form of quality of life measures, treatment acceptability or something similar. These are termed secondary outcome measures, which are also useful in the overall evaluation of a treatment. An example is illustrated in Figure 10.3.

The illustration is hypothetical, as yet there is no clear evidence that larval therapy (the use of maggots) to clean wounds and progress wound healing is effective, but it is useful to show how a primary outcome measure may demonstrate that an intervention is useful, but if 80% of the people who it could benefit might refuse to use it then practitioners need to take this into account

IDENTIFY A SEARCH STRATEGY

A comprehensive search strategy is key to locating research studies that address the review question. The aim of this stage is to maximise the number of relevant papers for

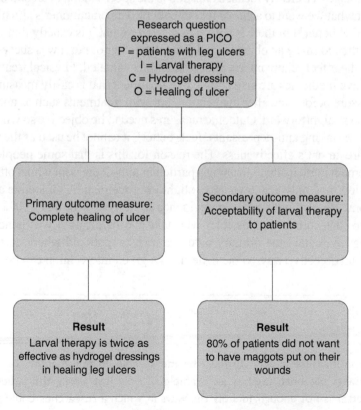

Figure 10.3   Larval therapy for the debridement of leg ulcers

evaluation whilst filtering out the irrelevant ones as efficiently as possible. In addition to formally published literature, the search should encompass relevant institutional and technical reports, as well as conference proceedings. These papers are not exposed to peer review; that is, read independently and anonymously by another expert in the field. In addition, these studies do not come under editorial control which ensures that the papers published in their journals comply with specific rules, models and guidelines. Literature of this nature is referred to as **grey literature** and to exclude it altogether would expose the review to publication bias. For example, there has been a long standing issue in the medical literature where only the positive outcomes, that is showing that an intervention works, are published, whilst similar studies demonstrating negatives are rejected by journals. If *all* the literature on a topic is not included, the review may reach an incorrect conclusion.

THINK POINT ACTIVITY   10.2

Choose a paper on a topic you are interested in, it should be a study involving a randomised controlled trial. Browse the Internet for a critical appraisal tool for RCTs that you are most comfortable with and use it to evaluate your chosen article.

As language develops so people use different words for the same thing, see the example for older adults illustrated in Figure 10.4. Some of the adjectives such as geriatric, now considered pejorative, have been replaced with more respectful terms such as older adult, but if the search is to capture all potential papers including those written when the term geriatric was in common use, then this has to be included in the search strategy. As the search for literature should be worldwide, transatlantic differences in spellings also need to be taken into consideration, labor/labour and pediatric/paediatric, for example. The term worldwide needs to be taken literally and not be limited to English language papers, developed countries or places where health care systems are similar. The search strategy also needs to contain a timeline but it is a common misconception that searching should be confined to a five- or ten-year period preceding the current search, when it should extend back to the origins of research on a particular topic. We know for example that the human immunodeficiency virus (HIV) has existed in the United States since at least the mid to late 1970s. In 1982 public health officials began to use the term 'acquired immunodeficiency syndrome', or AIDS and formal tracking (surveillance) of AIDS cases began that year in the United States. Research on HIV/AIDS emerged around this time and so a search of this literature would extend back to this date.

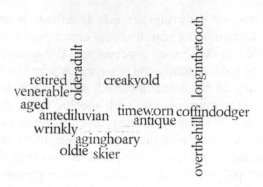

Figure 10.4 Synonyms for the older adult

All of the components of the strategy need to be in place before the search is executed and each element of the PICO should be specified in detail to focus the question further. The use of an explicit search strategy should produce a list of publications which then needs to be sifted to exclude papers that are irrelevant to the review question, or do not fit other criteria for inclusion for review.

STUDY SELECTION CRITERIA AND PROCEDURES

Following the literature search there needs to be a clear description of the processes that will be used to decide if a primary study will be included or excluded from the review. This will initially depend on whether it matches the PICO specified.

For the population, the types of participants need to be specified so that only papers that have researched this group would be included.

The type of intervention needs to be identified, for reviews of a medication for example, the drug, its preparation, route of administration, dose, duration, frequency would be stated. For non-drug interventions such as an educational intervention, defining the intervention can be a bit more difficult and there is a need to consider exactly what was done, how often it was done, who did it, were they trained and so on.

The types of counter intervention (comparison) need to be considered alongside the intervention. For a medication, an included paper might need to compare the medication with a placebo or similar medication for example. Other comparisons might involve whether the intervention is a novel treatment to be compared against standard treatment.

For types of studies consideration of the design is needed, for example, which design will best answer the question and whether included studies will be restricted on the basis of language, date or publication status. For a quantitative systematic review, papers using only randomised controlled trials or cohort designs would be included.

Included papers need to have the specific primary outcome measure identified in the PICO. If a secondary outcome measure is stated, that also needs to be evident in the paper but additional outcomes found in the paper that do not relate to the proposed review can be disregarded and it does not mean that the paper should be excluded.

In summary, the search, retrieval and filtering of papers forms the initial part of the systematic review process and, although it may appear a daunting process, the actual amount of work involved depends upon the number of papers retrieved from the literature search and how efficiently they are managed. It is not necessary to read all the papers that are found from the initial search, the PRISMA (Preferred Reporting Items for Systematic Reviews and Meta-analyses website provides a framework for filtering included and excluded papers.

Website activity 10.1

It is important to record as much information as possible from the search and to search each database separately. Hand searching and other methods of retrieving potential papers are described in Chapter 13.

ASSESS THE QUALITY OF THE INCLUDED PAPERS

The final papers that are suitable for inclusion in the review can number from many to none! A systematic review can still be produced by professionals even if there are no findings as it establishes that there is no evidence. The example on larval therapy in Figure 10.3 is a case in point (see further reading). A failure to find research on a particular topic also provides a very good justification of the need for research which can support the case for grant funding, so this part of the process should not be regarded as a waste of time. More often than not there will be past research in the form of papers that can be reviewed, but the review needs to establish the quality of this research. If the standard of design and reporting is poor or contains significant bias, then the findings cannot be relied upon to support practice. To determine whether a study is of good quality the reviewer needs to scrutinise the paper carefully and use a critical appraisal tool (CAT) to assess whether it conforms to accepted current standards. Critical appraisal tools can be found on the Internet and there are severable available that provide a framework to help evaluate studies. Visit the accompanying website for an example. See also on the companion website (https://study.sagepub.com/harveyandland) the CONSORT 2010 statement, which provides a standard tool for reporting randomised controlled trials. In addition to the quality of the study design, there needs to be an evaluation of whether bias has been introduced. Publication bias (explained earlier) is not the only type of bias; others include whether the study has randomised participants or whether it has made efforts to blind the intervention, and a variety of other issues can inadvertently skew the results of the research. This stage of the review process is one of the most intensive as it requires the reviewer to scrutinise all aspects of the research very carefully and make an overall evaluation of how robust each individual paper is.

DATA EXTRACTION

Once their quality has been assessed, the main elements contained in each paper need to be pulled out or extracted, so all the essential details from each study can be placed on one form. This is to allow comparison between articles that are in different formats and use different styles of reporting. As discussed earlier in the chapter the search strategy may have revealed relevant studies spanning over decades, and styles of reporting have become more sophisticated and more standardised. This means that more current studies contain far more detailed information than earlier ones, which makes data extraction more difficult. Standardising the results aids pattern recognition and ultimately helps to detect whether a clear answer to the systematic review question can be found. As with critical appraisal tools, there are several instruments on the Internet which will serve as a guide to the elements that should be extracted from a research study, or in some cases it may be necessary to design a form that is fit for purpose.

THINK POINT ACTIVITY   10.3

Using this chapter, go to the Cochrane Library and locate a systematic review on a topic of your choice. Identify the stages of the review to gain a better understanding of how systematic reviews are constructed.

META-ANALYSIS

Website activity 10.2

The point of a quantitative systematic review is to collate research papers on a clearly focused question. Different studies, even when conducted in a similar way, may come up with different conclusions and it is impossible to judge which contains the best evidence. The aim of a systematic review is to resolve these therapeutic dilemmas not only by reading all the relevant papers but by combining the data from them into one data-set as if it were one large study. These data are then statistically analysed to see if the findings yield a clearer result. This process is called a meta-analysis (*meta* coming from the Greek, meaning 'after' or 'beyond'), which can improve the estimation of how effective a treatment is. It is essential that the data in the individual studies are similar enough to be combined so that a meta-analysis can be performed.

For example, five papers report a reduction in blood pressure using a new anti-hypertensive but five other papers disagree. All ten studies collect data that record changes in blood pressure using millimetres of mercury (mmHg). A meta-analysis can be performed because the data are in the same form.

In a different scenario, five papers report a reduction in depression following cognitive behavioural therapy, but five others disagree. Within the ten studies, three different types of rating scales are used to measure patients' depression before and after treatment. Although the purpose of the scales is the same they are constructed differently and the scores cannot be combined in a meta-analysis.

If meta-analysis is not possible as in the example above, it is still possible to assess the components of each paper and reach some objective conclusions. This is sometimes called a qualitative systematic review, even though the papers included contain *quantitative* studies. This should not be confused with systematic reviews of *qualitative* studies (also called qualitative systematic reviews), which are explained earlier in this chapter.

SUMMARY

Systematic reviews represent quite a complex set of processes and usually involve two or more people who verify each other's work at every stage. The purpose of this chapter has been to outline this process so that the reader can appreciate this and show that findings from a systematic review can provide clear evidence on which to base their practice.

FURTHER READING

Boland, A., Cherry, G. and Dickson, R. (2017) *Doing a Systematic Review. A Student's Guide*. London: Sage Publications.

An easy-to-follow practical guide for student looking to actually do a systematic review.

Edwards, J. and Stapley S. (2010) Debridement of diabetic foot ulcers. *Cochrane Database of Systematic Reviews*, Issue 1, Art. No.: CD003556. DOI: 10.1002/14651858.CD003556.pub2.

A good example of a systematic review that examines a common nursing problem.

Hemingway, P. and Brereton, N. (2009) What is a systematic review? www.medicine.ox.ac.uk/bandolier/painres/download/whatis/syst-review.pdf (last accessed 1 June 2016).

This is a very good summary of systematic reviews.

Don't forget to visit https://study.sagepub.com/harveyandland to watch videos, take quizzes and to follow specially designed web activities.

11

RESEARCH DESIGN

This chapter builds upon Chapters 4, 5, 7, 8 and 9 and provides an overview of the research designs commonly used in nursing and midwifery studies. In this chapter we will:

- establish the difference between research method and research design
- provide an overview of the most commonly used experimental and non-experimental research designs
- identify factors to consider to ensure the selection of the most appropriate research design for a study.

RESEARCH DESIGN OR RESEARCH METHOD?

As we have identified in previous chapters, the research world abounds with the use of a variety of terms which refer to the same thing. In addition, some research terms are used inappropriately, usually because the meaning of a particular term is misunderstood. Unfortunately both these situations can be identified when we step into the world of research design. Later in this chapter we will explore the designs most commonly used in nursing and midwifery research and we will see that several designs have a number of different names. It is also important to note that the term 'research design' is sometimes used inappropriately when researchers are actually referring to the 'research method'. This is therefore an appropriate point at which to clarify the difference between these two terms.

As we have seen in Chapters 4, 5, 7, 8 and 9, the research method is the specific way in which a study is conducted and it reflects the key principles of the methodology to which it is allied. A research method includes the following characteristics: an underpinning philosophy (research paradigm), a strategy for recruiting participants, method(s) of data collection, method(s) of data analysis, and strategies for facilitating reliability and validity (quantitative methods) or trustworthiness (qualitative methods). In Chapters 4 and 5 we identified a number of different research methods such as randomised controlled trials, surveys and phenomenology. By contrast, the research design is the overall plan which identifies the way in which the study will be carried out. The design could therefore be regarded as being a framework, model, blueprint or even a map which identifies what is to be done when and how (Robson, 2011; Bryman, 2012).

As we will see, some research methods can be carried out in a number of different ways. In other words having selected the research method, the researcher sometimes has a range of options to choose from regarding which design to use. All research designs have strengths and weaknesses and the researcher should select the most appropriate design for the particular study that they are planning. It is important to note here that in most cases we will be reviewing research designs in the context of quantitative research. As identified in Chapter 8, a key feature of qualitative research is the use of flexible, evolving designs. Therefore, whilst the qualitative researcher may set out with a plan, the very nature of this type of study means that the plan may alter as the study progresses. Consequently, the design can often only be described in retrospect. In addition, in Chapter 6 we reviewed different models of mixed methods research which could be regarded as being designs. In this chapter, we will therefore explore fixed research designs that are used in quantitative research. To facilitate this process we will review designs that can be classified as being either experimental (interventional) or non-experimental (observational) designs (Besen and Gan, 2014).

EXPERIMENTAL RESEARCH DESIGNS

Experimental research is a good example of a method that can be carried out in a number of different ways (Bench et al., 2013). The researcher, having decided to use the experiment method, must therefore next decide which design to use. Whilst there are many options, some of which are complex, we will consider the five most commonly used experimental designs here. You will recall that the three essential elements of a true experiment are:

- randomisation
- manipulation (of the independent variable)
- control.

The designs that we will consider here all include these fundamental elements but the way in which the study is configured varies. The experimental designs that we are going to describe can be classified into three main groups: **between-participants design**, **within-participants design** and **matched pairs design**.

BETWEEN-PARTICIPANTS DESIGN

This is the most basic and most commonly used experimental design (Bench et al., 2013) and it involves two separate groups of participants. There are three between-participants designs that are commonly used.

BETWEEN-PARTICIPANTS: POST-TEST ONLY DESIGN

This design is sometimes called the **after-only design**. When using this design, participants are randomised into either the experimental or control group. The experimental group receives the 'new' treatment or intervention (the independent variable), whilst the control group receives the conventional treatment or intervention. The impact of both the experimental and control interventions are then measured (the dependent variable) (see Box 11.1).

Website
activity 11.1

BOX 11.1   EXAMPLE OF A POST-TEST ONLY DESIGN

We are planning to conduct a study with the following hypothesis:

> Preterm babies who receive developmental nursing care gain weight faster than preterm babies who receive conventional nursing care.

In order to carry out this study, we plan to recruit 100 preterm babies; 50 will be randomised to the experimental group and 50 will be randomised to the control group (see Figure 11.1). The experimental group will receive developmental nursing care whilst the control group will receive conventional nursing care. The impact of the two styles of nursing care on the babies' weight will then be measured.

100 preterm babies are recruited and randomised into the experimental or control group:

Experimental group	**Independent variable**	**Dependent variable**
50 preterm babies ⟶	Developmental nursing care ⟶	Weight

Control group		
50 preterm babies ⟶	Conventional nursing care ⟶	Weight

Figure 11.1   Between-participants: post-test only design

Whilst this is the most basic design and therefore probably the most straightforward to conduct, this design has limitations. The most fundamental weakness is that account has not been taken of pre-intervention dependent variable data; in our example this would be the babies' weight at the start of study. Also, differences in the dependent variable (weight gain) may be caused by individual differences between the two groups of participants rather than the independent variable. So, for example, in our study, despite randomisation the experimental group may include more girls (who generally do better than boys) or babies who had a higher birthweight in the first place.

There are strategies that can help to reduce the impact of individual differences. These include identifying specific, predetermined criteria for participant inclusion in the study and the involvement of a large number of participants.

BETWEEN-PARTICIPANTS: PRE-TEST, POST-TEST DESIGN

This design is sometimes called the **before and after design** and may be regarded as being the traditional experimental design. To some extent, it addresses the weaknesses of the **post-test only design**. The **pre-test, post-test design** involves the collection of dependent variable data before the independent variable is introduced. This pre-test data is sometimes referred to as baseline data (see Box 11.2).

BOX 11.2   EXAMPLE OF A PRE-TEST, POST-TEST DESIGN

Website activity 11.2

We are planning to conduct a study with the following hypothesis:

Drug A is more effective than drug B in reducing hypertension in adults.

To carry out this study, we aim to recruit 200 adults (see Figure 11.2). Following recruitment participant blood pressure levels will be monitored to provide baseline data. Participants

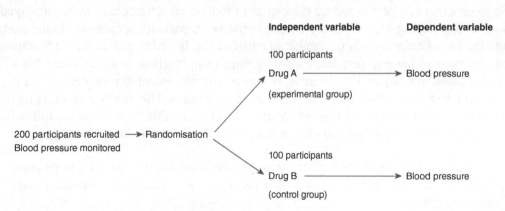

Figure 11.2   Between-participants: pre-test, post-test design

(Continued)

(Continued)

will then be randomised to the experimental or control group. The experimental group will receive drug A (the new treatment) whilst the control group will receive drug B (the conventional treatment). The impact of the two drugs on participant blood pressure (the dependent variable) will then be measured. We can compare the blood pressure levels of the two groups as a whole (those receiving drug A and those receiving drug B) and also the blood pressure levels of individual participants pre- and post-administration of the drug.

Whilst this design addresses some of the limitations of the post-test only design, it does have weaknesses. The problem of individual differences between the two groups of participants remains. Consequently, differences in the dependent variable may be caused by individual differences between the two groups of participants rather than the effect of the independent variable. So in our example, despite randomisation the experimental group may include more men and more smokers.

THINK POINT ACTIVITY   11.1

Make a list of the possible differences between the two groups of participants that may impact on the dependent variable (blood pressure).

Strategies that can help to reduce the impact of individual differences can be employed, such as identifying specific, predetermined criteria for participant inclusion in the study and the involvement of a large number of participants. In addition, statistical adjustment can be made to the post-test data for both groups using analysis of covariance (this will be discussed in Chapter 19). There is, however, another potential weakness of the pre-test, post-test design that will be relevant in some studies. This is when conducting the pre-test impacts upon the dependent variable. To illustrate this we will use the following example. We are planning to conduct a study with the following hypothesis:

Nurses working in palliative care settings who attend staff support groups cope better with work related stress compared to nurses who do not attend a staff support group.

If we were using the pre-test, post-test design for our example, we would measure staff stress before the intervention is implemented. However, doing the pre-test may reveal to some nurses just how stressed they are. This in turn may cause them to implement their own additional coping strategies or may cause them to become even more anxious. Either response may influence the dependent variable regardless of the implementation of the independent variable. The following research design overcomes the potential impact of the pre-test.

BETWEEN-PARTICIPANTS DESIGN: SOLOMON FOUR DESIGN

This somewhat strangely named design minimises the possible effect of collecting dependent variable data before the intervention is introduced. It is a variation of the pre-test, post-test design. However, pre-test data are not collected on all of the participants. Following recruitment, participants are randomised to one of four groups:

1　Participants in this group have the pre-test and receive the experimental treatment/intervention.
2　Participants in this group have the pre-test and receive the conventional treatment/intervention.
3　Participants in this group do not have the pre-test, but receive the experimental treatment/intervention.
4　Participants in this group do not have the pre-test and receive the conventional treatment/intervention.

The **Solomon Four design** enables the researchers to compare the two groups who received the experimental treatment (groups 1 and 3) and the two groups who received the conventional treatment (groups 2 and 4). They can then determine the impact of the pre-test.

　　This design can be complicated to set up and the problem of individual differences between participants remains. Identifying specific, predetermined criteria for participant inclusion in the study and the involvement of a large number of participants may help to minimise the impact of any individual differences (see Box 11.3).

WITHIN-PARTICIPANTS DESIGN

This experimental design is sometimes referred to as the **cross-over** or **repeated measures design**. This design overcomes the problem of individual differences between participants in the intervention and conventional treatment groups in the between-participants designs. During the course of a study using the within-participants design, each participant is exposed at some point to both the experimental and control treatment (Coates, 2011). In other words, participants act as their own control. Once participants have been exposed to both the experimental and control treatment the two groups can be compared as a whole and the researchers can also compare the differences in individual participants' responses (see Box 11.4).

Website
activity 11.3

BOX 11.3   EXAMPLE OF A SOLOMON FOUR DESIGN

Using the hypothesis involving nurses working in palliative care settings, 200 nurses are recruited and randomised to one of the four groups listed above (see Figure 11.3). The stress levels of the nurses allocated to groups one and two are measured. Groups one and three then attend a newly established staff support group (the independent variable) whilst groups two and four continue to access conventional sources of support. After a predetermined period of time, the stress levels of the nurses in all four groups are measured (the dependent variable).

200 nurses are recruited and are randomised into one of four groups:

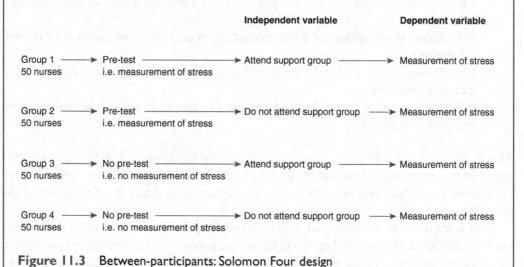

Figure 11.3   Between-participants: Solomon Four design

Website
activity 11.4

BOX 11.4   EXAMPLE OF A WITHIN-PARTICIPANTS DESIGN

We are planning to conduct a study with the following hypothesis:

Non-uniformed nurses establish a better rapport with adults with learning disabilities in comparison to the rapport they develop with them when wearing uniform.

To carry out this study we plan to recruit 50 nurses working in care settings with adults who have learning disabilities (see Figure 11.4). Following recruitment, nurses are randomised to a number from 1 to 50. During the first phase of the study, nurses numbered 1 to 25 wear their uniform to work whilst nurses numbered 26 to 50 are non-uniformed. After a predefined period of time the second phase of the study begins whereby nurses numbered 26 to 50 wear their uniform to work whilst nurses numbered 1 to 25 are non-uniformed.

50 nurses are recruited and are randomised to a number between 1 and 50:

Phase one

Nurses 1–25 uniformed (independent variable) ⟶ Measure rapport (dependent variable)

Nurses 26–50 non-uniformed ⟶ Measure rapport (DV)

Phase two

Nurses 1–25 non-uniformed ⟶ Measure rapport (DV)

Nurses 26–50 uniformed (independent variable) ⟶ Measure rapport (DV)

Phase three

Comparison of findings

Figure 11.4   Within-participants design

Randomisation therefore determines the order in which participants encounter the experimental treatment or intervention (Polit and Beck, 2014). A key advantage of this design is that a smaller number of participants may be required and this in turn can be advantageous in terms of time and cost.

In the real world there would be a number of limitations conducting a study such as the example we have given. However, we have deliberately used this to illustrate the key weaknesses of the within-participants design. The main factor that could detrimentally affect the findings is **order effect**, sometimes known as **practice effect**. This is when whatever is done first influences the final findings of the study (Polit and Beck, 2014). In our example, this would mean the rapport (good or bad) that develops between nurses and clients in the first phase determines the final outcome of the study and therefore the effect of the second phase is negligible. Whether or not order effect has an impact on the dependent variable (rapport in our example) can sometimes be determined by statistical analysis of the order of treatment and outcome. In some studies a **wash-out period** may be added between the first and second phases to allow the effect of the first treatment to diminish. The length of this period will be determined by the individual study. There are, however, other weaknesses in this design. For example, participants may drop out of the study after the first phase. The other important factor is the need to ensure consistency in all aspects of the study across both phases to reduce the impact of other variables.

THINK POINT ACTIVITY   11.2

List the factors that the researcher should endeavour to ensure remain consistent across both phases of the study to reduce the impact of other variables on the dependent variable (rapport).

MATCHED PAIRS DESIGN

In many respects, this is regarded as being the ultimate or gold-standard experimental design as it attempts to address the weaknesses of the between-participants and within-participants designs. Within the matched pairs design, participants in the experimental and control groups are matched as closely as possible (Robson, 2011). One member of each pair is randomised to either the experimental or control group. The closer participants are matched the better because the intention is to minimise the impact of individual differences between participants in the experimental and control groups.

Website
activity 11.5

BOX 11.5   EXAMPLE OF A MATCHED PAIRS DESIGN

We are planning to conduct a study with the following hypothesis:

Children who have a pre-surgery hospital visit experience less post-operative pain in comparison to children who do not have a pre-surgery visit.

We plan to recruit 500 children. They will be matched as closely as possible into 250 pairs and then randomised to either the experimental or control groups (see Figure 11.5). One child from each pair will have a newly established pre-surgery hospital visit (independent variable) whilst the matched child does not (the control group). Following surgery each child's post-operative pain will be measured (the dependent variable). We will then compare post-operative pain between the two groups (pre-hospital visit and no pre-hospital visit) and between individual pairs of children.

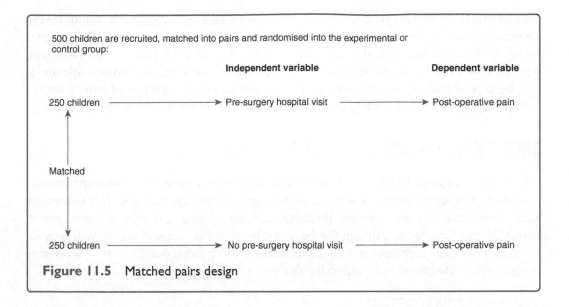

500 children are recruited, matched into pairs and randomised into the experimental or control group:

Independent variable   **Dependent variable**

250 children ⎯⎯⎯⎯⎯⎯⎯→ Pre-surgery hospital visit ⎯⎯⎯⎯⎯⎯⎯→ Post-operative pain

Matched

250 children ⎯⎯⎯⎯⎯⎯⎯→ No pre-surgery hospital visit ⎯⎯⎯⎯⎯⎯⎯→ Post-operative pain

Figure 11.5   Matched pairs design

In some studies, matching takes place retrospectively, as for example in the study by Goelz et al. (2013). So in our study children would be recruited and randomised into either the experimental or control group and they would be matched into pairs once data collection was completed.

THINK POINT ACTIVITY   11.3

List the variables that a researcher could match in children in this study.

Of the five experimental designs that we have reviewed, the matched pairs design is the most powerful and robust but it is also the most complicated. Matching can be difficult and time consuming and this in turn makes this design costly (Polit and Beck, 2014). If the study involves rare conditions or participants with uncommon characteristics, then matching can be even more challenging. The researcher should also be cautious not to try to 'over match' participants for irrelevant variables. So in the example we have given for this design, researchers could spend unnecessary time matching the children's shoe size, height and weight.

Sometimes possible participants have to be excluded from the study if an appropriate 'match' cannot be recruited. Researchers may also have to face the logistical problem when one half of a matched pair withdraws from the study, although statistical analysis can determine the impact of these factors. Despite very careful matching there may still

Website
activity 11.6

be individual differences between participants. Some studies endeavour to minimise the chances of this by recruiting identical twins, with one twin being in the experimental group and one in the control group, for example the study by Greene and Naughton (2011). However, the availability of appropriate participants may be problematic and it can be argued that any study involving the comparison of two groups of human beings will never be able to completely eradicate individual difference between participants.

NON-EXPERIMENTAL RESEARCH DESIGNS

We will now explore the fixed designs that are commonly used in other non-experimental quantitative research methods such as quasi experiments and surveys. The researcher using these methods has a number of choices regarding research design so should aim to select the most appropriate design for the study. In the following section, we will provide an overview of the four most commonly used non-experimental designs: **cross-sectional**, **longitudinal**, **Delphi** and **retrospective designs**.

CROSS-SECTIONAL DESIGN

This is sometimes referred to as the **one-hit** or **one-shot design** and it is the most common non-experimental design (O'Leary, 2014). A study using this design involves the collection of data either at one point in time (Besen and Gan, 2014) or a number of times over a very short time period (for example, hourly for 24 hours). This design

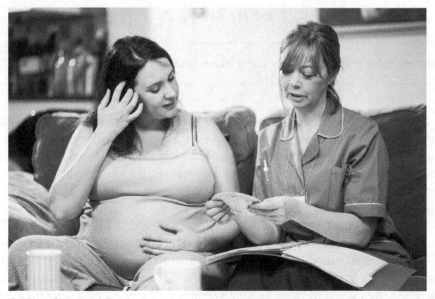

© MartinPrescott / iStock

often involves a representative cross-section of a defined population which means that the researcher can investigate a large number of participants at different stages of development simultaneously (see Box 11.6).

BOX 11.6   EXAMPLE OF A CROSS-SECTIONAL DESIGN

We are planning to conduct a survey of community midwives working in the UK about their job satisfaction using questionnaires which are posted to the participants. The sample will include midwives who have been qualified for varying lengths of time with a range of community experience. In accordance with the cross-sectional design, data will be collected from the midwives on one occasion, including time allowed for the follow-up of non-returners.

Website activity 11.7

LONGITUDINAL DESIGN

This design is most commonly used in surveys (sometimes referred to as **panel design**) and cohort studies (sometimes known as **trend** or **follow-up design**). It involves the repeated collection of data at pre-specified intervals from the same sample over a set or on-going period of time (LoBiondo-Wood and Haber, 2014). The longitudinal design is used in health care research to identify patterns and trends and to measure changes because over time the researchers are able to compare the data of individuals and the group as a whole (O'Leary, 2014) (see Box 11.7). In this way, researchers gain detailed insight into the issue under investigation, particularly the longer term impact. This means that over time, the researchers may be able to make links between the variables that they are measuring. This in turn may enable researchers to identify associated risk factors. The UK has a long-standing history of running cohort studies, particularly those which follow-up children from birth such as the 'Millennium Cohort Study' (Connelly and Platt, 2014) and the 'Life Study' (Stewart, 2014).

Website activity 11.8

BOX 11.7   EXAMPLE OF A LONGITUDINAL DESIGN

To illustrate this design we can use the example of investigating community midwives' job satisfaction that we gave previously. If using the longitudinal design we would regularly collect data from the same group of midwives over an extended period of time, for example annually for ten years. This would enable us to detect patterns, trends and changes both in the job satisfaction of individual midwives and the whole group.

Website activity 11.9

DELPHI DESIGN

We must acknowledge here two points of contention about the Delphi design. Firstly, it is sometimes referred to as the panel design (see above). However, because there are a number of issues that are specific to the Delphi design, it warrants separate consideration here. The second point of dispute is that some regard it as a method rather than a design. However, we maintain the view that it is a design which is usually used with the survey method of research.

The origins of the Delphi design can be traced back to ancient Greece where the Priestess at Delphi was consulted about actions to be taken such as when to declare war on enemies. She was said to be able to predict the outcome of events and therefore her opinion was consulted. As a consequence she became known as the Delphi Oracle. The Delphi design was first developed for research purposes in 1950s in the United States when a panel of experts was consulted to identify industrial sites that were likely to be most at risk of Soviet attack (Keeney et al., 2011). It has evolved as a research design since then and it is increasingly used in health care research (Vernon, 2009). The design starts with the recruitment of a panel, the members of which the researcher considers to be experts in the topic under investigation. The aim of this design is to reach agreement (consensus) about the topic and data are collected from participants during a number of rounds of data collection. In round one, participants are asked to respond to broad key questions about the topic and their responses are collated. In round two, participants consider more focused questions which are based on the collated responses from the first round. Participants can add, alter or retract information during the second stage (Keeney et al., 2006). The rounds continue until consensus is reached (see Box 11.8). The Internet is an asset to this design because participants can be anywhere in the world and their anonymity and confidentiality can be maintained (Vernon, 2009). However, it must also be acknowledged that unless strategies are put in place, researchers cannot be absolutely certain about who is actually participating in the study.

Website
activity 11.10

BOX 11.8   EXAMPLE OF THE DELPHI DESIGN

A group of mental health nurses wish to identify the three most important nursing research priorities in order to inform future research funding. They therefore recruit senior clinical nurses working in the speciality in the UK. In the first round of the study participants are asked to identify aspects of nursing care that they feel should be researched. Data analysis of the first round identifies that the participants have identified 30 potential topics. As the rounds progress, the list of potential topics is refined until the group finally agrees on the three most important nursing care issues to be researched (see Figure 11.6).

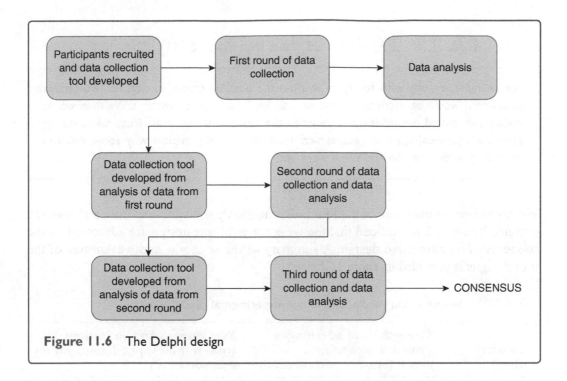

Figure 11.6   The Delphi design

RETROSPECTIVE DESIGN

Probably the most famous study using the retrospective design is Richard Doll's work, which identified a link between smoking and lung cancer (Doll and Hill, 1950). This is sometimes known as **ex post facto, after the fact** or **correlational design** and it is most commonly seen in case-control studies and historical research. As the name suggests, using this design involves the collection of data retrospectively whereby the dependent variable (the effect) has already been affected by the independent variable (the cause) (LoBiondo-Wood and Haber, 2014). The aim of this design is therefore to link the present situation with what has happened in the past. Participants with a particular condition, problem or characteristic are recruited (the cases) and compared with participants who do not have the condition, problem or characteristic (the control). Differences between the two groups give the researcher an indication of the likely causes of the condition or problem (see Box 11.9).

An increasingly popular way of capturing retrospective data about patients and clients is by accessing clinical databases. Whilst researchers have to acquire the appropriate permissions and approvals to access a database and in some cases may also be charged per data-set to do so, databases nevertheless provide a ready-made data source (Loke, 2014).

Website activity 11.11

BOX 11.9   EXAMPLE OF THE RETROSPECTIVE DESIGN

For example, we may wish to try to find out the possible causes of cleft lip. Two groups of children would be recruited: those with a cleft lip and those without. We then would endeavour to find out differences between the two groups such as drugs taken during pregnancy, parental age and geographical location that may explain why some children were born with a cleft lip and some were not.

We have given an overview of the four most commonly used non-experimental research designs. You may have noticed that the weaknesses of one design are addressed by the strengths of an alternative design. A summary of the strengths and weaknesses of the four designs is provided in Table 11.1.

Table 11.1   Strengths and weaknesses of non-experimental research design

Research design	Strengths and advantages (may not all apply, dependent on method used)	Weaknesses and limitations (may not all apply, dependent on method used)
Cross-sectional	• Economical: time, money, resources and effort • Does not require on-going commitment from participants • Findings are available promptly • Can use large samples	• Extraneous variables may impact on the findings, particularly between different groups of participants. Care therefore needs to be taken about inferences that are drawn • Low response rates may impact on findings • Risk that extreme views/findings can be obscured because the findings are often reduced to averages • Provides only a snap-shot of the here and now • Data can be superficial
Longitudinal	• Identifies trends, changes and developments over time • Identification of trends, changes and developments may enable the researcher to make predictions about the future • Provides detailed and extensive data	• Can be costly: time, money and effort • Requires high levels of researcher/participant commitment • Risk of participant drop out (attrition) • Over time participants become aware of the variables that the researchers are interested in

Research design	Strengths and advantages (may not all apply, dependent on method used)	Weaknesses and limitations (may not all apply, dependent on method used)
	• Reduces the effect of recall bias • Can infer causal relationships between variables	• The research team may change over time • Following up participants may be a complex process • If there is a high drop out, the findings may become biased • Findings may not be available for some time • Blinding may not always be possible* • Cannot conclude causal relationships
Delphi design	• Utilises the expertise of participants • Participants do not need to meet, they can be located anywhere in the world • Economical: time, money, resources and effort • Participant anonymity and confidentiality can be maintained • Encourages participant honesty • Enables participants to consider issues and information that they may have overlooked • It is democratic, it prevents an individual participant dominating the responses	• Potential for bias in the selection and recruitment of experts • There is no agreement over the ideal panel size • Aiming to reach consensus may mean that diverse opinions are lost • Participants may drop out over time, particularly if there are a number of rounds or their responses appear to be overlooked • If high drop out, the findings may become biased • Can be time consuming • There is no clear definition of consensus • There is no evidence to suggest that a different group of experts would reach the same agreement
Retrospective	• Can collect extensive data • Realism is high because events have actually occurred • Can infer causal relationships • Economical: time, money and effort	• Can be susceptible to faulty interpretation • Accessing retrospective data can be problematic • Risk of recall bias • Cannot conclude causal relationships

*This is specific to cohort studies where a group of participants are followed up. Ideally the research team doing the follow up assessments should not know which intervention participants have received, but over time this can be difficult to conceal.

Website
activity 11.12

SELECTING THE MOST APPROPRIATE DESIGN

In situations where researchers need to choose which design to use, they should select the most appropriate design for the study. This will facilitate the collection of valid and reliable data and will consequently provide the best possible evidence. The hypothesis or research question should inform the choice of design, as should the aims and objectives of the study along with the findings of the literature review (Coates, 2011). In order to determine which design to use researchers should also consider the amount of time, funding and resources available.

When carrying out experimental research there are a number of specific questions the researcher should consider which will help determine which of the designs to use:

- Are individual differences between participants likely to detrimentally affect the findings? If so, use a within-participants or matched pairs design.
- Is order effect likely to be a problem? If not use a within-participants design. If yes, use matched pairs or between-participants design.
- Is carrying out a pre-test likely to cause a problem? If yes, use a post-test only or Solomon Four design.
- How many participants are you likely to recruit? If only a small number, use a within-participants design.
- Do you need to measure the impact of the independent variable and the control treatment or intervention in the same people? If so, use a within-participants design.
- Is matching likely to be problematic? If so, if using the matched pairs design, consider carefully which variables to match or do not use this design.

When deciding which non-experimental design to use, the amount of time, funding and resources that are available are very important factors for the researcher to consider. Again, the purpose of the research should ultimately determine which design the researcher selects. To help make their decision the researcher should consider:

- Are data required from participants on more than one occasion? If so, use a longitudinal, Delphi or retrospective design.
- Is participant commitment likely to be problematic? If so, use a cross-sectional or retrospective design. If use of a longitudinal or Delphi design is required, ensure participants know the proposed timeframe at the start of the study.
- Are the findings required promptly? If so, use a cross-sectional or retrospective design.

SUMMARY

In this chapter we have established the difference between research method and research design. We have reviewed the most commonly used experimental and non-experimental research designs and the way they might be used. We have also shown that understanding the key features of the different designs, and particularly their strengths and weaknesses, helps researchers to select the most appropriate design for their study.

FURTHER READING

Creswell, J.W. (2014) *Research Design: Qualitative, Quantitative and Mixed Methods Approaches* (4th edn). London: Sage Publications.

A straightforward overview of research designs covering a wide range of methods and methodologies.

Gray, J.R., Grove, S.K. and Burns, N. (2012) *The Practice of Nursing Research* (7th edn). St Louis: Elsevier Saunders.

See Chapter 10, 'Understanding quantitative research design' and Chapter 11, 'Selecting a quantitative research design'.

> Don't forget to visit https://study.sagepub.com/harveyandland to watch videos, take quizzes and to follow specially designed web activities.

PART III

USING RESEARCH METHODS AND DESIGN: THE PRACTICE

12

THE RESEARCH PROCESS

This chapter summarises the research process. It deals briefly with the definition of research, describes the sequence of activities known collectively as the research process and draws attention to the techniques required to carry out these activities. In this chapter we will:

- identify the steps in the research process
- explain what is involved in each of these steps
- refer to the chapters that explain these steps in full.

Research is a planned, systematic search for information for the purpose of increasing the total body of knowledge (Clamp et al., 2004). 'Information', in this context, is taken to mean the data collected and analysed in the course of the research. Knowledge is the understanding which can develop as a result of studying research findings in the light of previous information and experience.

Research involves looking for information which is not at the time readily available, or for which there is no generally accepted evidence. There are different kinds of research, depending on the kind of question which is asked and the methods used to find an answer. It is not always easy to classify the different types satisfactorily because they overlap one another. The use of research depends upon the type of data and how they are collected. It may be used to describe a particular situation, to explain why certain events occur, or to predict what is likely to happen under specific conditions.

THINK POINT ACTIVITY   12.1

Browse Chapters 5 and 6 to familiarise yourself with the type of research methodologies used in health research.

THE STEPS OF THE RESEARCH PROCESS

Whatever the purpose of the investigation or the methods used, the whole research process consists basically of several steps and related activity (see Figure 12.1). These steps constitute a way of thinking which is not confined to research in the strict sense of the word, but can be applied to many kinds of problem-solving, such as managerial decision making. At each step, certain activities must be completed before proceeding to the next. In practice, some of the steps may have to be repeated and some consist of a number of different tasks.

IDENTIFY A PROBLEM, QUESTION OR HYPOTHESIS

A research problem often begins with a discrepancy, the perception of a difference between two states of affairs or an uncomfortable feeling about things as they are. In practice it may boil down to a feeling of 'why do we do it like that?'

Our clinical practice is a good source of potential research questions, see Table 12.1 for some examples. In reality there are a whole host of topics that could be investigated, which might come from experience, the literature, theory developed from professional practice or theory derived from other disciplines.

A workable question has to be narrow enough to allow a fruitful investigation in the library, on the Internet and/or in the field. Many interesting questions are too immense – the research they would require would take years, not the time you have available, for example, 'How is the climate of the earth changing?' or 'Why does poverty exist?' As you consider your question, think carefully about whether it is one that you could answer within your time and length constraints. You should also consider whether your question is *too* narrow. If you restrict your topic too far, for example, 'How did John F. Kennedy's maternal grandfather influence the decisions he made during his first month as president?', it may be impossible to find relevant sources.

A question may also be so narrow that it becomes uninteresting – avoid questions that can be answered with a simple yes or no or by stating a few statistics, for example, 'Are there more African American students than Hispanic students in the freshman class

Table 12.1   Examples of questions that might arise in practice

Interventions	Is kangaroo care for babies more effective than incubator care?
Communication	Should terminally ill patients be told of their diagnosis?
Targeting	Which men need to be told of testicular self-examination?
Timing	At what age should school children have sessions on sexual health?
Management	Should young people with a moderate learning difficulty be taught in mainstream schools?

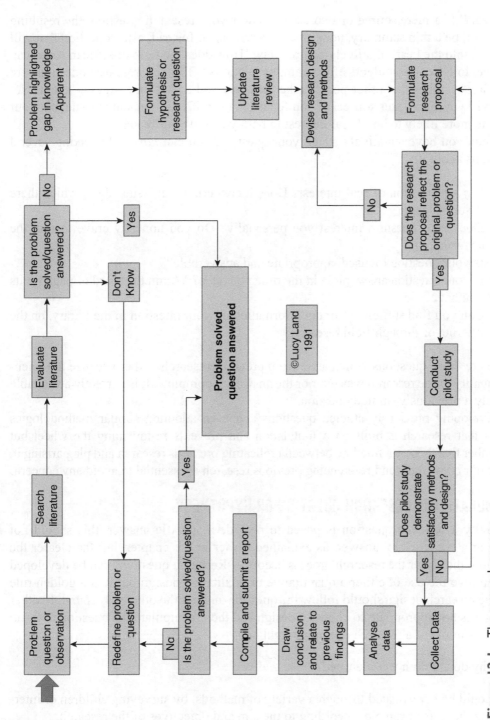

Figure 12.1 The research process

this year?' If a mere source or two could answer your research question, the resulting paper will be a thin summary, not a true research paper. Instead, ask a question that will lead you into the heart of a lively controversy: 'How does the ratio of African American students to Hispanic students affect campus relations?' The best research questions are those about issues that other people take seriously and spend time arguing about. Not only will you find better sources if you focus on a significant, debatable issue, but your paper is more likely to be of real interest to both you and your readers.

When you have tentatively stated your question, you can *hone* it by asking several questions about it:

- Is your question of real interest? Does it concern a real issue, about which there is some debate?
- Does your question interest you personally? Do you honestly crave to find the answers to it?
- Is your question focused, appropriate and answerable?
- Is your question answerable in the time you have? Within the word or page limits you have?
- Can you find sufficient, timely information on your question in the library, on the Internet or through field research?

There are those questions which arise from previous research, either because the scientific quality of the research was poor or the answers incomplete. It is perfectly acceptable to study a previously studied question.

Developing previously studied questions and even adopting similar methodologies means that research is built on a foundation and prevents re-inventing the wheel but remember that there is a fine line between replicating previous research and plagiarising it. Using our own words and referencing previous research is essential to avoid any concern.

FORMULATE THE RESEARCH QUESTION OR HYPOTHESIS

Generally a research question is posed to provide a specific answer, this should not result in a 'yes' or 'no' answer, as explained earlier in the chapter, but the clearer the question, the easier the research process becomes. Research questions can be developed that involve the use of either a quantitative or qualitative design but it is a golden rule that the research design should follow the question and not the other way round. In other words it is not appropriate to choose a design and then manipulate the question to fit it.

An example of a research question might be:

'Why do children wet their bed?'

This could be investigated through a variety of methods, by surveying children or interviewing them, for example, according to the aim and objectives of the research.

The hypothesis is a formal statement that proposes a cause and effect relationship between two variables and possesses key characteristics. It must be testable, that is it must contain a stated outcome measure. See the chapter on experimental design for an example of a hypothesis and how it is constructed. A hypothesis should also be falsifiable; that is, we must be able to reject the hypothesis if the data do not support it. A good hypothesis is simple and precise as well as useful and the structure of a PICO (explained in Chapter 2) provides an excellent way of developing one.

THINK POINT ACTIVITY   12.2

For the following research topic:

  Nocturnal enuresis in children

Generate five potential qualitative research questions and five different hypotheses.

RESEARCH TITLES

One of the most frustrating things about literature searching is locating a paper that you think is going to be very useful only to find when it arrives that the content bears no resemblance to the title. On the other hand it's tempting to give your work an 'appealing' title, for example:

  'The hand that rocks the cradle'

when you are investigating the extent of Munchausen's by proxy amongst first time mothers. By doing this you are seriously reducing the number of people who could locate the work you publish.

SEARCH AND EVALUATE THE LITERATURE

A search of the relevant literature needs to be made before any study is designed and executed. It should then be evaluated (reviewed) in respect of the problem to be studied. This step is essential to find results of previous research and indeed the existence of research which answers our research question. Similarly we may discover previous research that has partly done so, in which case we may decide to revise our problem slightly. We may be disappointed to find that our question has already been answered satisfactorily, but it does save time, effort and resources in finding evidence we already have.

The background to and the methods used in previous research should also be reviewed. It ensures that you have a comprehensive knowledge of the subject to be investigated, or at least an appreciation of the extent of the knowledge which is required for such research. Defining what is to be done and reviewing the literature, are very closely linked. Many people who contemplate doing research are already to some extent familiar with published material on the subject. Chapters 10, 13 and 14 provide a more in-depth explanation of this step.

DEVISE THE RESEARCH DESIGN AND METHODS

All the stages of the investigation must now be thought through in order to decide the appropriate method, and to find out whether the whole thing is feasible. This involves:

- deciding the type of research designs and methods that are most appropriate to the investigation
- identifying the type of data needed
- identifying the population and sample
- choosing the techniques to be used for data collection
- determining how the data will be analysed and presented
- determining how the report will be structured.

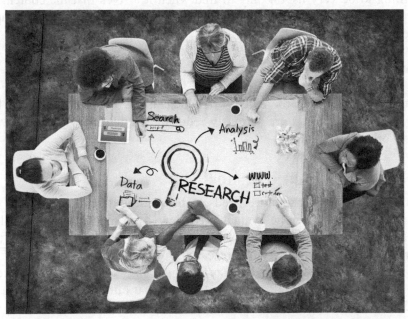

© Shutterstock

THINK POINT ACTIVITY   12.3

For each of the bullet points above, locate the relevant chapters in this book that relate to this and make notes on potential methods you might use in your research.

TEST THE PROPOSED METHODOLOGY BY CARRYING OUT PILOT STUDIES

When the plan is finalised a pilot study is often needed. This means using a small sample as similar as possible to the sample to be used for the main study, and working through each stage of the research process. Almost inevitably the study will be modified. If major alterations have to be made, more than one pilot study may be needed.

COLLECT DATA

When pilot studies are satisfactory, full-scale data collection can be carried out, keeping strictly to the method planned. A wide variety of data collection methods exist and good care should be taken when choosing a particular type to ensure that it is in a form that is most likely to answer the research question. See Chapters 16 and 17 for the most often used.

CONDUCT DATA ANALYSIS

Data analysis involves using particular techniques to make sense of the data we have collected and it is important to adhere to the conventions of each type. If employing a qualitative approach using observation or interviews, for example, it may involve grouping, classifying and coding the data according to a pre-arranged system. In the broadest sense, a quantitative approach involves 'counting' the data: finding out how many times a particular response occurred, or how often a particular event took place; subjecting the data to statistical analyses by using the techniques decided beforehand. See Chapter 18 regarding the analysis of quantitative data and measures of **clinical effectiveness**.

DRAW CONCLUSIONS AND WRITE A REPORT

The purpose of a research report is to make known the findings and to inform people how the study was carried out so that they can assess the value of the work. Transparency is critical so that readers can verify the quality of the work, so the report should be as detailed as possible. It also allows readers to decide whether to use similar methods for their own research if they wish to do so and therefore limitations of the study should also be acknowledged so that others can avoid similar mistakes, the structure of a research report is illustrated in Table 12.2. A report should be clearly written, bearing in mind the purpose for which the research was carried out and the people who will be reading it.

Table 12.2   The structure of a research report

Heading	Content
Introduction	An introduction to the topic, the rationale for undertaking the study and a statement regarding the purpose of the study
Literature review	A critical evaluation of the relevant literature that demonstrates a need for the research
Methodology	A statement of the research question/hypothesis and a detailed description of its design and methodology
Study sample	Information about the population studied, the method of sampling and the size of the sample
Data collection	A description of the method used for collecting data together with a rationale for its use
Data analysis	A description and justification for the methods used to analyse the data
Ethical issues	An explanation of the ethical issues involved in the research and evidence of ethical approval of the study
Pilot study	A description of pilot studies and any major changes which were made as a result
Findings	The findings, including the data from which the conclusions were derived
Discussion	A discussion of the findings in relation to previous research and to recent developments
Limitations	An account of any major difficulty encountered and how it was dealt with
Conclusions and recommendations	A summary of the main findings and an indication of how they might be used
References	A complete list of references, acknowledgement of all source material
Appendices	Copies of all data collection instruments where appropriate such as questionnaires or interview schedules used in the main study Any other documents used in the study

---

THINK POINT ACTIVITY   12.4

For your chosen research topic:

- Identify a formal research question of hypothesis using a PICO
  - What type of research design would best help answer that question?
  - What sort of data would you need to collect to answer the question?
  - Where would you get these data from?
  - How would you analyse the data?

Website activity 12.1

SUMMARY

Familiarising yourself with the research process will help you in later chapters to structure you own research, particularly when you are writing your dissertation.

Ultimately, the success and quality of a research study is directly related to the amount of time and effort invested in the development of your research ideas. Thorough planning and design will help facilitate data collection and analysis and reduce research stress during the next phase of the research process.

FURTHER READING

Thomas, G. (2013) *How to Do Your Research Project* (2nd edn). London: Sage Publications.

The first chapter, 'Your introduction: starting points', will get you started quickly and efficiently; the fourth chapter, 'Decide on your question – again', is helpful in focusing your project and fine-tuning your question or hypothesis.

Don't forget to visit https://study.sagepub.com/harveyandland to watch videos, take quizzes and to follow specially designed web activities.

13
LITERATURE REVIEW: IDENTIFYING AND SOURCING THE LITERATURE

To produce any piece of academic work it is essential to identify and source relevant literature to establish the evidence base for the paper and to support critical analysis for the arguments presented. In this chapter we will:

- establish the need for the inclusion of robust literature in academic writing
- identify different sources of literature
- describe the process of searching the literature
- identify methods of recording the results of a literature search.

One of the most frequent questions asked by students who have been given an essay to write, is to ask 'how many references do I need?' The most frequent answer to this is a corny, 'how long is a piece of string?' The most successful essays, that is, the ones that get a high grade, are ones that have used the literature to its best effect; tutors don't count the number of them. There is also a tendency amongst students to want to try and cram in all the literature they have found regardless of its relevance, to illustrate how hard they have worked. This may lead the student to wander off the subject and lose marks rather than gain them. The art of searching the literature for an assignment or a research study involves sacrificing material that, although painstakingly found, does not meet the requirements of the paper being written.

Fraser and Dunstan (2010) estimate that there are now 25,400 journals in science, technology and medicine, and their number is increasing by 3.5% a year, whilst the Cumulative Index to Nursing and Allied Health Literature (CINAHL) provides indexing for around 3,075 nursing and allied health journals. This information explosion together with technological innovation, specifically access to infinite Internet sources, means that enormous amounts of information are literally at our fingertips. The availability of literature does not guarantee its quality so literature searches need to be conducted using a critical approach. It can also make us lazy and neglectful of traditional sources of information that can be found in the physical recesses of the library or using only full text sources. The key to good literature searching has the following elements:

- defining the key concepts and potential themes
- planning a search strategy, allowing enough time to search using as many sources as practically possible
- discarding irrelevant and poor quality material
- keeping a comprehensive record of the literature retrieved.

Knowing what we want to look for is a key element of literature searching, which can sound bizarre – if we know what to look for then surely we know already what we're going to write! Well not exactly. Knowing what to look for is actually about understanding the concepts, key words, opposing views and on top of all this understanding the quality of the literature on the subject. In the first instance we need to read around the subject to provide a more complete understanding. If we are going to write a paper on an intervention in diabetes care, for example, it would be reasonable to have a good understanding of what this condition is and how it affects people. Essential and background reading usually provides an understanding of the key definitions and concepts that we want to work with, even if this reading is not actually used in the final paper, but it does give us the ability to write with greater confidence. Background reading can also provide us with a certain amount of material from which we can cite definitions and concepts and use as a platform from which to start searching for more specific literature and this will give us a clue about generating key words that we can build into a search strategy.

Suppose we are given the question:

'What influence can the environment have on a child's life?'

Hopefully essay questions you receive will not be as vague as the example above, but there are still decisions to be made as to what needs to go in it. Some students choose a 'scattergun approach', which involves trying to use as many different themes and sources of literature as they can in the belief that it shows that they have made the effort to read widely. This often results in remarks by the marker about superficial understanding. On the other hand another high-risk strategy is to concentrate on a seminal (influential) piece of work. Whilst this can be persuasive if there are no contrary arguments, it doesn't reflect breadth of reading. Another way of ensuring a low grade is to quote references within references known as secondary referencing. Experienced markers can see this quite clearly, particularly if they can see that the secondary reference would probably be difficult for the student to access.

BACKGROUND READING

Reading background literature should give us a handle on what sort of things we might investigate on this topic, which could be unfathomably broad, for example we could focus on any of the sub-topics identified in Table 13.1 using the above title.

Each of these topics could again be broken down into sub-categories that could quite easily produce yet more papers. Using this question we could generate a similar question which focuses on the effect of a particular environment on the child.

Evidence-based practice demands that we focus our research questions as accurately as possible by using a structured question or PICO (refer back to Chapter 2 for an explanation of a PICO). Once your background reading is complete, you should be able to formulate a PICO if using a quantitative approach or a well-formulated research question if using a qualitative approach.

Table 13.1   Topics that could address the question, 'What influence can the environment have on a child's life?'

The nature/nurture debate
Quality of life, health and wellbeing
Family life
Psychosocial wellbeing
Socialisation and occupation
Education and personal development
The built environment
Technological and scientific innovation
Aesthetics

KEY DEFINITIONS AND CONCEPTS

Whether or not we include definitions and the key concepts of our topic in our essay depends largely on what is required of the piece of work we aim to produce.

Website
activity 13.1

THINK POINT ACTIVITY   13.1

Locate the following article on the Cochrane Library database:

> Dumville, J.C., Webster, J., Evans, D. and Land, L. (2015) Negative pressure wound therapy for treating pressure ulcers. *Cochrane Database of Systematic Reviews*, Issue 5, Art. No.: CD011334. DOI: 10.1002/14651858.C D011334.pub2.

Read the sections 'Description of the condition' and 'Description of the intervention'.

Systematic reviews of the literature always include a basic explanation of the problem or condition as well as a description of the proposed intervention.

SPECIFYING KEY WORDS AND RELATED TERMS

If we take the question of the influence of the environment on a child's life as an example, what concepts do we need to galvanise in order to be able to make a discussion? If we take the nouns in the question sentence, define each and identify synonyms we can find potential words to use as search terms in order to maximise the amount of literature we might find (see Table 13.2 for an example). Dictionaries, an encyclopaedia and a thesaurus are useful tools for this; all of these can be found online if preferred. This may over-simplify the context of what we are looking for, but by doing it we can

Table 13.2 Potential key words

Noun	Definition	Synonym
Influence	Power over persons or events Determining factor	Affect Move Strike Impress Touch
Environment	Surrounding, external physical, psychological or social and cultural conditions	Environs Setting Location Surroundings Milieu Atmosphere

(Continued)

Table 13.2   (Continued)

Noun	Definition	Synonym
Child	An infant or baby Immature or childish Offspring or descendent	Youngster Kid Young person Teenager Teen Adolescent
Life	State or condition, a being; physical, mental or spiritual existence	Existence Being Time Living Days Years

see what is likely to come up if we enter key words as search terms, then we can filter inappropriate terms out of the search in order to concentrate on likely literature.

THREE STEPS TO SEARCHING

Step 1: Write out your search as a sentence.

Step 2: Identify the important words and concepts.

Step 3: Think about ways you could limit your search.

You might find too many references on your topic, so think about ways you could limit your search. Most databases will allow you to limit your search in these ways:

- *Date*: do you only want items published after a certain date?
- *Language*: do you only want references in English?
- *Geography*: do you want information about a specific place or published in a particular country?
- *Type of publication*: do you only want references to journal articles, books or theses, for example? This might influence your choice of database.

See Table 13.3 for the types of information you might access.

Website
activity 13.2

METHODS OF SEARCHING

Databases are not as intelligent as we may think. If we type wound care into a health database you will retrieve thousands of hits. This is because the database will look for 'wound care', 'wound' and 'care'. To overcome this you could place quotation marks (' ') around your phrase, for example, 'wound care'. More often we need to find all

Table 13.3   Type of information in specific data sources

Type of publication	Where to find them	What sort of information	Advantages	Disadvantages
Books	Identify from reading list Browse library shelves Search library catalogues Look at publishers' catalogues	Background and supplementary reading	Useful if reader is new to the topic and needs to learn basic concepts A valuable source of supplementary help, e.g. skills books, methodology Reference books provide a quick insight into issues that could be studied in depth using other publications and papers	Not as dynamic as journal articles for up to the minute thinking
Journal articles	Suggested reading Databases including library and online sources indexes and abstracts By browsing the reference list of articles retrieved	A very wide range from personal opinion, literature reviews, research, education and debate, methodological pieces and much more	If the subject is known about it will have something written about it Generally up to date, it can provide a wealth of information to support academic writing	Beware of variable quality: just because it's published doesn't mean it's good Opinion articles particularly are liable to personal bias
Media articles	Newspapers Magazines Online media sources	A wide range of topics that are relevant to current issues	Can spark an idea or debate, can support arguments about popular ideals and beliefs	Not an academic source of literature. Views may represent the 'colour' of the media. Open to bias, inaccuracy and poor reporting
Research articles	Suggested reading Databases including library and online sources Indexes and abstracts By browsing the reference list of articles retrieved	Structured scientific or social reports that demonstrate the methods used to answer a specified question Requires some skill in appraisal to make appropriate judgements	Can provide a definitive or persuasive answer to a focused question	May be of questionable quality, methodologically unsound

words that could be relevant to your search, so if you type 'child' – the database just searches for exactly what you type in. Wild card symbols enable you to overcome this limitation. These symbols can be substituted for letters to retrieve variant spellings and word endings and will help you to widen your search and ensure that you don't miss relevant information, for example, 'child?' will find child and children.

A truncation symbol retrieves any number of letters, which is useful to find different word endings based on the root of a word, for example, 'environment*' will find environmental and environmentally.

You will need to check the online help screens for details of the symbols recognised by the database you are searching – not all databases use the ? and * symbols.

SEARCH OPERATORS

Search operators combine your search words and include synonyms. Also known as **Boolean operators**, search operators allow you to include multiple words and concepts in your searches.

AND retrieves records containing both words. In our example, records with both children and environment in the text would be retrieved.

OR retrieves records containing either word. In our example the records with child or environment, or both words in the text would be retrieved and broadens your search and you can use this to include synonyms in your search.

NOT retrieves your first word but excludes the second. In our example we could specify child NOT teenager to limit the papers retrieved to those involving children under 13. Using this operator you might exclude relevant results because you will lose those records which include both words, so some caution is needed.

Once you have identified your key terms and limits you can construct a search strategy.

THINK POINT ACTIVITY   13.2

Browse your library databases, read the description of databases *not* allied to health and make a note of any you find useful.

Locate your college/university library resources page to find an example of how a search strategy is constructed.

ALLOWING TIME FOR SEARCHING

Wherever the starting point for literature searching is – either from the comfort of our own computer or in the library, we need to allow enough time to make a proper search. If we grab 15 minutes or half an hour here and there we will waste more time than we gain because it is impossible to execute a search strategy in this time. A piece-meal approach is counterproductive as we can get very frustrated as we have not had time to find anything useful. If we do find something useful and then run out of time for photocopying it we end up having to go back and locate it again, which quite often results in going over the same ground on subsequent searches.

It makes sense therefore to take time out for this activity, usually about three hours (more than that and 'searching fatigue' may set in). This time should include time for recording the citation for each paper found. Simple as it sounds we also need to have had something to eat and drink so that we know we can spend a decent amount of time searching without distractions.

WHERE TO SEARCH FOR LITERATURE

ELECTRONIC SEARCHING OF DATABASES

Most electronic databases are bibliographic, which means that they contain details of publications, such as books, journal articles, conference papers, theses and so on. Your college or university will subscribe to a wide number that you can access. It is useful to note that whilst there are databases dedicated to your particular field, there are social science, education, law and business databases as well as a host of others that could also provide useful resources. Database searching can be done before you get to the library providing you have access to a computer with an Internet connection and good off-campus library links. Some databases also provide full-text articles, for example CINAHL and Science Direct.

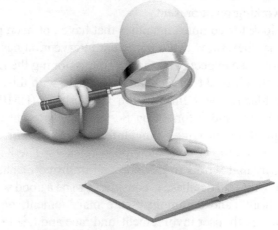

© Palto / Shutterstock

Website
activity 13.3

PHYSICAL ACCESS TO THE LIBRARY

Decide which library you need to visit according to the type of material you need to retrieve. The most obvious will be linked to what and where you are studying, which will contain the specialist subject information you are likely to need and, in particular, specialist or professional journals and publications on your subject. If you need local information and statistics, you might also want to search your public library. There are also local and national collections of published and unpublished works to be found in specialist and museum libraries. For all of these you need to be aware of the opening or more importantly the closing times; there is little sense in arriving half an hour before closing time. Work out ahead of time what activities you really need to go to the library for so that you make best use of your time there.

HAND SEARCHING AND THE GREY LITERATURE

To make sure that you find all sources of literature, you may need to do this manually, which is called a hand search. For example, you may look at documentary records or official publications that cannot be found on databases or in the comfort of our own surroundings. Hand searches also include looking at the list of references at the end of a paper you have retrieved. Using this method it quickly becomes clear that you have exhausted your search if the references you have discovered keep appearing.

To carry out a thorough search of the literature – in particular to do a systematic search – you would be expected to identify work that has not been published in conventional books and journals. This material is referred to as grey literature. This term includes reports, working papers, theses and dissertations, newsletters, many official and governmental publications, together with conference papers. Looking for unpublished material is a way of counteracting publication bias.

Key researchers in your field can also be useful and you could contact them to find out what they are working on at present.

You might also look for completed studies that have not been published – they may be significant because they show that a particular intervention has no effect, or because their results were not those expected by those commissioning the research. In health and medicine, checking the clinical trials registries will help with this.

The Healthcare Management Information Consortium (HMIC) database contains records from the Library and Information Services department of the Department of Health (DH) in England and the King's Fund Information and Library Service. It includes all DH publications including circulars and press releases. The King's Fund is an independent health charity that works to develop and improve management of health and social care services. The Ovid database is considered to be a good source of grey literature on topics such as health and community care management, organisational development, inequalities in health, user involvement, and race and health (www.ovid.com/site/catalog/databases/901.jsp).

Other databases that provide cover for grey literature include PsychEXTRA (www.apa.org/psycextra/) and OpenSIGLE (opensigle.inist.fr).

THINK POINT ACTIVITY   13.3

Browse the Internet using the term 'clinical trials registry' and make a note of the location of registries that might be useful to you.

RETRIEVAL OF MATERIAL

At the beginning of the chapter we identified that it is tempting to use all the material we have located, which can be time consuming and costly. Also some students find it really difficult to gauge when to stop searching, convinced that if they continue they will find the one piece of work that will be perfect for their assignment. In reality the perfect paper does not exist and it's really only a delaying tactic to avoid starting that essay.

A smarter way of working is to use the PRISMA method, which involves a series of steps.

Step 1: Execute the search strategy and using the PRISMA flow diagram (see Figure 13.1) and record the *total number* of records identified from the strategy.

Step 2: Decide which records to discard using *only the title of the paper* and keep a note of the number of remaining papers.

Step 3: Read the *abstracts* (not the full paper) of the remaining papers and discard irrelevant papers, again make a note of the number of papers kept.

Step 4: Read the remaining papers and discard irrelevant ones recording the number of final papers for inclusion.

In this way you only need to read the papers you have found relevant to your work.

The literature you decide to retrieve may be in the form of a hard copy or electronic (PDF) format and you need to decide how you are going to keep this information so that you can locate it easily when needed.

MANAGING REFERENCES

Recording and storing the information (the reference or citation) from a paper that you intend to include in your work is vital.

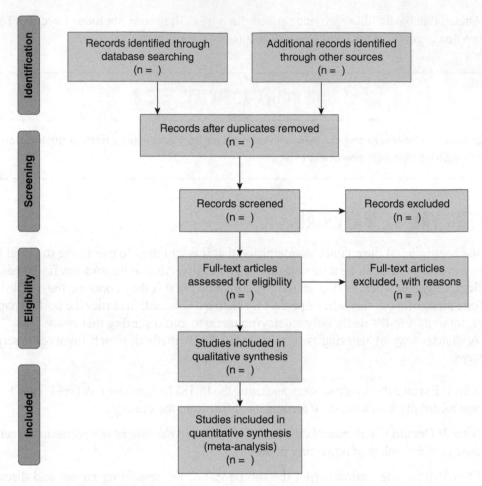

Figure 13.1   The PRISMA flow diagram

WHY RECORD REFERENCES?

It really is worth the time and effort to make a separate note of all your references at the end of your search. The value of this only becomes evident the night before (or worse in the early hours of the morning) when you are due to hand in the essay, after you have spent hours turning the world upside down trying to find one paper because you need the complete reference for the reference list. It is also worth taking the trouble to make a brief note of the main themes or arguments in the paper so that you can identify it easily again if needed.

METHODS OF RECORDING AND STORING REFERENCES

The method you use to record and store the references from the papers you have found doesn't really matter, the important thing is that you are able to locate them when you need them, particularly if you are writing large pieces of work such as dissertations or thesis. It depends upon how much time you have and how technologically competent you feel.

There is nothing wrong with an old fashioned approach such as hand writing index cards and filing them in a box using your chosen filing system, although this may take time.

Typing all the references into a word-processing document *before* writing your paper means that you can cut and paste the reference to your reference list as you cite it, which is easier than stopping every time you cite a reference to type it in at the bottom.

Electronic spreadsheets or databases could also be used to organise your references. There are a number of citation or reference managers that are extremely useful. A reference manager is the software you use to handle references, full-text documents and citations whilst writing. References can be handled manually as well, but the reference manager allows for greater flexibility and efficiency. The scientific disciplines vary in how references are written and consequently in how references are managed. Therefore, some reference managers may be preferred within your discipline. Other factors are personal preferences and work style. Choose a reference manager that adapts easily to your way of working and lets you establish an efficient workflow. There are several reference managers to choose from, Mendeley, for example, is free to download. ENDNOTE® and REFMan® or similar software are often available through your educational institution. If you decide to use a reference manager make a habit of storing all useful references to research literature as you come across them. This practice will save time later when you are writing. Building your reference collection can be done in several ways and you will probably use them all at some point:

- registering the reference manually: this is mostly done for older material not readily available online, especially books and grey literature
- transferring from reference databases like Web of Knowledge or Pub Med: here you may transfer large sets of references
- downloading a reference at the journal home page
- downloading references from Google Scholar
- pulling reference data from the PDF of the article.

Always check references for accuracy; proofreading references directly saves time later and allows you to focus on writing when you use the reference.

SUMMARY

Other than devising a well-constructed research question, searching the literature is one of the most important parts of the research process. The more organised you are during this process the better, it will save you time and ensure there are fewer mistakes.

FURTHER READING

Power, A. and Siddall, G. (2015) Ensuring practice is based on the best evidence: masterclass on literature searching. *British Journal of Midwifery*, 23(5): 356–358.

Easy to follow advice from experts.

Ridley, D. (2012) *The Literature Review: A Step by Step Guide for Students*. London: Sage Publications.

This book will take you through each step of the process in a logical and useful order.

Don't forget to visit https://study.sagepub.com/harveyandland to watch videos, take quizzes and to follow specially designed web activities.

14

LITERATURE REVIEW: REVIEWING THE NARRATIVE DATA

A narrative literature review refers to the works we consult in order to understand and investigate a specific research problem. In this chapter we will:

- discuss the purpose of a narrative literature review
- distinguish between systematic literature reviews and narrative reviews
- explain the structure of a narrative literature review.

A literature review is not just a summary of a particular topic, but a conceptually organised synthesis of the results of a literature search. It must organise the information we have located and relate it to the research question we are developing. The aim is to synthesise the results of our search into a summary of what is and isn't known. It can be defined as follows:

> A literature review is an objective, thorough summary and critical analysis of the relevant available research and non-research literature on the topic being studied. (Hart, 1998: 13)

THE PURPOSE OF A NARRATIVE LITERATURE REVIEW

Every research project should reflect the outcome of previous thinking and research in the chosen area, and a narrative review places our planned study in the context of previous work and requires a critical examination of the related literature, strengths, weaknesses and gaps. The objective is not to rack up points by listing as many articles as possible; rather, we want to demonstrate our intellectual ability to recognise relevant information, and to synthesise and evaluate it according to the guiding concept we have determined regarding our research question. The reader of a review not only wants to know what literature exists, but also requires an informed evaluation of it.

To meet both of these needs, we must employ two sets of skills:

- information seeking
- critical appraisal skills.

Chapter 13 gives guidance on scanning the literature efficiently using manual or computerised methods to identify a set of potentially useful articles and other work we might include in our review. We also need to develop critical appraisal skills, that is, the ability to apply principles of analysis to identify those studies which are unbiased and valid. Readers want more just than a descriptive list of articles and books and it's usually a bad sign when every paragraph of a review begins with the names of researchers. Instead, a review should be organised into useful, informative sections that present themes or identify trends.

During this process it is necessary to identify controversy when it appears in the literature and, although we value 'unbiased' scientific research, the truth is that no author is free from outside influence, such as a particular **theoretical framework** or model, for example, a feminist examination of gender inequity in medical research; or the author's rhetorical purpose, for example, a researcher's reasons for advocating the effectiveness of a certain drug. It is a criticism of narrative literature reviews that experience-based rather than research-based literature is included, for example, the belief that one approach to pain management is more effective than another.

QUESTIONS TO ASK YOURSELF ABOUT YOUR REVIEW OF THE LITERATURE

Website
activity 14.1

- Will my literature review help to define my research question and the issues surrounding it?
- Am I looking at issues of practice or theory or potential methodologies?
- What types of publications should I be using? For example, journals, books, government documents or popular media.
- What discipline am I working in? For example, nursing, psychology, sociology, medicine.
- Is there a specific relationship between the literature I've chosen to review and the problem I've formulated?
- Have I critically analysed the literature I use? Do I just list and summarise authors and articles, or do I assess them? Do I discuss the strengths and weaknesses of the cited material?
- Will the reader find my literature review relevant, appropriate and useful?

Not all of these questions need to be asked about a single review, but they do help to focus on its purpose. It may include reading basic writings in the field as well as writing of key thinkers (seminal works), even if they are not used in the final review. This way we can examine others' points of view and learn to understand their arguments.

When writing the review it is important to distinguish between summaries of the work of others and your own point of view. Grammatically, reviews are written in the third person, which some students find difficult and employ the phrase 'the author' to denote their views. For example, 'The author concludes that this study is of high quality'. But in a literature review this can be confusing as it won't be clear whether it is you or the author of the paper you are reviewing that is making the conclusion, so instead we should write, 'In conclusion, the study appears to be of high quality'.

AVOIDING PLAGIARISM

Plagiarism is the practice of taking someone else's work or ideas and passing them off as one's own, which often carries serious penalties for any scholar or student attempting to do this. Summarising other's work in a narrative review needs to be done carefully to avoid this. All work commented on needs to be referenced and although we sometimes find it difficult to paraphrase a sentence or paragraph, it is worth the effort. The alternative would be to quote from the paper directly and place the sentence or paragraph in quotation marks with an accompanying reference. It is, however, worth remembering that if direct quotes are used too often it breaks up the flow of the review as well as making it descriptive rather than analytical. One of the best ways to avoid plagiarism

© docstockmedia / Shutterstock

is to put the review through originality software, often provided free by your university or college.

NARRATIVE REVIEWS VERSUS SYSTEMATIC REVIEWS

As discussed in Chapter 10, systematic reviews are a form of primary research using research studies rather than participants. They follow a very strict protocol so that the outcome of the review is clear and transparent. Narrative reviews provide the context for proposed research by demonstrating that the research question is worthy of study, but in recent years they have become less popular than systematic reviews for quantitative research studies for several reasons. Narrative reviews can be seen as subjective or potentially biased in that they rely on the reviewer's decision about which studies they include. In the past, narrative reviewers weren't explicit about the studies that they included. This can be addressed by using a systematic approach to searching and retrieving studies in a similar fashion to systematic reviewing. By providing a clear audit trail of which studies were included or excluded, the accusation of subjectivity can be redressed. A further criticism of narrative reviews is that included studies are not treated differently, that is, that research studies and opinion articles (the rhetorical purpose identified earlier in the chapter) are given equal weight, which introduces further bias. To avoid this it is wise to include only research studies where possible. Narrative reviews are also said to be obscure in process, methodology and generation of conclusions. All of these perceived disadvantages can be minimised by adopting a systematic *approach* to reviewing the literature.

THE STRUCTURE OF A NARRATIVE REVIEW

Like all essays the review should have a beginning, middle and an end. The following headings can be used as a guide for structuring a review.

TITLE

This should be a concise and precise reflection of what the review is about. It is a good idea to formulate this before the review is written and keep it in sight whilst reviewing so that you can remain focused.

ABSTRACT

The abstract is a concise summary of the literature review, yet it must be comprehensive enough for the reader to become acquainted with the content of the body of the review. The abstract should not exceed 150 words and must contain a clear statement of the purpose of the review, together with a brief outline of how the review was conducted. It should include the main findings of the review, followed by its conclusions. Key words can be added here so that readers can determine the relevance of the review.

INTRODUCTION AND RATIONALE

This section must be written to convince the reader that the research question, and therefore the review, is worthwhile. This is an opportunity to define the concepts that surround the question as well as the extent to which the problem/issue is placed in a national and local context. It might include a description of the problem. If, for example, you are writing about gestational diabetes, your introduction might include a physiological explanation of this, which could be supported by references from textbooks or articles. The scale of the problem can be identified such as what proportion of women are diagnosed with gestational diabetes, again supporting statistical literature can be used here. The overall impact of this section relies on the ability of the student to 'sell' the research question.

MAIN BODY OF THE REVIEW

The actual heading of the main body of the review will depend on your topic and how you organise your content, but it will begin with making yourself familiar with

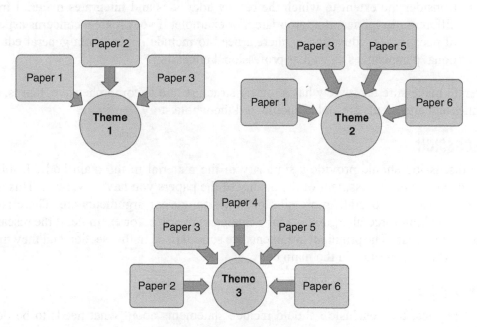

Figure 14.1   Organising the themes for the literature review

the literature you intend to include. Read each paper thoroughly, using an appropriate critical appraisal tool to assess the quality of the research (see Chapter 10). As you read you should begin to observe the emergence of similar ideas and arguments and possibly opposing views on interventions, for example.

Make additional notes on each paper, idea, intervention or recommendation that you think is useful for inclusion in your final review. Do not be afraid of discarding some papers here if they do not fit with your overall review, they will only weaken your review. As you make notes you should be able to identify themes, see Figure 14.1 for a diagrammatic representation of how this might work.

Organise your themes in a logical order and begin to write. As you write remind yourself of the following:

- Question the relevance of the material you are including. It is tempting if you have located an interesting article to work it into your review when it doesn't really add to the discussion; don't be afraid to discard it. A balanced review relies on accurate reporting of findings from other studies even if they are contrary to your arguments, to leave them out would introduce bias.
- Avoid an in-depth evaluation of each piece of research included in the review. Instead your critical appraisal should focus on an evaluation of the themes and arguments as a whole.
- Consider the extent to which the review addresses and integrates material from different disciplines, if appropriate. For example, if your review concerns aspects of pedagogical education, is there a need to include papers from general educational perspectives as well as professional education?

Website
activity 14.2 Overall, make sure the review has a logical structure and is comprehensive, that is, the themes and arguments presented should 'tell the whole story'.

DISCUSSION

The discussion should provide a summary of the material in the main body. It might include an overall assessment of the quality of the papers you have reviewed. This will give the reader an overall impression of how strong your arguments are. There is no point in making forceful arguments for a change in practice, for example, if the research evidence is weak. The principal arguments are summarised in this section and they must reflect what was written in the main body.

CONCLUSION

As it implies, the conclusion should include statements about what needs to be done next. If the review suggests your research question should be pursued then that will be the main conclusion of your review. It may have also revealed a new way or method of conducting the proposed research and that should also be included. If the review was conducted to determine best practice, then recommendations for improvement or change could be summarised.

REFERENCES

Particular attention needs to be paid to referencing papers in a literature review. There is nothing more annoying than reading a review and coming across a paper you would like to read in full only to find that the reference is missing, incorrect or incomplete. See Chapter 13 about recording references.

The style of referencing you use is guided by the conventions of your university or college regulations. The most often used are:

- an alphabetical system (Harvard): the authors' names are placed in the body of the text and the reference list is compiled alphabetically
- a numerical system (Vancouver): a number is placed in the text at the point of reference and full references are listed numerically in the reference list.

THINK POINT ACTIVITY   14.1

Locate a narrative literature review that relates to an area of your interest. Using this chapter in general and this section in particular, assess the quality of the review.

The nature of literature reviews often means that references are grouped together when a point is made by two authors or more. Using an example from the assisted conception paper in Website activity 14.1, which includes multiple references, the Vancouver method would involve putting consecutive numbers in the text:

The possibility of an increased risk of major malformations in children conceived via assisted conception has been widely discussed.[1][2][3][4][5]

Using the Harvard method the references would look like this:

The possibility of an increased risk of major malformations in children conceived via assisted conception has been widely discussed (Hanson et al., 2005; Ludwig, 2005; Van Voorhis, 2006; Paulson, 2007).

Note that the authors are listed in the text in chronological order of publication, not alphabetically.

> ## THINK POINT ACTIVITY 14.2
>
> Locate a copy of your institution's library guide to referencing and make a note of its conventions.

SUMMARY

The prospect of writing a literature review can seem daunting, but in fact they are not much different from writing an essay on a topic, they just tend to be longer in length and more focused. Narrative reviews are extremely useful to clinical practitioners as they provide an up-to-date summary of a topic, which saves the time and energy taken to research the topic.

FURTHER READING

Ridley, D. (2012) *The Literature Review: A Step by Step Guide*. London: Sage Publications.

This provides good suggestions for developing and using narrative reviews in your research.

Snyder, H. and Engström, J. (2016) The antecedents, forms and consequences of patient involvement: a narrative review of the literature. *International Journal of Nursing Studies*, 53: 351–378.

This paper provides a good example of a narrative literature review.

> Don't forget to visit https://study.sagepub.com/harveyandland to watch videos, take quizzes and to follow specially designed web activities.

15
SAMPLING

Whilst there has been some discussion about sampling in previous chapters, here we will
explore sampling issues in depth and in doing so we will:

- clarify terminology commonly used in relation to sampling, such as total population,
  sample, generalisability, representativeness, data saturation, probability and non-probability
  sampling
- review the different types of sampling methods used in qualitative and quantitative research
- explore the factors that the researcher should consider when deciding which sampling
  method to use
- consider how sample size and configuration are determined
- explore factors the researcher should consider when recruiting a sample of participants
  to a study.

In previous chapters we have considered different methods of research. In the discussions
about a particular research method, we have identified the sampling strategy commonly
used. In this chapter we will explore in more detail the decisions a researcher has to
make about which sampling strategy to use, what size the sample should be and how it
should be configured. We will also take the opportunity in this chapter to discuss issues
the researcher needs to make decisions about when recruiting a sample because the strategies adopted can impact on the eventual size and format of the sample.

CLARIFYING TERMINOLOGY

As is the case with other aspects of the research process, sampling abounds with terminology and in some cases different terms can mean the same thing. Furthermore, some
sampling terms are more closely associated with quantitative research than qualitative, or
vice versa. Whilst some definitions have been given in earlier chapters, it seems prudent
to take this opportunity to clarify the meanings of terms commonly used in association
with sampling, which will be used in this chapter.

TOTAL POPULATION

This is sometimes referred to as the study's population, target or wider population. The population is all possible cases or participants who are eligible to take part in a study. The cases could be people, objects, places or events, and they will all have at least one variable or characteristic in common in order to make them suitable for the study. For example, the population could be all children's nurses working in the United Kingdom, all community midwives working in Scotland or all critical care nurses working in Europe. Note that in the context of a research study, the term 'population' should not be confused with the general population of an area or country because they are not usually the same thing.

A study's total population may consist of thousands of cases (such as all qualified nurses working in the State of Victoria in Australia) or a small number (e.g. parents of a child with a rare genetic disorder living in Wales). The characteristics of the study's total population should be clearly defined. In some studies it may also be possible to identify the size of the population. However, in other studies the size may be unknown, for example, the number of people living in Europe with a particular respiratory problem.

SAMPLE

The sample is part of, a selection from, a sub-group or a sub-set of the total population. The sample is the participants or cases who actually take part in the study.

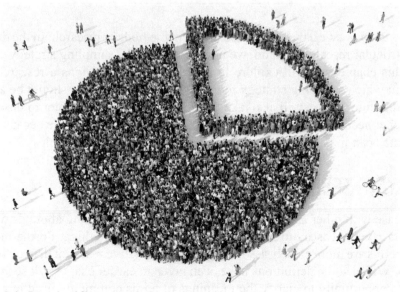

© Arthimedes / Shutterstock

REPRESENTATIVENESS

This term is commonly associated with quantitative research. The intention is to ensure that the participants who take part in the study have the same characteristics as those in the study's total population. In other words, the sample is as close as possible to or is representative of, the population. This representativeness enables the researcher to generalise the study findings to the population (see below) (Grubs and Piantanida, 2010). In qualitative research, rather than representativeness the phrase that is often used is that the characteristics of the participants in the sample 'reflect' those of the study population. In qualitative research representativeness is not required because the findings can only relate to the participants in the study (see below).

GENERALISABILITY

This is another term closely associated with quantitative research. This is when the study findings are generalised or applied to the study's total population. In order to generalise the findings, the sample must be representative of the population (Casey and Devane, 2010) (see Box 15.1).

BOX 15.1   EXAMPLE OF STUDIES WHERE THE FINDINGS CAN AND CANNOT BE GENERALISED

The findings from a survey of oncology nurses in the United Kingdom which involved graduate level, female nurses, working in an oncology care setting who are 30 years of age or younger should not be generalised to all oncology nurses working in the United Kingdom. However, the findings could be generalised to graduate level, female nurses aged 30 years or younger who are working in an oncology care setting in the United Kingdom.

Representativeness and generalisability therefore go hand-in-hand. Generalisation requires representativeness. However, we can sometimes fall into the trap of making faulty inferences about the findings of a research study. Before generalisation of a study's findings can be made, it is important that we ensure that the sample was representative of the population to which we are applying the findings.

TRANSFERABILITY

This is a term closely associated with qualitative research. Whilst it is not possible to generalise the findings of a qualitative study, it may be possible to make inferences if participants in the sample 'reflect' those of the wider population (see Chapter 21).

DATA SATURATION

This is a term used in association with qualitative research and grounded theory in particular. It is when no new data or information is discovered both in terms of the depth and breadth of the data (Casey and Devane, 2010). Whilst the point at which saturation is reached can usually only be pinpointed in retrospect, it is often used to determine the size and configuration of a sample.

HOMOGENEOUS SAMPLE

This is a sample which includes a single or narrow range of characteristics.

HETEROGENEOUS SAMPLE

This is a sample which includes a wide range of characteristics.

SAMPLING STRATEGIES

Before deciding which sampling strategy to use the researcher first needs to decide if it is feasible to involve the total population, or if a sample of the population is required. In most studies it would be unusual to include the whole population unless it was a very small or precise group such as nurses working on a specific ward or mothers attending a particular antenatal clinic. Another example of the total population being involved in a study is the national census in the United Kingdom. However, in most studies it is not practical to involve the population primarily due to resource restrictions such as insufficient time or money. It may also be unethical to involve the whole population in a study if the findings can be confirmed by involving just a sample of the population. In most studies, therefore, the researcher must decide which sampling strategy they will use.

There are two broad sampling strategies, which are allied to the two main types of research: probability sampling (quantitative) and non-probability sampling (qualitative). We will explore these two broad sampling strategies and the most common strategies that they both encompass. We will also explore systematic sampling, a strategy that uses both probability and non-probability approaches. In reviewing these different strategies, for consistency we will refer to the person undertaking the recruitment and sampling of participants as the 'researcher'; however, note that in some studies someone may be undertaking these activities on the researcher's behalf (we will discuss the pros and cons of this later in the chapter).

PROBABILITY SAMPLING

This is the selection of a proportion of the population using random procedures. It is important that random sampling is not confused with the random assignment of treatments and interventions in experiments. Random sampling means that everyone in the study's total population has an equal chance of being included. In this way, the sample is representative of the population, which means that the findings can be generalised to the total population. Probability sampling is generally used in quantitative research (Kandola et al., 2014). There are three commonly used probability sampling strategies: **simple random**, **stratified random** and **cluster sampling** (see Figure 15.1).

SIMPLE RANDOM SAMPLING

This is the most basic type of probability sampling (Kandola et al., 2014). Each potential participant has an equal chance of being included in the sample (Figure 15.1). Selection of the sample from the total population is now usually done using a computer program or a random table. However, in the past this could have been done by drawing names or participant numbers from a hat. Whichever way it is done, it is essential that the sample is selected randomly. However, it is important to note that this sampling strategy may not obtain representation of the full range of characteristics within the population as is the case in the example given in Figure 15.1.

Website activity 15.1

STRATIFIED RANDOM SAMPLING

This strategy overcomes the shortfalls of simple random sampling. Using stratified random sampling the population is divided into strata or sub-groups from which the sample is selected randomly (Figure 15.1) (Polit and Beck, 2014). Examples of strata could include age, gender, ethnic group or geographical location. Using this strategy means that the configuration of the sample can be more representative of the total population than a sample that has been created using simple random sampling (Kandola et al., 2014).

Website activity 15.2

CLUSTER SAMPLING

This is when the study population is divided into sub-groups or clusters such as academic institutions training nurses or maternity hospitals. The clusters are then selected randomly (Figure 15.1) (Casey and Devane, 2010). Either the whole cluster participates in the study or participants may be randomly selected from the cluster. This sampling strategy is particularly useful for large-scale geographically spread and international studies. However, researchers must be cautious about the generalisation of the findings as they may only be applicable to that particular cluster.

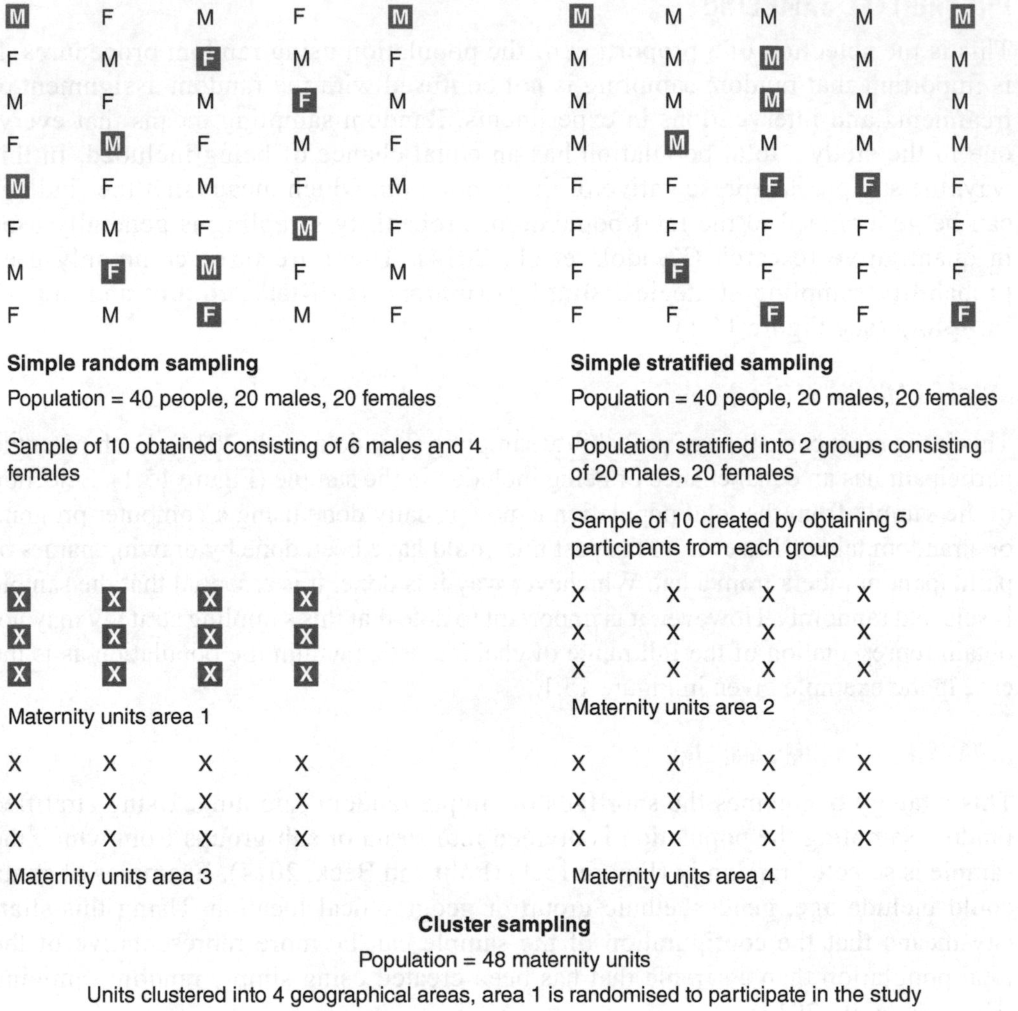

M	F	M	F	M
F	M	F	M	F
M	F	M	F	M
F	M	F	M	F
M	F	M	F	M
F	M	F	M	F
M	F	M	F	M
F	M	F	M	F

M	M	M	M	M
M	M	M	M	M
M	M	M	M	M
M	M	M	M	M
F	F	F	F	F
F	F	F	F	F
F	F	F	F	F
F	F	F	F	F

Simple random sampling

Population = 40 people, 20 males, 20 females

Sample of 10 obtained consisting of 6 males and 4 females

Simple stratified sampling

Population = 40 people, 20 males, 20 females

Population stratified into 2 groups consisting of 20 males, 20 females

Sample of 10 created by obtaining 5 participants from each group

X	X	X	X
X	X	X	X
X	X	X	X

Maternity units area 1

X	X	X	X
X	X	X	X
X	X	X	X

Maternity units area 2

X	X	X	X
X	X	X	X
X	X	X	X

Maternity units area 3

X	X	X	X
X	X	X	X
X	X	X	X

Maternity units area 4

Cluster sampling

Population = 48 maternity units

Units clustered into 4 geographical areas, area 1 is randomised to participate in the study

Figure 15.1   Three types of probability sampling

THINK POINT ACTIVITY   15.1

How does probability sampling, whichever specific strategy is adopted, help the researcher to achieve the fundamental principles of quantitative research? You may wish to refer to the research examples given in Chapters 4 and 7.

NON-PROBABILITY SAMPLING

This is the selection of participants from a population using non-random procedures (Kandola et al., 2014). This strategy is used in qualitative research where there is no intention to generalise the findings to the study population. In most qualitative studies the researcher does not know at the outset exactly how many participants will be recruited. Sample size is usually determined by data saturation. This can be problematic for research-ers endeavouring to acquire ethics committee approval for their research because this is likely to be the sort of information that the committee will ask for (see Chapter 18). There is also the view amongst some, traditionally the proponents of quantitative research, that non-probability sampling is inferior to probability sampling because it is perceived to be biased and the findings of such a study therefore unscientific (Grubs and Piantanida, 2010). However, if undertaken in a transparent way, a non-probability sample can be as robust as a probability sample. Whilst for all studies using non-probability sampling strategies the findings only apply to that particular sample, it may be possible to make inferences to the wider population by determining the **transferability** of the findings (see Chapter 21). There are five commonly used non-probability sampling strategies: **convenience**, **purposive**, **quota**, **snowball** and **theoretical sampling**.

CONVENIENCE SAMPLING

This is sometimes referred to as **accidental** or **opportunistic sampling**. Using convenience sampling the researcher recruits the most readily available participants who meet the study's inclusion criteria (Casey and Devane, 2010). A classic example of convenience sampling is when academics recruit their students to take part in their research. Convenience sampling is probably the most commonly used non-probability sampling strategy but it is also the weakest (Robson, 2011) and it is probably what gives non-probability sampling and, as a consequence, qualitative research a bad name. This is because there is a risk that the sample will not reflect the characteristics of the population. Whilst primarily associated with quali-tative research, convenience sampling may be used in more quantitative approaches such as pilot studies and surveys (Bryman, 2012).

PURPOSIVE OR PURPOSEFUL SAMPLING

This may also be referred to as **judgement sampling**. This sampling strategy is com-monly used in the early phases of a grounded theory study or a phenomenological study. Using this strategy, participants are recruited who meet the study's inclusion criteria, who the researcher judges have knowledge or experience of the topic under investigation and will be therefore be the most informative for their study (Kandola et al., 2014; Polit and Beck, 2014). During the course of the research, the researcher should constantly monitor the configuration of the sample and should attempt to recruit individuals to address any shortfall in the sample. However, it can be a challenge for researchers to recruit participants with an appropriate range of experience of the problem or topic under investigation. For example, in a study of fathers' experiences of being present during the resuscitation of their baby it was important that the sample included fathers who had been present during different types of delivery and newborn resuscitation (Harvey and Pattison, 2012).

QUOTA SAMPLING

Using this sampling strategy the researcher pre-specifies the required characteristics of the sample to ensure the final sample includes a certain number with each characteristic (Casey and Devane, 2010). This strategy is used when probability sampling is not possible. For example, in a survey of critical care nurses' experiences, a researcher may endeavour to recruit a predetermined number of nurses working in paediatric intensive care, adult intensive care and emergency care units.

SNOWBALL SAMPLING

This is sometimes called **chain**, **network** or **nominated sampling**. This involves the identification of potential participants through referrals from earlier participants (Sadler et al., 2010). This strategy is a useful way of accessing otherwise difficult-to-reach participants and may be used in studies of particularly challenging topics. Whilst there may be legitimate concerns about the potential for bias within the sample (Polit and Beck, 2014), there may simply be no other way for a researcher to access potential participants.

Website
activity 15.3

THEORETICAL SAMPLING

In contrast to other research methods, researchers using grounded theory sample concepts and ideas rather than participants (Corbin and Strauss, 2015). Theoretical sampling is the method used in order to do this and it enables the researcher to collect data from a range of sources (e.g. people, photographs or documentation) in order to gather ideas and concepts, which in turn will refine or challenge the theory that they are developing (Grubs and Piantanida, 2010). Concurrent sampling, data collection and data analysis facilitate theoretical sampling. The evolving theory therefore determines the researcher's sampling of subsequent data sources (Bryman, 2012) and theoretical sampling continues until the theory has been finalised. The researcher does not therefore know the nature and extent of the sample at the beginning of the study (Grubs and Piantanida, 2010). Corbin and Strauss (2015) describe theoretical sampling as being concept driven, open, flexible and responsive. However, theoretical sampling can present some challenges. Not knowing exactly who, what or how many will be sampled where and when, at the outset of a study can be problematic for researchers endeavouring to acquire ethics committee approval for their research (see Chapter 18). In addition, novice grounded theorists can sometimes lose focus as they chase new ideas and concepts that do not inform their developing theory.

Website
activity 15.4

THINK POINT ACTIVITY   15.2

How does non-probability sampling, whichever specific strategy is adopted, help the researcher to achieve the fundamental principles of qualitative research?

Think about the different non-probability sampling strategies and how they may be used in the different qualitative research methods. You may wish to refer to the research examples given in Chapters 5 and 8.

SYSTEMATIC SAMPLING

This strategy combines elements of both probability and non-probability sampling and is sometime referred to as **list sampling** because the strategy starts with the generation of a list of all participants in the population (see Box 15.2). The selection of the first participant is undertaken randomly (non-probability sampling). From then on, every nth participant is selected for the study (Polit and Beck, 2014). Therefore a participant's inclusion is determined by their position on the list (non-probability sampling).

BOX 15.2   EXAMPLE ILLUSTRATING SYSTEMATIC SAMPLING

A list consisting of 100 potential participants is generated and 20 participants are required for the study. Firstly 100 is divided by 20, which equals 5. To find the first participant, a number less than 5 is randomly selected and in our example, number 3 on the list is chosen. Every 5th participant from the list from number 3 onwards is then recruited to the sample (Figure 15.2). Note that the way in which the list is compiled, and perhaps by whom, may have an impact on the configuration of the final sample. In the example we have given here, only the first four people had a truly random chance of being involved, from that point on inclusion is determined by the participants' position on the list. Hence elements of both probability and non-probability sampling are evident.

CHOOSING A SAMPLING STRATEGY

The choice of specific sampling strategy may in some studies be evident, for example, purposive sampling in phenomenology. However, in other studies it can be less obvious and the researcher may have choices to make. The researcher will first need to decide if a

Website activity 15.5

X	X	**X**	X	X	X	X	**X**	X	X
X	X	**X**	X	X	X	X	**X**	X	X
X	X	**X**	X	X	X	X	**X**	X	X
X	X	**X**	X	X	X	X	**X**	X	X
X	X	**X**	X	X	X	X	**X**	X	X
X	X	**X**	X	X	X	X	**X**	X	X
X	X	**X**	X	X	X	X	**X**	X	X
X	X	**X**	X	X	X	X	**X**	X	X
X	X	**X**	X	X	X	X	**X**	X	X
X	X	**X**	X	X	X	X	**X**	X	X

100 potential participants and 20 are required for the study. 100 is divided by 20, which equals 5.
A number less than 5 is randomly selected and in our example, number 3 on the list is chosen. Every
5th participant from the list from number 3 onwards is then recruited to the sample

Figure 15.2 Systematic or list sampling

probability or non-probability sampling strategy is required. Having made that decision, the researcher can then decide which specific strategy to use. In making this decision, there may not be an obvious choice and the researcher must decide which strategy will enable them to answer the research question most effectively using the resources that they have available to them. The choice of sampling method should be determined by a number of factors:

Is there an intention to generalise the findings? The answer to this question should be found in the study's aim(s), objective(s), hypothesis and/or research question. If the answer is yes, then a probability sampling strategy is required. If the answer is no, then a non-probability sampling strategy can be used.

Does the research method/design dictate which strategy is used? Some sampling strategies are allied to particular methods, for example, probability sampling used in RCTs or purposive followed by theoretical sampling in grounded theory.

Are there resource restrictions? Whilst we might like to include all of the total population in our study, time and money restrictions will usually prevent this. In any case it may not be ethical to include the whole population in a study. The researcher must therefore decide which sampling strategy will enable them to answer the research question most effectively.

Website activity 15.6

Whichever sampling strategy the researcher decides to use, it should be well defined in the research report and a clear rationale given.

CONFIGURATION OF THE SAMPLE

Another important question that the researcher must consider before the research begins is who should take part in the study, or perhaps more importantly, who should not (see Box 15.3). Being clear about this will save time, money and effort in the long run and will increase the likelihood that the research aims and objectives are addressed. Clarity will also save the unnecessary disruption that might be caused to people who turn out to be ineligible for the study. The required characteristics for participants may include factors such as age, gender, ethnic group, occupation or medical condition. There may also be other more general requirements such as the ability to give informed consent or take part in interviews in English if the researcher does not have access to an interpreter. The researcher may also devise exclusion criteria so that people who have encountered difficult or challenging situations are not further distressed by being approached about the study. For example, a study of parents' experiences of neonatal intensive care may exclude parents whose baby has died.

Deciding who should or should not take part in the study should be determined by the study's aim(s), objective(s), hypothesis and/or research question.

The required characteristics of participants are usually summarised as inclusion and exclusion criteria, which are generally presented in table format with an accompanying rationale. Sometimes the configuration of the sample is determined by the research method and the setting used. For example, in action research or ethnography the sample will be determined by the people involved in that particular setting.

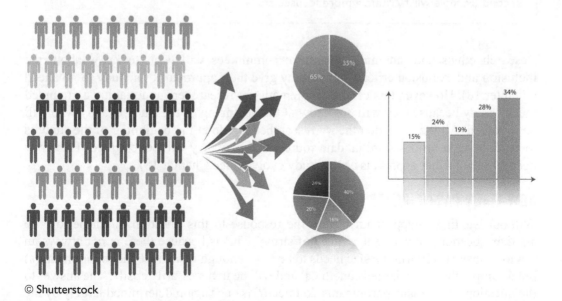

© Shutterstock

BOX 15.3   EXAMPLE ILLUSTRATING THE WAYS IN WHICH A RESEARCH QUESTION INFORMS A STUDY'S INCLUSION AND EXCLUSION CRITERIA

Jason plans to carry out a phenomenological study using interviews. His research question is 'what are the experiences of nurses working in a hospice'. A broad research question such as this would mean that any nurse, of any age, gender or level of experience could potentially take part in the study. 'Nurses' may also be widely interpreted, because Jason might plan to include health care assistants in this group.

A more specific research question such as 'what are the experiences of female, recently qualified nurses of working in a hospice' will necessitate the following inclusion/exclusion criteria:

Inclusion	Exclusion
Female nurses	Male nurses
Registered nurses	Non-registered nurses
Less than two years since qualified	Qualified two years or more

The first example may provide Jason with the findings he is interested in. However, the second example will facilitate a more focused study.

Research ethics and indemnity insurance committees will want to know about the inclusion and exclusion criteria before they give their approval for a study to go ahead (Chapter 18). However, this can be problematic for researchers undertaking a grounded theory study because they will not know at the beginning of the study exactly who will be involved. All the grounded theory researcher can do at the beginning of the study is to describe their proposed initial data sources and how they will be recruited. They may need to seek further approvals as the study evolves (see Chapter 18).

HOW MANY PARTICIPANTS DO I NEED?

Without wanting to appear unhelpful, the response to this question might be to pose another question, how long is a piece of string? This is because there is not always an obvious answer. The sample size needs to be large enough to achieve the research aim(s) but a sample that is too large is unethical and will be unnecessarily costly. The answer to the question, 'how many participants do I need?' is once again determined largely by the study's aim(s), objective(s), hypothesis, research question and/or the research method used. There is also a clear difference between quantitative and qualitative research when the sample size is determined. In quantitative research the sample size is always established prospectively, in other words, before the study starts, whilst in qualitative research, the sample size is usually determined as the study evolves.

In quantitative research it can generally be assumed that the larger the sample, the more accurate the findings and therefore the more generalisable the findings (Casey and Devane, 2010). The required sample size for most quantitative studies and certainly all experimental research should be determined by a power calculation. This is usually undertaken by a statistician on behalf of the research team. The calculation is undertaken to ensure that the sample size is sufficient to demonstrate statistical differences between the experimental and control groups and to reduce the chances of type I and type II errors (see Chapter 19) (Bench et al., 2013). The calculation is based on outcome measures, measurement tools used, expected differences between the experimental and control groups, expected rates of non-compliance and withdrawals from the study, and the likelihood of achieving complete data-sets. In large-scale studies where there is more than one outcome variable, the sample size is usually calculated using the primary or main outcome (Peat, 2002). Most studies aim for 80% or 90% power. In other words, there is an 80% or 90% likelihood of detecting a true difference between the experimental and control groups (Bench et al., 2013). However, the greater the power the larger the sample size is required.

For qualitative research, sample size is usually determined by data saturation (Casey and Devane, 2010). This means at the start of the study the qualitative researcher can usually only indicate the likely number of participants based on the traditions and conventions of that particular method. However, determining the point at which data saturation is reached is not always straightforward. Sometimes other factors such as running out of research time and money can be influential (Corbin and Strauss, 2015). In some types of qualitative study the sample size is decided by the research method and the setting used. For example, in action research or ethnography the sample size will be determined by the number of people involved in that particular setting who consent to take part.

HOW DO I RECRUIT PARTICIPANTS FOR MY STUDY?

Having decided which sampling strategy to use, the inclusion and exclusion criteria and required sample size, the researcher must now decide how participants will be recruited. We will explore some key factors for the researcher to consider here. Some of these overlap with issues we will discuss in more detail in Chapter 18. However, we are including this here because failure to consider these issues may have a negative impact on the successful recruitment of participants. In some cases, there are no right or wrong answers to the questions we pose below. The researcher must weigh up the pros and cons and provide a rationale for the strategy they adopt so that they are able to obtain the necessary approvals for the study and recruit the required number of participants in the shortest time possible.

QUESTIONS FOR THE RESEARCHER TO CONSIDER

1 *Who will recruit the participants?*

This could be the lead researcher, a member of the research team or someone external to the research undertaking recruitment on behalf of the researcher or research team.

THINK POINT ACTIVITY   15.3

Using the example of Jason's phenomenological study of the experiences of nurses working in a hospice, what are the pros and cons of:

- Jason recruiting the participants?
- A member of Jason's research team recruiting the participants?
- Someone external to the research such as the team leader at the hospice recruiting the participants?

---

2 *How will the person recruiting the participants know who to approach?*

Sometimes the person recruiting participants needs help to identify potential participants who meet the inclusion criteria. For example, this might be a person working in that care setting or someone who has a list of the names of qualified nurses or midwives working in a particular trust (see point 3).

3 *Do I need permission to access potential participants?*

The answer to this question is almost certainly yes. This is something that the researcher should establish early on and if necessary obtain written confirmation of permission. The person giving permission may, for example, be the senior midwife at a trust, the dean of an academic institution or the team leader of a group of health visitors.

THINK POINT ACTIVITY   15.4

Using the example of Jason's study, whose permission will he need in order to access nurses for his study? What factors may influence their decision?

4   *What other permissions or approvals do I need?*

Ethics committee and indemnity insurance committee approvals should always be in place before recruitment of participants begins (see Chapter 18).

5   *What is the best way to make contact with potential participants?*

A number of options are available. These may include face-to-face discussion, letter, telephone call, email, word-of-mouth (snowball sampling), posters displayed in venues where potential participants will see them or notices on websites or in journals. Note that if letters, telephone calls or emails are used, the researcher will need permission in order to access the contact details of potential participants.

Website activity 15.7

6   *Where should potential participants be recruited?*

This will depend on where the participants are situated. If they are located in clinical settings (whether patients/clients, staff or relatives) the person doing the recruitment may need an honorary contract (Chapter 18).

7   *What information do potential participants require?*

Potential participants need sufficient information about the study and any possible risks involved to enable them to make an informed decision about their participation. It is unethical to withhold information about a study and this is something that ethics committees are particularly vigilant about. Information about the study is generally presented in a participant information leaflet (PIL) of which there is usually a required format (Chapter 18). Note that for some participants this information may need to be in a language other than English or in another format (such as an audio tape).

8   *How much time should potential participants be given to decide?*

The key issue is that participants have sufficient time to decide. Some participants will say straight away that they want to take part in a study. The person undertaking the recruitment will need to be happy that the potential participant has had sufficient time to think about it. However, it must be noted that in some studies such as those in critical care situations there may only be a few hours or even minutes for decisions to made about participation (Chapter 18).

Website activity 15.8

SUMMARY

In this chapter we have considered the decisions a researcher has to make about sampling strategy, sample configuration and sample size. We have also introduced some issues that the researcher needs to make decisions about when recruiting a sample. These will be further explored in Chapter 18.

FURTHER READING

Casey, D. and Devane, D. (2010) Sampling, *The Practising Midwife*, 13(1): 40–43.

This provides more detailed discussion and application to practice.

Kandola, D. Banner, D. O'Keefe-McCarthy, S. and Jassal, D. (2014) Sampling methods in cardiovascular nursing research: an overview, *Canadian Journal of Cardiovascular Nursing*, 24(3): 15–18.

A useful example of the impact and importance of sampling.

Polit, D.F. and Beck, C.T. (2014) *Essentials of Nursing Research* (8th edn). Philadelphia: Wolters Kluwer Health, Lippincott Williams & Wilkins.

See in particular, Chapter 10 'Sampling and data collection in quantitative studies' and Chapter 15 'Sampling and data collection in qualitative studies'.

Don't forget to visit https://study.sagepub.com/harveyandland to watch videos, take quizzes and to follow specially designed web activities.

16
QUANTITATIVE METHODS OF DATA COLLECTION

This is the first of two chapters in which we explore methods of data collection in depth. In this chapter we will explore quantitative methods and questionnaires specifically, and we will:

- review the factors the researcher should consider when deciding to use questionnaires
- explore issues the researcher should think about when designing a questionnaire
- explore strategies the researcher can use to facilitate the collection of robust, relevant and usable data when using questionnaires.

Whilst a number of methods of data collection are available to the researcher, the ways in which these methods may be employed will vary in accordance with the type of research (quantitative or qualitative). In this chapter we will explore the practical, logistical and research governance issues that the researcher should think about when deciding to use questionnaires and when designing the data collection tool.

QUESTIONNAIRES

It is easy to think that questionnaires are not much trouble and it is only asking a few minutes of peoples' time, but health care workers lead busy lives, patients and clients have their own problems and carers are busy caring. So, questionnaires that do not appear to be important to these people can be thrown away without a second thought. This wastes everyone's time.

It is essential to make sure that if people do take the time to fill in questionnaires we take care over their construction. If the question is important enough to require an answer, then it must be important enough to get the right answer. Good information improves our ability to make better decisions and this is the basic premise for using questionnaires as a method of data collection.

THINK POINT ACTIVITY   16.1

What influences your decision whether to fill in a questionnaire? (Think about consumer surveys, magazines or on-the-spot surveys in the street.)

CREATING TRUSTABLE DATA

Website activity 16.1

Most problems with research using questionnaires can be traced back to the design phase of the project (or more likely the *lack* of design phase). These design faults usually surface when it is far too late to correct them, that is, when we come to analyse the data. The best way of avoiding this is to state a clear overall research aim and identify the objectives that will achieve that aim. The most useful objectives contain statements that can be measured, that is, ones that actually have a real-life outcome. This means deciding how you intend to use the information you are gathering, it sounds obvious but it is a trap researchers often fall into. After all why do research, if you are not going to use the results?

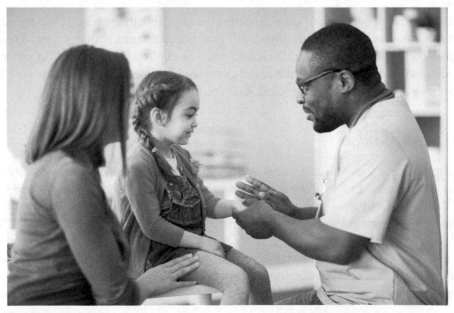

© shironosov / iStock

QUESTIONS TO ASK YOURSELF ABOUT QUESTIONNAIRES

For any proposed study you should ask yourself whether you could construct a rational, logical argument as to why you should use questionnaires as opposed to any other form of data collection. For instance, think in terms of feasibility, cost, time and the people who might participate in your study.

If the advantages of using a questionnaire for a proposed study outweigh its disadvantages then it is likely to be the right choice for data collection. Before settling finally on questionnaires as a method of data collection thought needs to be given to the whole research process. The research question or hypothesis and the research design must be clear, only then will it be obvious whether the questions in a questionnaire are suitable and likely to yield the information needed.

Questionnaires should *not* be used where you want to find out how often people do things (wash their hands, drink alcohol, smack their children) – they lie! Neither should they be used for self-reports involving status or ability, quite often people either overestimate or underestimate these. If you need to gather performance data, think of another method such as observation. If at the end of all this it is clear that questionnaires are the method of choice, then finding one is the next step.

USING EXISTING QUESTIONNAIRES

It is advisable wherever possible to use ready-formulated questionnaires. There are a huge amount of these on an even larger subject range, reinventing the wheel sacrifices reliability and validity. These terms are the key words in making sure information is accurate and stands the tests of time and situation (see Chapter 21).

Validity in a questionnaire involves collecting the data that actually answer the question. For example, if you ask how old someone is you expect him or her to respond by giving their age in years. This concept is easier to understand if using a measure such age, weight or other physical measurement, it is not so easy if you are looking at more sophisticated concepts like mood, character traits and personality. The more complex the concept, the more likely it is that a range of questions are required to demonstrate evidence of that concept in order to establish validity.

Reliability in a questionnaire provides an indication that the questionnaire will give the same results when filled out by like-minded people in similar circumstances. You would expect answers to be consistent. If using bathroom scales, for example, you would expect to remain roughly the same weight over a number of weeks given that you were taking in a similar amount of calories and expending a similar amount of energy each day. As with validity, the more complex the measurement the wider the variety of questions that are needed to make sure that the concept is properly examined.

Researchers go to a lot of trouble to make sure their questionnaires are valid and reliable so if you were choosing a topic where appropriate questionnaires exist, you would have to make a very good case for not using them.

QUESTIONNAIRE DESIGN

Website
activity 16.2

However, not all topics have ready-made instruments so sometimes it is necessary to construct your own. The first rule of design is to keep your questionnaire as short as possible; long questionnaires are more likely to end up in the rubbish bin. The response rate is important and you should do everything you can to maximise it.

MUST, SHOULD AND COULD

The most obvious questions to ask are those that will fulfill the aims and objectives of your research, these are *must* questions. For example, if your research aims to determine job satisfaction amongst work colleagues, you need to ask a specific question or set of questions to answer it. The more complex the concept, the greater the range of questions needed to validate the responses.

Should questions are usually those that support the research topic and often include demographic data or socio-economic status. These questions are ones that might provide a context for your research; using the above example you might want to know your colleagues' length of service because the number of years worked might have a bearing on how happy they are.

Then there are the *could* questions – avoid them! These are the questions you want to ask just because you think the answers might be interesting. They rarely have anything to do with your research and you cannot think of a good reason for including them. If you put them in regardless, remember, you have to find ways to analyse the responses and then have to think how to fit them into your results and conclusions. It is far easier to discard them.

WHAT TYPE OF QUESTIONS?

There are basically two types of questions, closed and open.

CLOSED QUESTIONS

Closed questions are those that usually require a short affirmative or negative answer and there are several types of these (see Table 16.1). Closed questions are quick to answer and easier to code for analysis. People do not need to be very articulate to answer these types of questions. They do have disadvantages, however; the questions are researcher defined and therefore the participants can be easily led. The questions can often contain researcher bias and the responses cannot be qualified by the participant, for example, 'Yes, but it depends'.

OPEN QUESTIONS

Open questions ask the participant to write a longer answer, or in some instances to reply to an interviewer using a schedule of questions. There is an obvious blurring of

Table 16.1   Types of closed questions

Type of closed question	Example
Dichotomous	Yes/No
Multiple choice	a) Less than once a month b) Once a month c) Twice a month d) More than twice a month
5/7 point Likert type scale	Very strongly agree Strongly agree Agree Neither agree nor disagree Disagree Strongly disagree Very strongly disagree
4/6 point Likert type scale Omits the neutral stance to force a choice	Very strongly agree Strongly agree Agree Disagree Strongly disagree Very strongly disagree
Semantic differential Bipolar words, participant selects point on the line which corresponds with intensity of feeling	Fat ——————————— Thin Old ——————————— Young Rich ——————————— Poor
Word association Words presented one at a time the participant gives the first word that comes to mind	Teacher 'excellent' Scenery 'beautiful' Kitchen 'sink'
Rank order List in order of preference	Blue Green Red
Numeric Absolute value	How many children do you have?

boundaries between where a questionnaire ends and an interview begins. There are several ways in which this can be done (see Table 16.2).

Open questions allow a greater freedom to respond but do depend upon the participant's ability to articulate their feelings and the time they have to fill them in. It is best not to use this type of question if the respondent cannot write reasonably well. They do,

Table 16.2   Types of open question

Type of open question	Example
Sentence completion	One of the highlights of my career was when …
Story completion	I looked at the patient lying there, pale and clammy, I took her hand …
Unstructured Allows unlimited response	Tell me about the time you …

however, allow the participant to respond exactly how they feel and qualify any answers they have given. This makes it very time consuming to code and the research can easily misinterpret the responses, but the responses should contain a wealth of information.

BASIC RULE OF DESIGN

Explain clearly what you want from participants and give as much detail as you can about why you want it. If you are using some kind of psychometric test, you will not want to give away the exact nature of the test, but response rates will be affected if people are suspicious of your reasons for asking for the information.

BOX 16.1   EXAMPLES OF THE WORDING OF QUESTIONS IN QUESTIONNAIRES

- Use short affirmative sentences, for example:

  Always follow the safety instructions

  not

  Do not ignore the safety instructions

- Use an active voice rather than passive voice, for example:

  Read the instructions carefully

  not

  The instructions should be read carefully

It is important to make sure that both the instructions and the questions in your questionnaire are pitched at a fairly easy level to accommodate all levels of readers. Use simple familiar words; if people cannot understand what you are asking for, they will not respond so you need to cater for the lowest reading ability. Avoiding the vernacular is also important, for example, if you want to give a questionnaire out to adolescents about their attitudes on sexual activity it might be tempting to use their slang, but in fact it will seem embarrassing and patronising.

QUESTION WORDING

Avoid ambiguity, ask one question at a time. For example, asking 'Have you a wife and children?' does not allow for people to say yes I have a wife but no children, or vice versa.

Use a natural sequence. Most questionnaires you see will start with simple demographic details such as age, marital status, length in post. The most difficult or sensitive questions are placed in the middle and the questionnaire will end with simple, non-intrusive questions as a way of 'debriefing' the respondent.

DO NOT USE CAPITALS because this is the written form of shouting.

Leave enough space for the answers. There is nothing more irritating than having to squeeze your thoughts into the margins or on the back if you are suddenly filled with the desire to disclose. Leave plenty of space on the questionnaires for people to add other thoughts, you may not use them in your analysis but it may allow someone to provide further information or explanation.

Avoid leading or presuming questions. For example, you would not say 'What is the worst thing about your job?' or 'When did you stop keeping up to date with current research?' (see Box 16.1).

PRINT LAYOUT

Decisions have to be made about how to set out the questionnaire. Avoid commercial logos on the front of the questionnaire where possible, for example, if the questionnaire is about breastfeeding then apparent sponsorship by a powdered milk company could have an effect on the respondent's views of who is conducting the research. Leave plenty of room for participants to write comments; even if that is not the point, they are more likely to feel motivated to contribute.

INSTRUCTIONS

If you are using a self-completion questionnaire, make sure the instructions for completing it are clear. The type of instruction varies with the format and context used for the questionnaire. For example, if you are posing questions to a participant face to face as opposed to a postal or email questionnaire, the instructions should be tailored to suit the format.

General instructions are needed to help the participant understand what to do with the questionnaire. That is, the practicalities of completing and returning. Specific question instructions are needed to tell the participant how to fill in the questionnaire, for example, 'tick one box only', or 'describe below ...'.

Routing instructions are used where the questions do not always apply to participants, for example, if the questions in section 5 do not apply, skip to section 6. This prevents 'completion fatigue', a situation where respondents fail to complete the questionnaire because it is too arduous.

RETURNING THE QUESTIONNAIRE TO THE RESEARCHER

Returning a completed questionnaire to the researcher should be made as easy as possible to maximise return rates (Edwards et al., 2002). The questionnaire should also have the name and contact details of the researcher so that queries and complaints can be made directly. Questionnaires can take many forms and the form chosen may impact on the number of returned completions. The media format of the questionnaire will affect the type of language and authoring style that will be used, as well as the question order and grammatical construction. A live, person-to-person or telephone delivery of a questionnaire will be conducted very differently from an online or mail version and different again if questionnaires are distributed in a real environment such as the workplace, hospital, theme park or community.

Website activity 16.3

SUMMARY

In this chapter we have explored the use of questionnaires in health care research. We have considered the practical, logistical and research governance issues that the researcher should think about when deciding to use questionnaires and when designing a data collection tool. To summarise:

- Only use questionnaires when you are sure that it is the best method for gathering data from your proposed sample.
- Effort upfront saves a lot of work later.
- There are many types of questions, choose those that will yield the best data for your study.
- Make sure the design and layout is user friendly and appealing to fill in.
- Test your questionnaire before using it.
- Make sure you know how your data will need to be analysed.

When using questionnaires, it is essential that data collection is undertaken in a rigorous and consistent way. This issue will be explored in greater depth in Chapter 21. In the following chapter we will explore qualitative methods of data collection. This will include interviews, observation, focus groups and diaries, and other less commonly used methods. We will also consider in the following chapter factors the researcher should consider when deciding which method of data collection (quantitative or qualitative) they should use.

FURTHER READING

Fowler, F.J. (2013) *Survey Research Methods* (5th edn). Thousand Oaks, CA: Sage Publications.

A good resource for anyone trying to do applied survey research. It includes material on typical errors, shaping questions and ethics.

Gobo, G. and Mauceri, S. (2014) *Constructing Survey Data*. London: Sage Publications.

A thorough introduction to the challenges of constructing survey questions and using survey data.

Don't forget to visit https://study.sagepub.com/harveyandland to watch videos, take quizzes and to follow specially designed web activities.

17

QUALITATIVE METHODS OF DATA COLLECTION

This is the second of two chapters in which we explore methods of data collection in depth. In this chapter we will explore data collection methods that take a more qualitative approach. In doing this we will focus on interviews, observation, focus groups and diaries. We will also consider less commonly used methods of data collection such as vignettes, Q-sort and art-based methods. In this chapter we will:

- review the factors the researcher should consider when using qualitative methods of data collection
- explore issues the researcher should think about when designing qualitative data collection tools
- explore strategies the researcher can use to facilitate the collection of robust, relevant and usable data when using qualitative methods of data collection
- identify factors the researcher should consider when deciding which method of data collection they should use.

Whilst a number of methods of data collection are available to the researcher, interviews, observation, focus groups and diaries are commonly used. Whilst the ways in which these methods may be employed can vary in accordance with the research method, the tools themselves usually take a qualitative approach. In this chapter we will explore the practical, logistical and research governance issues that the researcher should think about when deciding to use a qualitative data collection method and when designing a data collection tool. We will also consider less common but increasingly used methods of data collection such as vignettes, Q-sort and art-based methods.

INTERVIEWS

Although often associated with qualitative research, interviews may also be used in quantitative studies. However, the type of research (quantitative or qualitative) will influence the format of the questions and the way in which the interview is conducted.

INTERVIEWS IN QUANTITATIVE STUDIES

In quantitative research a pre-planned list of questions will be devised which will mainly consist of closed questions, where for example a 'yes' or 'no' answer is required. This structured interview schedule will therefore look very much like a structured questionnaire as discussed in the previous chapter. The researcher asks the participant the questions in the order that they appear on the interview schedule and there will be little or no opportunity for the participant to provide any additional information or explanation to support their responses. Consequently this type of interview can be quite brief and could be conducted by telephone, via the Internet or face to face.

INTERVIEWS IN QUALITATIVE STUDIES

Interviews are more commonly associated with qualitative research, particularly phenomenology and grounded theory. Although usually conducted face to face, qualitative interviews can also be undertaken via the telephone or Internet. In qualitative studies the researcher will use a semi-structured or unstructured interview schedule or, as it is more commonly known, a topic guide.

THINK POINT ACTIVITY   17.1

Have you ever taken part in an interview for a research study? What are your reflections on the participant's perspective that could inform any interviews you conduct for a research study in the future?

DEVELOPING AN INTERVIEW SCHEDULE OR TOPIC GUIDE

Whether the interview is taking a qualitative or quantitative approach, when it comes to developing the interview schedule or topic guide, the principles are the same. The starting point for the researcher should be consideration of what it is they want to know. This may seem obvious, but the researcher should avoid annoying participants by asking them seemingly irrelevant questions and having data that do not fulfil the aims and objectives of the research. Probably the easiest way to generate questions for an interview is to develop a mind-map of the topics or issues to be addressed. From this, the researcher can then devise the questions. Whatever the questions are about, they should be brief and simple, avoiding the use of jargon and complicated terminology.

The interview schedule used in quantitative studies should be designed in the same way as a structured questionnaire as discussed in the previous chapter.

By contrast, the topic guide used in qualitative studies should consist of key open questions which are worded in such a way as to trigger the discussion and enable the participants to respond as comprehensively as possible. The topic guide should also include possible probing, or follow-up questions, which the interviewer may use to further explore issues initially raised by the participant in order to yield clearer, deeper and richer descriptions (Johnson, 2000; Baker, 2006).

The opening question of the topic guide should be broad and will often include a phrase such as 'tell me about' or 'can you describe'. It is difficult for a researcher to determine in advance the exact format of the subsequent questions for a topic guide because of the flexible nature of the interview process (Kvale, 2007). Usually, therefore, the researcher develops a loose set of open questions and possible probes. However, this can be problematic for the researcher when trying to acquire ethics committee approval for their study (see Chapter 18). If the interview is likely to focus on difficult or delicate topics it is important not to end the interview with an emotionally sensitive question (Corbin and Morse, 2003; Rogers, 2008). To avoid this and to ensure all aspects of the

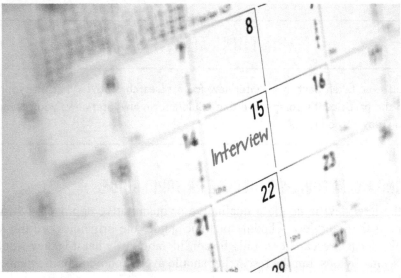

© Masuti / iStock

participants' experiences are covered, the last question on the topic guide usually asks the participant if there are any other issues that they wish to raise.

CONDUCTING AN INTERVIEW

In a quantitative interview the researcher asks the participant the questions in the order that they appear on the interview schedule. In a semi-structured or unstructured interview in a qualitative study the interview begins with the initial broad opening question. For the remainder of the interview, the researcher may not follow the order of the questions as they appear on the topic guide. This is because the second or subsequent questions should be influenced by the participant's response to the initial question. In this way, the interview becomes more akin to a conversation. In order to cover all of the topics on the topic guide, the researcher must be extremely vigilant throughout the interview to ensure that by the end, all of the questions on the topic guide have been addressed. The flexible nature of semi-structured and unstructured interviews means that the format of these types of interview undertaken in a study will not be exactly the same (see Box 17.1).

BOX 17.1 EXAMPLE ILLUSTRATING THE FLEXIBLE NATURE OF A SEMI-STRUCTURED INTERVIEW

Rachel is conducting an interview with Laura about her care following a road traffic accident. Rachel's opening question asks Laura about the accident. Laura gives a lengthy response which includes the description of a particular nurse who supported her throughout her time in the Emergency Department. Rachel had planned to ask Laura about members of the health care team later in the interview. However, in order to enable Laura to give a full and seamless account, Rachel's second question focuses on the nurse that Laura mentioned. Rachel asks the remaining questions on the topic guide later in the interview.

The flexibility of a semi-structured or unstructured interview enables the participant to retain a level of control over the discussion and therefore reduces the likelihood of power imbalance occurring between themselves and the interviewer (Rogers, 2008). However, probing questions should be used judiciously because although they can have benefits, they can also have limitations. Probing questions enable the researcher to explore issues in greater depth and can be used to draw the participant back to the phenomena under investigation. They also help the participant to understand the nature and depth of information the researcher is seeking. However, probes may limit the boundaries of what is discussed by narrowing the focus (Johnson, 2000). They may also disrupt the participant's narrative (Corbin and Morse, 2003) and if inappropriately applied, the participant can feel as though they are being interrogated (Manning, 2004).

FACTORS TO CONSIDER WHEN CONDUCTING INTERVIEWS

Usually interviews are conducted face to face. If this is the case, they should be carried out in a quiet, private, comfortable location where participants will feel safe and at ease (Brinkmann and Kvale, 2015). If the venue is a location where other colleagues are not immediately accessible to the researcher, such as the participant's home, then lone worker policies should be implemented (see Chapter 18). If appropriate, refreshments should be provided in order to make the participants feel comfortable, relaxed and valued. At the very least a drink should be available because talking can be thirsty work. It may also be sensible to ensure tissues are to hand if it is possible that the participant will become upset during the interview. The interviewer may also need to consider what he or she wears, as it may not be appropriate for clinical uniform to be worn.

Interviews are generally audio-recorded to facilitate transcription and data analysis, and unobtrusive, inexpensive digital recorders are readily available. In some cases, interviews may be videoed. Participants must consent to the recording whatever the format and their consent should be reaffirmed immediately prior to the interview.

The usual procedure before the interview begins is to reassure participants of their right not to answer specific questions and to tell them that they can temporarily pause or discontinue the interview at any time (Corbin and Morse, 2003). Participants should also be reassured that their comments will be anonymised and any names they use identifying people and places will be replaced with a code in the transcript. It is also usual to reassure participants before the interview begins that confidentiality will be maintained. However, this may be problematic if participants reveal issues of concern during the interview (Rogers, 2008). If the interviewer is a nurse or a midwife then he or she will be duty bound by the code of conduct (Nursing and Midwifery Council, 2015a) as well as the law. There may therefore be situations where the researcher has a moral, professional or legal obligation to disclose information to others (Manning, 2004). This issue will be explored in more depth in Chapter 18.

It is important that a level of trust is established between the researcher and the participant particularly when the interview is likely to encroach on difficult or sensitive subjects (Kvale, 2007). The researcher must therefore find a way of establishing a good rapport and being responsive to the participant's accounts (Creswell, 2014). Maintaining eye-contact, if the participant appears to be comfortable with this, is one way that the researcher can demonstrate interest in the participant's account. The researcher must also decide if they will take notes during the interview. This can be distracting to both parties and it may disrupt attempts to establish a rapport (Brinkmann and Kvale, 2015). However, it may be necessary if the participant has declined audio- or video-recording.

It is important to thank participants at the end of the interview and it may be relevant to provide information, usually in the form of a debriefing sheet, identifying potential sources of support (see Chapter 18) (Baker, 2006; Rogers, 2008). This is because the participant may become anxious and distressed when reflecting on their feelings and experiences. The actual process of being interviewed can also cause participant anxiety. However, individuals who think they will be unduly upset or are uncomfortable about being interviewed usually decline participation in the first place (Corbin and Morse, 2003). Sometimes participants reveal additional information once the interview has ended. However, any information provided by the participant outside the interview should not be used in the study without the participant's permission.

Participants are generally well protected during research. However, researchers are often not well supported. This may become an issue when they conduct interviews addressing sensitive or emotionally challenging topics (Rager, 2005; Lalor et al., 2006). If there is the potential for the interviewer to be adversely affected, then strategies should be put in place to support them. This will be discussed in more depth in Chapter 18.

The researcher should reflect on the interview as soon as possible afterwards. Issues to consider include the way in which the interview was conducted, ways in which questions and probes could be refined and the presence of any power issues (Brinkmann and Kvale, 2015). Inevitably some participants will be more articulate and focused than others (Corbin and Morse, 2003). The researcher should consider if the way in which they worded questions and probing questions had an impact on the participant's responses. However, Brinkmann and Kvale (2015) offer reassurance about this, suggesting that less articulate accounts usually reflect the complex nature of the phenomenon under investigation. Rather than being adversely affected, participants often report that an interview has been a positive experience (Corbin and Morse, 2003; Rager, 2005) and participants appreciate an interest being taken in their experiences.

TELEPHONE INTERVIEWS AND INTERVIEWS VIA THE INTERNET

Most of the issues described above apply when interviews are conducted via the telephone or Internet. However, there are also some obvious differences. The researcher and participant cannot see each other during a telephone interview. Therefore the interviewer needs to have highly developed listening skills in order to carry out the interview effectively. There may be pros and cons of this method of data collection, particularly when compared to face-to-face interviews, see Table 17.1.

It might also be assumed that participants will be reluctant to discuss difficult and sensitive topics over the telephone. However, a number of studies have demonstrated that this is not the case (Préau et al., 2009; Stringer et al., 2010; Letourneau et al., 2011). Whilst it may be more difficult to provide participants with information about on-going support after a telephone interview, strategies can be put in place to ensure appropriate support is available (see Chapter 18).

Website activity 17.1

Table 17.1   Advantages and disadvantages of telephone interviews

Advantages	Disadvantages
Participants may feel more comfortable revealing information than during a face-to-face interview	Participants may feel less comfortable revealing information than during a face-to-face interview
Telephone interviews tend to be more focused and concise	The more concise nature of the interview may mean that issues are not explored in depth
Telephone interviews can be more convenient for both parties	The interviews can be disjointed with both parties speaking at the same time
Telephone interviews may be less disruptive to the participant	There may be long pauses as each person waits for the other to speak
Telephone interviews are less expensive to conduct	The researcher is unable to take the participant's non-verbal cues into account
Telephone interviews avoid either or both parties having to travel	The interviewer may not be certain that they are speaking to the right person
Telephone interviews avoid lone worker issues arising	The interviewer will have access to limited information about the context
The researcher can make notes during the interview to remind them of issues they want to return to later in the interview	The researcher is unable demonstrate non-verbal cues that may encourage the participant to continue speaking

Interviews conducted via the Internet might be considered to include the benefits of face-to-face and telephone interviews. With the wider availability of packages such as Skype and FaceTime interviews conducted via the Internet are on the increase. Like telephone interviews they have the advantage of enabling participants anywhere in the world, time differences permitting, to take part in an interview.

WHO SHOULD CONDUCT THE INTERVIEW?

The person conducting the interview could be the lead researcher, a member of the research team or someone acting on behalf of the research team. The interviewer may be known or unknown to the participant.

THINK POINT ACTIVITY   17.2

List the advantages and disadvantages of the interviewer being known to the participant prior to the interview.

If more than one person is involved in conducting interviews for a study, the research team should consider how they will address consistency between the interviewers. If the interviews are to take place in a practice setting, then the interviewer(s) may require an honorary contract or research passport (see Chapter 18). Whilst interviews undeniably require a level of skill to be conducted appropriately, novice researchers who are nurses and midwives should note that discussing issues with patients, clients, relatives and colleagues forms the foundation of everything they do. Therefore, with some practice, nurses and midwives should not find interviewing as daunting as they may first anticipate.

Whatever the interview format, the data will be either in the form of a video, an audio-recording or the interviewer's notes, or a combination of all three. These will need to be transcribed into a word-processing document before data analysis can take place. Transcription and data analysis will be discussed in Chapters 19 and 20.

Website
activity 17.2

OBSERVATION

Observation enables the researcher to understand how people behave in particular situations and how they interact with others. This approach is based on anthropological methods whereby people are usually studied in the environment in which events occur (Silverman, 2015). Observation is most commonly associated with ethnography. However, this method of data collection may be used in research involving other methods such as grounded theory and surveys. One of the main advantages of observation is that it facilitates the direct collection of data regarding behaviours, interactions and events occurring in a natural setting. A first-hand account of what happened is therefore generated, which avoids inaccurate recollection. Direct observations undertaken in real time also provide essential information about the context. However, an important disadvantage of this method of data collection is that observations can be time consuming.

DIFFERENT APPROACHES TO OBSERVATION

There are a variety of ways in which the different approaches to observation have been classified. Observation can be undertaken covertly or overtly using participant or non-participant observation. Observations can also take a structured (quantitative) or semi-structured or unstructured approach (qualitative).

Overt observation is when participants are fully aware that they are being observed, and the researcher will usually be present in the setting with them.

By contrast, **covert observation** is when participants do not know that they are being observed. The classic ways in which this was done in the past was using two-way mirrors or hidden cameras. Another strategy would be for a researcher to temporarily join a group in order to carry out covert observation, for example, a researcher undertaking the role of agency nurse and joining a ward setting for a short period of time (Chapman, 1983). In recent years, concerns about covert observation have been raised and it is now very difficult for researchers to acquire the necessary research governance approvals for observation using this approach (see below).

Researchers using participant observation attempt to 'get back-stage' (Polit and Beck 2014: 293) whereby they take part in the activities and interactions being observed. In this way, the researcher endeavours to develop an understanding of the behaviours and experiences of the participants. It is the appropriate means by which to carry out unstructured observation in ethnographic research. A potential problem, however, is that the researcher becomes too familiar with the participants, risking a loss of perspective. Conversely, during non-participant observation, the researcher adopts a passive role and does not participate in activities and interactions. However, it has been argued that the overt non-participant researcher, by the very nature of their presence, has an impact upon the group (Robson, 2011).

WHO SHOULD CARRY OUT OBSERVATIONS?

The person carrying out the observations could be the lead researcher, a member of the research team or someone acting on their behalf. The observer may be known or unknown to the participant. If the observations are to take place in a practice setting, then the observer may require an honorary contract or research passport (see Chapter 18).

THINK POINT ACTIVITY   17.3

List the advantages and disadvantages of the observer being known to the participant(s) prior to an observation.

The observer who has an understanding of the language and practices of the participants has some leverage, whereby little time is required to become accustomed to the environment and the incidents that occur. It can also be argued that observation requires skills allied to those of nursing and midwifery. An observer with experiential understanding and skills may also be more acceptable to the participants than someone without relevant knowledge or experience. However, an observer who is familiar with the setting can be at risk of making assumptions about what is occurring.

DESIGNING THE DATA COLLECTION TOOL

Key issues for the researcher to consider before embarking upon observation include what will be observed, the tool to be used, the time frame and the method of data recording. Data collection may be unstructured (qualitative) or structured (quantitative) or a combination of both. Unstructured qualitative data recording provides the observer with flexibility and freedom, as there are no previously defined parameters. This facilitates the recording of data that are generally descriptive and have a greater depth and breadth than can be achieved when utilising a more structured approach (Polit and Beck, 2014). Unstructured observation is particularly appropriate when little is known about the phenomena being studied. However, the unstructured method is said to require greater skills because of the need to avoid becoming discriminating in the observation and recording (Feher Waltz et al., 1991). The tools for the researcher taking this approach may simply be a pen and a blank piece of paper (with perhaps a clipboard to lean on). The observer documents what they see in as much detail as they can manage. Alternatively a semi-structured approach may be taken whereby the researcher has identified a range of behaviours that they wish to describe.

Structured, quantitative data collection is regarded as being less complex (Polit and Beck, 2014). It is the most appropriate method of data collection when the aim is to record the nature, frequency, duration, context or outcomes of activities and behaviours. In structured observation, checklists and rating scales are commonly used and these tools must be devised and piloted before the study commences (see Chapter 21). The categories used in a structured schedule must be clearly defined and mutually exclusive. However, the structured approach can be too rigid and inflexible (Polit and Beck, 2014). Whilst pre-determined categories facilitate accurate and speedy recording, an extensive number can be difficult for the observer to remember. Therefore, the wrong category may inadvertently be documented. This problem can be overcome by recording a brief comment or description in conjunction with the category. In this way, the appropriateness of the allocated categories can be checked at a later date.

Whether taking a quantitative or qualitative approach to data recording, the researcher must decide the time frame. They may decide, for example, to record data over a defined period of time such as 15 minutes. Alternatively the data may be recorded at regular, timed intervals such as every two minutes. If taking the latter approach an unobtrusive ear piece attached to a device that signals at pre-set time intervals will be invaluable to the observer.

RECORDING THE DATA

Observations are usually carried out with the observer documenting data manually. However, hand-held electronic devices are available to facilitate this process. Alternatively audio- or video-recording may be undertaken with participant consent. This enables the researcher to capture events in a format that can be listened to, or viewed again at a later date (Caldwell and Atwal, 2005). However, the use of video cameras can restrict flexibility, they can be expensive, cumbersome and intrusive and they are difficult to use effectively. It can also be complicated trying to film when events occur in more than one setting (Robson, 2011). Protecting the identity of participants is also problematic (Caldwell and Atwal, 2005). In addition, some would-be participants may decline participation because they do not want to be filmed.

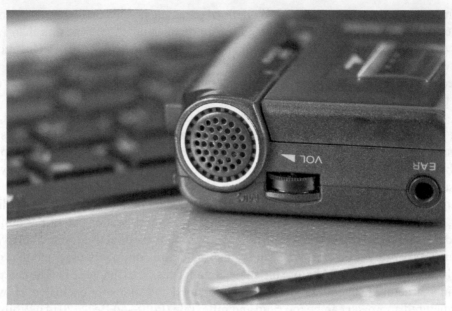

© Masterchief_Productions / Shutterstock

FACTORS TO CONSIDER WHEN CARRYING OUT OBSERVATIONS

The observer should endeavour to have a minimal effect on events, particularly when those being observed are undertaking psychomotor activities (Feher Waltz et al., 1991). Behaviour alteration in participants arising from the presence of an observer is known as **participant reactivity** (Polit and Beck, 2014). This phenomenon is sometimes referred to as the **Hawthorne effect** and was first described in a study at the Hawthorne plant of the Western Electric Company in the 1920s. The researchers in this study concluded that production levels changed when workers were observed (Roethlisberger et al., 1939). It might be assumed that whilst some participants may deliberately change their behaviour, others will feel uncomfortable such that their behaviour alters in a negative way (Rogers, 2008). However, there is no reason to assume one person will respond to being observed any differently from another. Participants soon forget they are being observed and therefore do not maintain a deliberate alteration in their behaviour (Walsh and Baker, 2004). However, it must be acknowledged that an observer cannot know how participants would have behaved had they not been present (Robson, 2011).

The justification usually given by researchers for covert observation is that this approach minimises participant reactivity (Polit and Beck, 2014). However, this strategy brings a range of ethical problems because observations are carried out without the knowledge of participants (Walsh and Baker, 2004). Deceitful, covert observation is therefore generally deemed ethically, morally and legally unacceptable, and ethics committees will require a very clear rationale before giving approval for research using this data collection method.

To reduce the effects of observer presence it has been recommended that the observer spends a period of time with the participants, before data recording commences. This helps the development of understanding between the parties concerned (Walsh and Baker, 2004). The length of time required for this settling in period can be as little as ten minutes (Feher Waltz et al., 1991). However, it must be questioned whether the development of a rapport in this way could lead to observer bias arising from preconceived ideas about the likely behaviour of participants.

An alternative strategy for minimising participant reactivity is for researchers to restrict observations whereby they spend intervals of time looking away, so participants do not feel they are being constantly monitored (Feher Waltz et al., 1991). However, this strategy risks the observer missing important activities or becoming distracted by other events. The ideal approach is for the observer to maintain a discreet distance but at the same time ensure they have a good view. The observer should try to ensure they do not interfere with events or make those being observed feel as though they are under the microscope.

A common concern of the observer is that they will miss something, particularly if several activities are occurring at the same time or when elaborate activities are occurring at a rapid pace; for example, imagine trying to observe events during a resuscitation or an emergency caesarean section. The observer can also be distracted by activities involving those not being observed, or environmental factors such as heat and noise (Polit and Beck, 2014). Observation can also be time consuming. Practice effects, as the observer becomes more experienced, reduce the risk of this problem occurring. The risk of recording errors should also be minimised by adherence to the observation schedule.

Sometimes observers experience role conflict during observations (Lalor et al., 2006). This may particularly be the case if the observer is a health care professional (see Box 17.2).

BOX 17.2   EXAMPLE ILLUSTRATING RESEARCHER ROLE CONFLICT DURING AN OBSERVATION

During an observation of a father during the birth of his baby, the midwife asks the researcher to press the emergency buzzer. The father is supporting his partner who is extremely distressed and the midwife is delivering the baby following a rapid second stage. No one else is present. Although it could be argued that if the researcher were not present the midwife would have dealt with the situation on her own, the researcher feels ethically and morally obliged to assist her in this emergency situation. The 'crash team' arrives instantly and the researcher continues the observations. (Harvey, 2010)

THINK POINT ACTIVITY   17.4

What do you think the researcher should have done in this situation? What are the possible implications of the different actions the researcher could have taken?

Whilst the observer should try to remain detached, there may be occasions when those being observed make direct comments to him or her. Usually this is general conversation and in most cases the observer will probably feel it would be rude not to respond (Robson, 2011). However, observers should try to minimise this type of interaction and this can usually be done by moving to a different part of the room. On more rare occasions, those being observed may try to influence what is recorded by pointing out particular behaviours or responses. The observer should not respond to this type of intervention and should ensure data recording continues in a consistent and robust way.

CONSENT FOR OBSERVATIONS

Whether overt or covert, observation risks invading the privacy of those involved. Holloway and Wheeler (2013) argue that when carrying out observations in care settings, consent should be obtained from all those who are likely to be affected. This should include all relatives and health care professionals. Others suggest it would not be possible to inform and obtain consent from every individual who may potentially be involved (Manning, 2004). Indeed some argue that people entering a public place should anticipate being susceptible to involvement in such activities (Johnson, 1992). Informed consent should definitely be obtained from those who are the focus of the observation. Whether or not informed consent should be obtained from all those who could potentially be involved should be determined by the ethics committee approving the study (see Chapter 18).

Website activity 17.3

However the observations are conducted, the data will be either in the form of a video-recording, an audio-recording or the interviewer's documentation or a combination of all three. These will need to be transcribed into a word-processing document before data analysis can take place. Transcription and data analysis will be discussed in Chapters 19 and 20.

Website activity 17.4

FOCUS GROUPS

Focus groups can be regarded as being a group interview and they are being increasingly used in health care research (Jayasekara, 2012). The intention of a focus group is that participants not only respond to the questions posed by the researcher, but they also discuss issues raised by fellow participants. Focus groups are primarily associated with qualitative research and are most commonly used in grounded theory and ethnography. There is less agreement about the appropriateness of using focus groups in phenomenology because the aim of this type of research is to explore the experiences of individuals (Bradbury-Jones et al., 2009).

In order to promote discussion, the ideal size of the group is between five and ten participants (Jayasekara, 2012). A focus group is therefore a time- and cost-effective way of collecting data from a group of people on one occasion. It may also yield deeper insight from participants as they respond to issues raised by fellow participants. In this way, participants may consider issues that they would not have thought of if they had been interviewed on their own. However, it should be acknowledged that a focus group will be more acceptable to some potential participants than others. Whilst some may find a focus group less intimidating than an interview (Shaha et al., 2011), others may feel the opposite.

CONDUCTING A FOCUS GROUP

A topic guide, which consists of key open questions and probes, is generated in the same way as we described for an interview. The researcher leading the focus group needs to be skilled in ensuring each participant has their say. This can be challenging if one participant dominates the discussion or has strong or contentious opinions about the topic. In these situations the researcher should invite other participants to contribute or suggest that others have a chance to speak. This, of course, needs to be done diplomatically. The researcher also needs to ensure that the discussion focuses on the topic under investigation. This can be difficult, because a participant may raise an issue that initially appears to be unrelated, but subsequent discussion within the group establishes that it is in fact relevant. There may therefore be occasions where the researcher allows the discussion to flow for a period of time but ultimately has to bring the participants back to the topic under investigation. The role of the researcher is therefore to unobtrusively guide the discussion.

As is the case for interviews, focus groups can be conducted face to face or via the Internet and they can be videoed or audio-recorded. It would be almost impossible for someone to document the discussion by note-taking alone. Potential participants should therefore be aware that the focus group will be recorded when consent is taken. Transcribing an audio-recording of a focus group can be a challenge as it can sometimes be difficult to distinguish between speakers. It therefore can be useful to have a second member of the research team present to document the first few words that each participant says as this will help the transcriber. This second member of the research team should sit out of sight of the participants so as not to inhibit the discussion. Another strategy that will help the transcriber is asking the participants before they start to try to not speak over each other. This is sometimes unavoidable when the discussion becomes established. Consequently the researcher may need to ask participants to repeat information for the benefit of the recording.

FOCUS GROUPS AND ETHICAL ISSUES

The very nature of a focus group may mean that it is not an appropriate method of data collection for some sensitive or challenging topics. However, informed consent requirements apply as they would in any research study and some potential participants may feel comfortable discussing difficult topics in this way. A way of facilitating confidentiality is for participants to use pseudonyms rather than their own name (Papastavrou and Andreou, 2012). However, this strategy will be negated if participants are already known to each other.

The particular ethical issue that arises in relation to focus groups is that potential participants must be aware that if they decide to withdraw from the discussion part-way through, it will not be possible to remove their contribution from the recording. Whilst their particular comments could be deleted it would render other participants' subsequent responses to those comments meaningless. Therefore, all participant contributions are required to provide a context. As a consequence, it is essential that potential participants are aware of this when their consent is taken. If a participant does decide to leave the focus group part-way through, a further benefit of having a second member of the research team present is that they could go with them if this seems appropriate.

Ground rules should be agreed by all participants before the focus group starts. The most important of these is maintaining confidentiality. It is imperative that the researcher reminds participants that all discussion 'remains within the room' and that participants do not repeat issues discussed during the focus group afterwards. The researcher should invite participants to suggest ground rules to which all participants then agree. Ideally the ground rules should come from the participants. However, suggestions that the researcher might make include:

- maintaining confidentiality
- allowing each other to have their say
- trying not to speak over each other
- acknowledging the differing views of others.

THINK POINT ACTIVITY   17.5

Are there any other ground rules you would suggest?

As the focus group draws to a close, the researcher should remind participants again about the need to maintain confidentiality. It may also be appropriate to suggest sources of support in relation to the issues discussed.

WHO SHOULD CONDUCT A FOCUS GROUP?

As was the case with interviews and observations, the person conducting a focus group could be the lead researcher, a member of the research team or someone acting on their behalf. This person may be known or unknown to the participants. If the focus groups are to take place in a practice setting, then the person conducting them may require an honorary contract or research passport (see Chapter 18).

THINK POINT ACTIVITY   17.6

List the advantages and disadvantages of the person carrying out the focus group being know to the participant(s) prior to the focus group taking place.

Data from the focus group will need to be transcribed into a word-processing document before data analysis can take place. Transcription and data analysis will be discussed in Chapters 19 and 20.

Website activity 17.5

DIARIES

When used in research, a diary is a tool that enables participants to record information within a time-based framework. Whilst the traditional written format can be used, more versatile ways in which participants can document information include audio, video and e-diaries and these are becoming increasingly popular. More diverse ways of documenting diary data are particularly useful for participants who are concerned about their writing skills (Välimäki et al., 2007). As a primary source of evidence, diaries enable the researcher to collect data over a defined period of time about activities and behaviours from a large group of people, from whom it could be difficult to gather the information in any other way. Diaries are a particularly useful way of collecting information from participants about sensitive topics (Way, 2011).

Diaries may be used in all types of research and can have a structured (quantitative), unstructured (qualitative) or semi-structured (qualitative and quantitative) format. The nature of the recordings within a diary therefore depends upon the purpose of the study. Information to be documented may include details of the participant's actions, behaviours, thoughts and feelings, and also the context in which the recordings are made (Breakwell, 2012). The period of time over which diaries can be used can vary from a few hours to years. Participants document information at regular intervals and this might range between every few minutes to annually. Structured diaries guide the participant

Website activity 17.6

to record specific information, which may be in the form of a checklist. By contrast, semi-structured or unstructured diaries enable participants to document information more freely about a broader range of issues (Phillips and Davies, 1995).

Information can be documented in a diary as, or soon after, events occur. This contemporaneous documentation is likely to produce more accurate data than those collected by other methods which rely on recall at a later date, such as interviews (Richardson, 1994). Nevertheless, potential problems are associated with the use of diaries. Inaccurate information may be recorded. This may be because the participant wishes to please the researcher, wants to be seen 'in a good light' (Robson, 2011: 268) or becomes bored with the process. The process of completing the diary may also change behaviour because participants may undertake the activities or behaviours identified within the diary, in order that they have something to record.

FACTORS TO CONSIDER WHEN USING DIARIES

Studies using diaries can have high attrition rates (Skirton et al., 2012), as participants fail to complete them over the required period of time. Unstructured diaries in particular often result in low response rates (Richardson, 1994). Completing a diary, particularly over a long period of time can be a burden, which can result in some prospective participants declining participation (Phillips and Davies, 1995; Välimäki et al., 2007). Maintaining participant motivation to complete a diary can therefore be a challenge. A strategy to promote engagement could be for the researcher to make contact with the participants periodically during the diary completion process (Skirton et al., 2012). This would enable the participants to clarify any queries or resolve problems that they may have regarding completion of the diaries. Providing participants with incentives to complete the task may be appropriate in some studies. However, this may raise ethical concerns (see Chapter 18).

The format of written diaries should be uncomplicated, with clear instructions about how to complete it, and there should be sufficient room for participants to record information (Robson, 2011; Breakwell, 2012). The researcher should also be aware when devising the diary that there probably will not be an opportunity for clarification (Richardson, 1994). It is therefore important that the diary enables the participant to record all the information that the researcher requires. The equipment for audio or video diaries should be straightforward to use. Whilst the participant may be given guidelines about what sort of things the researcher is interested in, the participant should retain control over what is recorded and when. The researcher should also ensure a secure means of returning the completed diary (in whatever format) at no cost to the participant.

As is the case with questionnaires, there are contrasting views over whether or not participants should provide written consent when diaries are used in a research study. In the past, the conventional argument was that if a participant completes the diary, their consent is implied. However, the consensus view is now that participants should provide written consent.

> ## THINK POINT ACTIVITY   17.7
>
> What do you think? Do you think that informed consent should be obtained from participants who are willing to complete diaries for a research study?

OTHER METHODS OF DATA COLLECTION

There are a variety of other, less commonly used methods of data collection which the researcher may consider using and we will give an overview of them here.

VIGNETTES

Vignettes or scenarios which describe a real or fictitious event can be used to elicit participant responses about how they would respond in that situation or their thoughts and feelings about the scenario. Participants may be given the whole scenario or the vignette may be revealed to them incrementally so that the participants can respond to each aspect of the scenario. Vignettes can be used in a structured way using pre-set questions or in an unstructured way whereby they provide a focus for discussion between the participant(s) and the researcher. An advantage of this method of data collection is that discussion of a hypothetical situation can be less intimidating for participants, particularly if the topic concerns a sensitive or challenging subject. However, a disadvantage is that it is difficult for the researcher to determine the extent to which the participant's responses reflect how they would feel or react when confronted with the situation 'in real life' (Bryman, 2012).

Website activity 17.7

Q-SORT

Q-sort is variously regarded as being a research method or a method of data collection. However, we are including it here because it is not covered elsewhere in the book. Q-sort is a quantitative method of data collection whereby participants are given predetermined statements about a particular topic on individual cards. They are then asked to sort or rank the cards, usually on a continuum that ranges between strongly agree and strongly disagree. The initial statements are often developed from the current literature. Alternatively they may be generated by an early phase of data collection in the study using qualitative interviews or focus groups.

Website activity 17.8

ART-BASED METHODS OF DATA COLLECTION

Art-based methods of data collection may be used, whereby participants draw, paint, take photographs, make collages or sculptures or collects objects that illustrate their thoughts, feelings and experiences (Driessnack and Furukawa, 2012). The art-work may be used as a stand-alone method of data collection or as way to facilitate discussion between the participant and the researcher. Art-work can be particularly useful in research with young children, participants for whom other methods of communication are difficult and participants who are already familiar with the art-form being used in the study (Harder et al., 2015). Art-based techniques can also be a way in which difficult or sensitive topics can be explored with participants.

Website activity 17.9

CHOOSING A METHOD OF DATA COLLECTION

Website activity 17.10

As we have identified in this and the previous chapter there is a vast array of data collection methods available to the researcher. When deciding which method of data collection to use, the most important factor to consider is the need to achieve the aim(s) and objective(s) of the research. The choice of data collection method should therefore be determined by the research question or hypothesis and the research method used. Whether or not a quantitative or qualitative approach, or a combination of both, is taken should also be determined by the research question or hypothesis. It is also imperative that the method of data collection is appropriate for the age and skills of the participants. A number of other factors may also impact on the final choice of data collection method. These include:

- time available
- the research setting
- researcher skills
- resources required/available
- cost (note that payment may be required to use previously validated questionnaires)
- acceptability to participants.

Website activity 17.11

To strengthen the findings of a study a combination of data collection methods may be used (Way, 2011).

SUMMARY

In this chapter we have explored the most commonly used qualitative methods of data collection in health care research. We have considered the practical, logistical and research governance issues that the researcher should think about when deciding which data collection method to use and when designing a data collection tool. Whichever methods of data collection are used, it is essential that data collection is undertaken in a rigorous and consistent way. This issue will be explored in greater depth in Chapter 21.

FURTHER READING

King, N. and Horrocks, C. (2016) *Interviews in Qualitative Research* (2nd edn). London: Sage Publications.

A simple to follow guide to planning and conducting interviews.

Silverman, D. (2013) *Doing Qualitative Research: A Practical Handbook* (4th edn). London: Sage Publications.

A comprehensive companion for researchers doing research. It has lots of examples from nursing and health and includes basic questions to help you plan your data collection.

Don't forget to visit https://study.sagepub.com/harveyandland to watch videos, take quizzes and to follow specially designed web activities.

18

RESEARCH GOVERNANCE IN CLINICAL RESEARCH: ADDRESSING ETHICAL ISSUES

In this chapter we will explore the ethical and legal issues and indemnity insurance issues that nurses and midwives should consider when conducting and reviewing research. In doing this we will:

- explore the development of ethical research both within the UK and internationally
- identify the research governance and legal requirements to be addressed when seeking approval to carry out a study in the UK
- explore the practical and logistical research governance issues to be addressed when designing a study
- consider the application of research governance requirements during a study.

Throughout this book we have emphasised that potential ethical and legal issues must be identified, considered and addressed before a study is carried out. These ethical and legal issues may, for example, impact upon decisions about which research method to use or the way in which data are collected. In this chapter we will explore research governance issues in detail. Whilst there will primarily be a UK focus to this chapter, particularly with regard to legislation and research governance requirements, the principles apply internationally. The chapter will begin by describing the origins of ethical research and the ways in which the lessons learned from past events have shaped current practice. We will then identify the research governance requirements that a researcher must address before undertaking a health care related study in the UK. Finally, we will explore the application of research governance requirements throughout the conduct of a study.

THE DEVELOPMENT OF ETHICAL RESEARCH

If we look through our twenty-first-century lens at health care research conducted in the past, we would see many examples of studies carried out in ways that would concern us. In many instances researchers in the past would have felt they were doing nothing wrong, their practice reflected approaches to research at the time. However, in other cases researchers must surely have known that what they were doing was inappropriate and in some instances illegal.

When an historical overview is given of the development of ethical research authors usually start with the Nazi atrocities carried out in concentration camps during the Second World War (1939–1945). While these crimes cannot be denied, research that we would now consider to be flawed was undertaken or commenced before that time, with researchers adopting a cavalier attitude to participants and to the research. This approach resulted in participants being involved in studies without their knowledge and therefore without their consent. Whilst in other past studies participants were not given complete information about the purpose of the research. For example, in the Tuskegee syphilis study (1932–1972) available treatment was withheld from 400 African American men with syphilis so that the natural progression of the disease could be investigated.

Nevertheless it was the Nuremberg Trials (1945–1949) which revealed the true horrors of the experimentation undertaken in concentration camps during the Second World War. Doctors attempted to justify what they had done by arguing that their actions were part of a clinical trial. However, interventions were undertaken without the participants consenting or even being aware that the 'treatments' they were being given were part of a trial. In addition, many of these interventions, such as deliberate exposure to mustard gas, malaria and iced cold water were known at the time to cause harm. However, these studies were undertaken because the doctors wanted to find out to what extent harmful interventions impacted upon humans. Many of the experiments resulted in the death or serious impairment of participants. The Nuremberg Trials paved the way for much of the research governance that is now in place internationally, the first of which was the 1949 Nuremberg Code which identifies ten standards regarding the conduct of research, which includes the need for voluntary consent from participants.

Website
activity 18.1

Other internationally endorsed codes and standards have been subsequently developed. Probably the most notable of these is the Declaration of Helsinki, which was first adopted in 1964 and was most recently revised in 2013. The key principles of the code include:

- protection of the participant
- the need for participant informed consent
- the need for independent approval for a study

- the need for a study having a scientific or medical basis
- the need for a study having an appropriate balance of risk versus benefit
- the wellbeing of the participant should take precedence.

Examples of other internationally accepted standards and guidelines include:

Website
activity 18.2

- The World Health Organization (2011) *Standards and Operational Guidance for Ethics Review of Health-Related Research with Human Participants.*
- The Council for International Organizations of Medical Sciences in collaboration with the World Health Organization (2008) *International Ethical Guidelines for Epidemiological Studies.*

RESEARCH GOVERNANCE AND LEGAL REQUIREMENTS IN THE UK

A number of research governance and legal requirements must be addressed before health care research can begin in the UK. Many of the research governance requirements have been put in place as a result of concerns raised about specific studies or aspects of research practice undertaken in the UK, such as the storage of tissue samples (Hall, 2001) or the Northwick Park study (Suntharalingam et al., 2006).

Researchers must put strategies in place to ensure the following requirements are met:

- Indemnity insurance approval (this will be reviewed in more detail below).
- Ethics committee approval (this will be reviewed in more detail below).
- Professional codes, standards and guidelines: these will be specific to the researcher's professional background and participant groups such as children or people with mental health problems.
- *The Research Governance Framework* (Department of Health, 2005): this provides guidance on the way in which research should be conducted. Whilst this is not 'law' it must be adhered to and therefore shapes the way in which health care research is conducted. This includes a shift away from 'doing research on' to 'doing research with'. The framework is currently being updated and is expected to be published in 2016.
- The law: for example, The Human Rights Act 1998; The Data Protection Act 1998, 2003; Freedom of Information Act 2000; The Human Tissue Act 2004; and the Mental Capacity Act 2005, 2007.
- Health and safety and European Union regulations.

THINK POINT ACTIVITY   18.1

Review the Nursing and Midwifery Council (2015a) *The Code: Professional Standards of Practice and Behaviour for Nurses and Midwives.*

What requirements are identified in the code that would apply to nurses and midwives who conduct or who are involved in the conduct of research?

Website
activity 18.3

It is essential however, that researchers remember that meeting these requirements does not only apply when a study is planned and designed. These requirements should also be addressed *throughout* the conduct of the study. The researcher therefore has the responsibility to ensure that, for example, the stipulations as identified in the research governance framework and their professional code of conduct are upheld throughout the research.

SEEKING APPROVAL TO CARRY OUT A STUDY

When undertaking research in the context of health care in the UK, two approvals are required: indemnity insurance and the approval of an ethics committee. The most important advice we can give about when, where and how to make an application for these approvals is to seek guidance from your employer or research supervisor/lecturer in the first instance.

INDEMNITY INSURANCE

Acquiring indemnity insurance was until recently referred to as getting 'sponsorship' or having a research 'sponsor'. However, these terms were sometimes misunderstood whereby researchers thought having a sponsor meant an organisation was going to fund their research. Sadly this is not the case. Having indemnity insurance approval means that, if necessary, compensation will be provided to anyone harmed by the study. Agreement that indemnity insurance will be provided must be in place before a study begins.

WHERE, WHEN AND HOW DO I APPLY FOR INDEMNITY INSURANCE?

Indemnity insurance is usually provided by the organisation that the chief or lead researcher works for, or the academic institution where a student is studying. Organisations and academic institutions will have an application process which will probably include the requirement to complete specific documentation pertaining to the study. Decisions about the provision of indemnity insurance are usually made by a committee on behalf of the organisation (see Box 18.1). If the application is approved the researcher will be issued with a letter of confirmation. Alternatively the researcher will be advised if they are required to provide further information or clarification before approval can be given.

BOX 18.1   EXAMPLES ILLUSTRATING WHICH INSTITUTIONS SHOULD PROVIDE INDEMNITY INSURANCE FOR SPECIFIC STUDIES/RESEARCHERS

Zoe is a midwife undertaking an MSc at her local academic institution. The academic institution will provide indemnity insurance.

Bob is a nurse lecturer at academic institution A. Bob is undertaking his PhD at academic institution B. Academic institution B will provide indemnity insurance for Bob's study.

Abigail is a midwifery lecturer at academic institution A. Abigail has acquired funding to undertake a study with students at the institution, which will provide indemnity insurance.

Tam is a Band 8a and has acquired funding to undertake a study in his clinical practice area. The NHS Trust will provide indemnity insurance.

Researchers should submit their application for indemnity insurance approval as and when they are ready. No aspect of the study, including participant recruitment, can begin until this approval is in place. Researchers should therefore pre-empt their application by finding out in advance from the institution where they will be making their application, what the process will be and what documentation they need to complete.

WHAT IS THE INDEMNITY INSURANCE COMMITTEE LOOKING FOR?

The purpose of the application for indemnity insurance approval is to enable the committee to assess the level of risk: to participants, the researcher, the study site and the institution providing the approval. The committee will therefore want to be reassured that the researcher has considered all potential risks and has put strategies in place to minimise the effect of these risks.

APPROVAL OF AN ETHICS COMMITTEE

A researcher must obtain ethics committee approval for their study before it can begin.

WHERE, WHEN AND HOW DO I APPLY FOR ETHICS COMMITTEE APPROVAL?

Approval will be provided in most cases either by an NHS or an academic institution's ethics committee. If the study is to be conducted in an NHS setting it is likely that NHS ethics committee approval will be required. However, in recent times some NHS committees have decided that their approval is not required for some types of study which they deem to be, for example, service evaluation or audit. The most straightforward way that a researcher can find out if they require NHS ethics committee approval is to contact the research and development office in the main study site for advice.

If a researcher is advised that approval by an NHS ethics committee is not required, they should be aware of two important issues. Firstly, if the research is being undertaken by a student or member of staff of an academic institution, the need for ethics committee approval is not absolved. They will need to acquire approval from the academic institution instead. Secondly, lack of NHS ethics committee approval may have implications for publication. This is because most editors, particularly the higher impact, international journals, will ask for evidence of NHS ethics committee approval and will not accept an academic institution's ethics committee approval as an alternative.

The NHS National Research Ethics Service (NRES) is managed by the Health Research Authority (HRA). NRES has an online application process called the Integrated Research Application System (IRAS) which includes the requirement to complete specific documentation pertaining to the study. Part of the application process includes the researcher assessing the level of risk, that is, whether or not the study is low risk. The researcher's assessment of risk is reviewed on submission. Low risk studies are reviewed 'proportionately'. This means that a sub-committee reviews the application and the researcher is notified of the outcome within 14 days. Higher risk studies require 'full' review and the researcher will be invited to attend a committee meeting to discuss their application. The researcher is notified of the outcome within 60 days. When an application (full or proportionate) is approved the researcher will be issued with a letter of confirmation. Alternatively the researcher will be asked to provide further information or clarification before approval can be given.

Website
activity 18.4

Academic institutions will have a similar application process for ethics committee approval, which will probably include the requirement to complete specific documentation pertaining to the study. Some institutions have similar arrangements in place to the NHS with regard to proportionate review. A committee will then review the application. If the application is approved the researcher will be issued with a letter of confirmation. Alternatively the researcher will be advised if further information or clarification is required before approval can be given.

As was the case for indemnity insurance approval, researchers should submit their application for ethics committee approval as and when they are ready. Researchers are sometimes surprised when they come to make their ethics approval application about the amount of detail and supporting documentation such as consent forms and participant information leaflets that are required. However, these are all issues that the researcher should have already thought about and if they have not, it suggests that they are not yet ready to make their application. Researchers should therefore pre-empt their submission by finding out in advance from the academic institution or NHS research ethics website what documentation they will need to provide.

WHAT IS THE ETHICS COMMITTEE LOOKING FOR?

Ethics committees want to be reassured that strategies have been put in place to promote the safety and wellbeing of research participants, researchers and the institution or organisation where the research is to take place. The purpose of ethics committee review is to determine whether any harm or risk associated with the research outweighs the benefits. In doing this, the committee will consider both short and longer term effects. The committee will look to see if the researcher has anticipated any possible adverse effects and outcomes and has put strategies in place should unexpected events occur. Sometimes researchers are frustrated when ethics committees focus on their research method and methodology rather than ethical issues per se. However, the ethics committee needs to be sure that what the researcher is setting out to do is realistic and achievable. For example, to conduct a study with an inadequate sample size or using a data collection tool that will not answer the research question(s) is unethical.

WHICH COMES FIRST, INDEMNITY INSURANCE OR ETHICS COMMITTEE APPROVAL?

Usually indemnity insurance approval is acquired first and the ethics committee will want to see written evidence that this approval has been given. However, in some organisations, particularly academic institutions, researchers make one application, completing one set of documentation which covers the application for both indemnity and ethics approval. The indemnity insurance committee will usually review the application first and, if approved, will pass the application on to the ethics committee for their approval a few days later. However, it is essential that the researcher ensures that they receive a letter confirming that they have been granted both indemnity insurance and ethics committee approval. In some institutions the researcher may receive a separate letter for each.

PRACTICAL AND LOGISTICAL ETHICAL ISSUES TO BE ADDRESSED

The documentation that a researcher is required to complete for ethics committee approval (whether academic institution or NHS) will indicate the sorts of issues that ethics committees will want to know that the researcher has addressed. The sorts of things that the researcher should consider are outlined below.

DO I NEED PERMISSION TO ACCESS POTENTIAL PARTICIPANTS?

The short answer to this question is 'yes'. The less straightforward question to answer is, 'from whom should I obtain this permission?' This depends on the location of the study and who the potential participants are. The researcher must therefore identify the gate-keeper and obtain their written permission to access participants. This should be obtained even if the researcher is an employee of the organisation where the study will be carried out and the potential participants are colleagues. The ethics committee will want to see evidence of this permission (see Box 18.2).

BOX 18.2   EXAMPLES ILLUSTRATING THE PROVISION OF PERMISSION TO ACCESS POTENTIAL PARTICIPANTS

Deborah is a researcher working for a private company. She plans to undertake research with student midwives studying at a specific academic institution. Deborah must obtain permission to access potential participants from the programme leader or head of school.

Jason plans to undertake research with the carers of adults with learning disabilities. Jason hopes to recruit participants via an organisation's website for carers. Jason must obtain permission from the organisation to display a notice about the study on the website.

Sanjay plans to undertake research involving adults with insulin dependent diabetes and hopes to recruit participants via the out-patient department at a local hospital. In order to do this, Jason must obtain permission to access potential participants from the NHS Trust.

If a study is to be undertaken in a clinical setting and the researcher does not work for that organisation, an honorary contract, research passport and/or Disclosure and Barring Service (DBS) clearance may be required. The researcher should seek guidance on this from the research and development office at the proposed study site(s) as quite often different sites require different things.

Similarly most trusts and NHS research ethics committees will require researchers to have successfully completed Good Clinical Practice (GCP) training before they can access a study site and research participants. This training is run by the National Institute for Health Research (NIHR), it is free and a certificate of confirmation is provided on successful completion. The NIHR offers a range of GCP training programmes some of which can be undertaken online. Website activity 18.5

Sometimes researchers want to use information that they have access to as part of their 'everyday' role, as data for a study. For example, a researcher may be involved in collating information on a database and wants to use this information in his or her study. Written confirmation of permission to access the information for research purposes should be obtained. The ethics committee will want to be assured that permission to use the data for research purposes has been granted (see Box 18.3).

BOX 18.3   EXAMPLE OF A RESEARCHER OBTAINING PERMISSION TO USE DATA FOR HIS RESEARCH

An NHS Trust is maintaining a database as part of the provision of care of patients with a pressure ulcer. Part of Sam's role is to maintain the database and he hopes to use some of the information for his study. Sam must, however, obtain permission from the NHS Trust before he can start using the data for research purposes.

CAN I GUARANTEE PARTICIPANT ANONYMITY?

Anonymity and confidentiality are often considered together and are sometimes regarded as being the same thing. However, whilst both can encompass the same issues, they can also present different challenges and so will be considered separately here.

Wherever possible researchers should reassure participants that they will remain anonymous and this should be stated on the participant information leaflet/sheet and consent form (see below). Being reassured about anonymity may increase the likelihood that a potential participant will agree to take part in a study. There are a number of strategies that a researcher can use to protect a participant's identity. These might include:

- minimising the number of people who have access to participant identifiers such as names and addresses – in many studies this information will be confined to only one member of the research team
- securely storing information about participants' names and contact details
- using codes to replace names and locations in the data
- careful use of direct quotes and data extracts in presentations and publications to minimise the likelihood of participants and locations being recognised.

However, guaranteeing anonymity can sometimes be problematic, particularly when a small-scale study has been carried out in a known location. Also, some data collection methods such as focus groups and observation mean that participants will know who else has taken part. In these situations the researcher should remind participants at the beginning and end of the data collection process not to disclose who has taken part in the

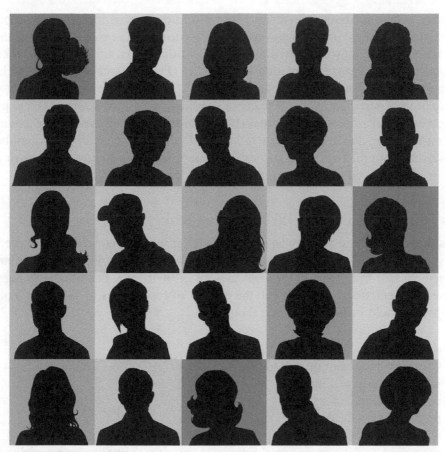

© aklionka / Shutterstock

research. However, if participants chose to disclose this information themselves, there is not much that the researcher can do.

CAN I GUARANTEE PARTICIPANT CONFIDENTIALITY?

Wherever possible researchers should reassure participants that the data they provide for the study will be confidential and any data used in presentations and publications will be anonymised. This should be stated on the participant information leaflet/sheet and consent form (see below). Being reassured about confidentiality may increase the likelihood that a potential participant will agree to take part in a study, particularly if the study is likely to touch on sensitive or challenging topics. However, there may be some situations where the researcher feels that they must breach confidentiality. This may particularly be the case for nurses and midwives, who must adhere to their professional code (Nursing and Midwifery Council, 2015a). For example, the researcher may have concerns about the safeguarding of children or vulnerable adults or may witness unsafe clinical practice during data collection. If the researcher thinks there is any possibility that they may need to breach confidentiality, this should be acknowledged on the participant information sheet/leaflet. The researcher should also have a plan in place for reporting their concerns. Whilst primarily these strategies are put in place to protect participants, the researcher should also be aware of the need to protect themselves and also their professional responsibilities. If the researcher encounters a situation that they do not know how to handle they should consult other members of the research team, their research supervisor, supervisor of midwives or the chair of the ethics or indemnity insurance committee.

WHEN AND HOW TO I OBTAIN INFORMED CONSENT?

As health care professionals, readers will be familiar with the concept of informed consent as it straddles all aspects of patient/client care. Midwives will be used to obtaining informed consent from women for many aspects of their care. The principles regarding informed consent are as applicable in the context of research as to any other. Potential participants should be fully informed about:

- the study
- why they have been invited to take part
- what the study will involve
- potential benefits for them
- potential risks for them
- what will happen if something goes wrong
- their right to withdraw from the study at any time without compromising themselves or their care
- strategies to facilitate their anonymity and confidentiality
- who is funding the study
- if the study is being undertaken as part of an educational qualification
- which organisations have approved the study.

This information is usually provided in a participant information leaflet or sheet. The researcher's academic institution or NHS Trust may have a required format for this. Alternatively, templates can be found on the NRES website. The challenge for the researcher is providing relevant information without making the information sheet too long because lengthy, complex information may impede understanding (Freer et al., 2009). Getting a peer review from someone who would meet the study's inclusion criteria can be helpful in terms of making appropriate amendments. Similarly ethics committees often request peer review particularly from user group representatives.

THINK POINT ACTIVITY   18.2

You have been invited to take part in a health related research study. What would you want to know about the study and the research team before you decide whether or not to take part?

When taking consent, the researcher must be sure that the potential participant fully understands what the study will involve. This is particularly important in randomised controlled trials in emergency or critical care situations where the person giving consent must understand that there is an equal chance that the participant will receive the conventional or placebo treatment. However, at times of acute anxiety, misunderstandings and misconceptions can occur. This has been particularly identified when parental consent is taken for a child's involvement in research (Needle et al., 2009; Kanthimathinathan and Scholefield, 2014).

DeMauro and colleagues (2014) have identified three conditions that must be achieved when health care professionals take consent. Whilst developed in the context of parents giving consent for neonatal research (DeMauro et al., 2014), these three principles can be applied to all health care research:

1   Health care professionals taking consent for participation must not have any concerns about the research.
2   Health care professionals taking consent must have an open and honest discussion with potential participants about the research.
3   Participants must make informed decisions about whether or not they participate in a study.

With respect to the last point, it is unusual for a study to achieve a 100% recruitment rate. It should always be anticipated that at least some potential participants approached about a study will decide not to take part.

The timing of consent can sometimes be problematic. Ideally participants should be allowed as much time as they need to decide whether they will take part. The usual practice is to give participants a minimum of 24 hours. However, in some situations such as emergency care, intensive care, maternity and newborn research, this length of time is not feasible. In these cases, the ethics committee must agree that consent can be obtained when those giving consent have a minimal amount of time to decide. An example of such a study is the 'Whole body hypothermia for the treatment of perinatal asphyxia encephalopathy; TOBY: Total Body Hypothermia Study' where babies had to be recruited and randomised within six hours of birth (Azzopardi et al., 2009). There may also be situations where researchers have to accept that the opportunity to obtain informed consent has been lost. For example, it may be inappropriate to seek consent from a woman who is in an advanced stage of labour (Harvey, 2010).

In many studies consent will be taken by the lead researcher or members of the research team. The indemnity insurance and ethics committees will need to be reassured that the person or people taking consent are adequately trained. For research undertaken in the NHS this may include successful completion of GCP training (see above). In some studies, taking consent may be devolved to other health care professionals. However, this can present challenges for researchers when seeking approval for their study and they may be required to provide training for all those who are likely to be involved. To facilitate this process, toolkits have been produced (Kenyon et al., 2013).

Both the person taking and the person giving consent should sign the consent form. The researcher should retain a copy of the signed form and a copy should be given to the participant. In some exceptional cases, ethics committees may approve a study in which participants give verbal assent, possibly by telephone before an intervention is implemented and written consent is obtained once the intervention is completed (Pushpa-Rajah et al., 2014).

An important factor for the researcher to consider is from whom consent should be taken. In most cases the research participant should be the person who consents to their involvement in the study. There are, however, notable exceptions such as babies, children and adults lacking mental capacity who are not able to consent for themselves.

HOW DO I OBTAIN INFORMED CONSENT FOR RESEARCH INVOLVING CHILDREN?

Website
activity 18.6

When the research involves babies and children under the age of 16, consent will be provided in most cases by the parents. However, it is good practice to provide age-appropriate information in a range of formats about the study for the child and obtain the child's assent (Kumpunen et al., 2012; Kanthimathinathan and Scholefield, 2014).

Obtaining consent from the parents is not always as straightforward as it may seem. There may be some situations where the mother does not have the mental capacity to give consent (see below). A father can only consent for his child if:

- he has the mental capacity to do so (see below)
- he is married to the child's mother *or*
- he is registered as the child's father on the birth certificate (if the child was born after 1 December 2003) *or*
- he has acquired parental responsibility (by formal agreement with the child's mother or by Court Order) *or*
- he has obtained a residence order.

Any of these situations may not be immediately apparent when a researcher approaches a father for his consent. For example, if the child is newborn, it is unlikely that the birth will have been registered. So in some cases the researcher will need to be sensitive and cautious when determining whether a father is able to give consent. Another potentially difficult situation is when one parent agrees to their child's participation in a study and the other parent declines. Whilst a clinician may be tempted to take consent from the parent in agreement, the long term implications of taking this course of action on both the child and the parents' relationship should be considered. Most clinicians in this situation would err on the side of caution and not enrol the child in the study. In this scenario, the child's views may be the deciding factor because whilst their consent is not required, their assent should be acquired if at all possible (Kumpunen et al., 2012) and researchers should be aware of situations where a child is being coerced to participate in a study against their will.

Another situation involving consent for babies and children that researchers may encounter is when a mother is under 16 years of age. She can consent for her child's participation in research, providing the person taking consent is assured that she understands what the research will involve. The researcher may elect to ensure the mother's parents (i.e. the baby's grandparents) are present when maternal consent is taken. However, in some families this may not be practicable or appropriate.

In some exceptional circumstances, when neither parent is able to give consent, this can be provided by the courts or a legally appointed guardian.

Website activity 18.7

HOW DO I ADDRESS ISSUES REGARDING MENTAL CAPACITY?

It is the responsibility of the researcher when taking consent, to assess whether the person giving consent has the capacity to do so. This applies in any situation and the researcher should not take consent if they feel the potential participant does not understand the research, what they are being asked to do and the possible consequences of the research. In some circumstances a personal, professional or nominated legal representative or consultee may consent on the participant's behalf. In these situations, consent can be given if the research is likely to benefit those lacking mental capacity without causing an unduly adverse effect on the participants. However, if it is clear that a participant does not want to take part in a study, then their wishes should be upheld.

If a participant regains capacity during a study, their consent should be taken for their participation in the remainder of the study. If a participant loses capacity during a study they should be withdrawn from the research and their data destroyed.

Website activity 18.8

CAN I INVOLVE VULNERABLE ADULTS IN MY RESEARCH?

Gaining ethics committee approval for research involving vulnerable adults can be problematic because the committee will want to be assured that participants will not be adversely affected. Whilst it might be argued that all patients and clients are vulnerable to some extent, in this context vulnerability may include those with altered mental health, physical health problems or learning disabilities, prisoners, those who have been bereaved and those who are marginalised or disadvantaged (Crowther and Lloyd-Williams, 2012). The ethics committee will want to be reassured that the researcher will take appropriate steps to ensure vulnerable participants have an equal opportunity to participate, that their involvement is meaningful and conversely that they will not be coerced to take part (Northway et al., 2015). Researchers should also be aware that involvement in the research may have an adverse impact on the participant's vulnerability and that therefore strategies should be in place to support them.

COULD POWER RELATIONSHIPS IMPACT ON THE RESEARCH?

In other words, is there any potential for someone, usually the researcher, to knowingly or unknowingly exert 'power', coercion or pressure over the participants? (Anderson, 2011). This may, for example, mean that participants agree to take part in a study although they do not really want to; they may feel obliged to respond in a certain way during data collection; they may feel concerned about disclosing personal information; or they may worry about the implications of agreeing or not agreeing to take part in a study (McNeill and Nolan, 2011; Larkin, 2013). Concerns about power relationships may also arise when someone else, for example a parent, consents to their child's involvement in a study (see informed consent above).

Most commonly power relationships occur when the researcher is known to those taking part in the study or is perceived to be in a position of seniority, authority or power by the participants.

THINK POINT ACTIVITY   18.3

Make a list of possible situations where a power relationship may exist (either perceived or actual) between a researcher and participants.

Examples of situations where possible power relationships might exist include where a module leader may ask students currently undertaking the module to participate in her study, a ward manager may ask his staff to take part in his study or a doctor caring for a group of patients may ask them to take part in his research. Whilst some participants will readily agree to taking part without any concerns, others may worry about the implications of their agreeing whether or not to be involved. Ethics committees will want to be reassured that the researcher has put strategies in place to minimise the risk or potential impact of power relationships.

There are a number of strategies that a researcher can put in place to minimise the impact of power relationships. Not all of the following may be appropriate, but could include:

- involving participant representatives in the design of the study to minimise the existence of power relationships
- not involving participants in a study who have had any prior interaction with the researcher
- stating in the participant information leaflet that a participant can decide not to take part and that doing this will not jeopardise their on-going situation in any way
- asking another member of the research team or a colleague to recruit participants (note the ethics and indemnity insurance committee must be made aware if this strategy is adopted as this may have implications in terms of research approvals)
- allowing participants sufficient time to decide if they want to take part in a study
- empowering the participants by being as flexible as possible in the conduct of the study, for example, the timing and location of participant interviews
- assuring participant anonymity
- using qualitative approaches and data collection methods that minimise the impact of power relationships such as semi-structured interviews or focus groups (Weaver and Olson, 2006; Anderson, 2011)
- involving another member of the research team in data collection (note the ethics and indemnity insurance committee must be made aware if this strategy is adopted as this may have implications in terms of research approvals)
- involving participants in checking the researcher's analysis of the data (see Chapter 20); however, note that participants may still feel obliged to agree with the researcher
- being vigilant about and acting upon the presence of any power relationships during the conduct of the study; this can be facilitated by keeping a reflective diary (Brinkmann and Kvale, 2015).

WHERE WILL DATA COLLECTION TAKE PLACE?

The answer to this question is not always as straightforward as it may seem. Clearly, for some studies the location for data collection will be determined by the research. For example, data collection for a randomised controlled trial will probably be undertaken whilst the participant is a patient in a clinical setting.

However, other studies may require the researcher to use facilities within a setting such as an out-patient department, a private room for interviews or a GP surgery.

If this is the case the ethics committee will want to be assured that the researcher has written permission to have on-going access to these locations. This confirmation should be obtained even if the researcher is an employee of the organisation concerned.

A preferred option may be to carry out data collection in the participant's home. This is likely to be more convenient for the participant and it avoids the need to reimburse their travel expenses. However, data collection in the participant's home is more costly for the researcher both in terms of time and travel. The most important factor to address in this situation is, however, the implications for the researcher of lone working. Whilst some health care professionals such as community midwives and health visitors are used to going to the homes of patients and clients on their own, researchers should not ignore the potential implications of lone working. Employers should have a lone worker policy and this should be implemented in the conduct of the research. Organisations such as the Suzy Lamplugh Trust also offer guidance and training for lone workers. Ethics and indemnity insurance committees will want to be assured that lone worker policies will be put in place if required.

Website activity 18.9

Online data collection methods are increasingly being used (Mahon, 2014). Whilst there are benefits associated with this method data collection such as convenience for the participant, it can present ethical challenges such as maintaining data security. One of the most serious challenges for the researcher using this approach is determining whether the participant is underage (Mahon, 2014) and that the person completing the data collection tool is who they say they are. The ethics committee will want to be assured that appropriate strategies are in place if this approach is adopted.

WHERE AND HOW WILL THE DATA BE STORED?

Indemnity insurance and ethics committees need to be reassured that data will be stored safely and securely. The requirements of the Data Protection Acts 1998 and 2003 should be adhered to at all times. The usual procedure is to store electronic data, including videos and audio-recordings, on a password protected encrypted memory stick or external hard drive. Data should not be stored on personal laptops and home computers. Hard copies of data, participant consent forms and participant contact details should be stored in a locked cupboard, ideally in a locked room. The researcher should seek advice from the indemnity insurance and ethics committees about how long data should be retained once the study is completed and how to safely destroy the data. There is a gradual move towards asking participants on the consent form at the start of a study if their data can be retained indefinitely. This facilitates further analysis and review of the data at a later date and, if appropriate, data sharing. However, institutions will need to ensure facilities are in place to store data in a secure way indefinitely.

SHOULD PARTICIPANTS BE PAID TO TAKE PART IN A STUDY?

> ### THINK POINT ACTIVITY   18.4
>
> Do you think research participants should be paid to take part in a study? Explain your point of view.
>   Under what circumstances do you think payment would be appropriate?
>   Under what circumstances do you think payment would be inappropriate?

This is an issue that provokes conflicting opinion. Payment may be regarded as coercion, even perhaps a bribe. It is also possible that some participants will volunteer for a study simply because they are going to be paid. However, offering payment acknowledges the time, effort and commitment that participants make to a study. Participants usually appreciate being offered payment (Harvey et al., 2014) and for some studies, offering payment may be the only way of recruiting sufficient participants. The participants certainly should not be left out of pocket and should, for example, be reimbursed any travel or child care expenses incurred. Organisations such as INVOLVE and the James Lind Alliance advocate financial redress for participants and provide useful guidance for researchers.

Website activity 18.10

Payment may take several forms. For example, rather than money, participants may be offered a gift, a voucher or a treat such as a day out somewhere. If payment is to be offered to participants, this should be costed and acknowledged on the application for ethics and indemnity insurance approval.

IS IT POSSIBLE THAT PARTICIPANTS WILL REQUIRE SUPPORT DURING OR AFTER THE STUDY?

As we have acknowledged in earlier chapters, some studies may involve participants talking about difficult or sensitive topics or may cause them to worry about something that they have not thought about for a long time, if at all. However, awareness of this possibility does not necessarily stop potential participants from agreeing to take part in such a study (Crowther and Lloyd-Williams, 2012). Researchers should therefore have strategies in place to support participants if and when such situations arise. This support should be provided by health care professionals and organisations external to the study. The researcher should be very careful not to confuse the role of researcher with that of a counsellor. If it is anticipated that it is possible that participants are likely to require on-going support, the researcher should develop an information sheet, identifying possible sources of support. This may include, for example, the participant's GP or health visitor, local or national support groups or charities. If the researcher intends to refer participants to specific organisations such as the staff counselling service in an NHS Trust or a local counselling service, then the ethics committee will want to see written confirmation that the provision of support will be available for participants. The ethics committee should also approve the information sheet for participants.

IS IT POSSIBLE THAT I (THE RESEARCHER) WILL REQUIRE SUPPORT DURING OR AFTER THE STUDY?

Quite often researchers become so focused on ensuring that participants are protected that they forget about themselves. However, it is possible that the researcher will face difficult, challenging and emotionally draining situations. Ethics and indemnity insurance committees therefore will want to be assured that the researcher and the research team are supported appropriately. In addition to the lone worker policy already discussed other strategies may include: keeping a reflective diary, periodically taking time out and regular discussion with a colleague, research supervisor or supervisor of midwives. Within any discussion or sharing of excerpts from their reflective diary, the researcher should ensure that participant anonymity and confidentiality are upheld.

APPLYING RESEARCH GOVERNANCE REQUIREMENTS

As soon as indemnity insurance and ethics committee approvals have been confirmed in writing, the study may begin. However, it is essential that the researcher constantly monitors the potential impact of any ethical issues or risk throughout the study. If an adverse event occurs which affects any aspect of the study or those involved, both committees should be notified and further guidance sought. Similarly, if a difficult or challenging event or incident occurs, the researcher may seek guidance from either committee about how to handle the situation. For example, a participant who having been told that their anonymity and confidentiality are assured then tells a researcher about something such as domestic abuse, which a researcher feels should be reported. Another potentially difficult situation is when a child discloses something to a researcher and asks them not to tell their parents.

THINK POINT ACTIVITY   18.5

What factors should a nurse/midwife take into consideration when a breach of confidentiality may be required? What would you do?

The researcher must also notify both committees of any planned changes to the conduct of the study. This could include, for example, using a different recruitment strategy or the addition of a new study site. Changes may also come about as a consequence of using a qualitative method such as grounded theory or action research. In these types of study the researcher will not know at the outset what the subsequent phases of the study will involve. Therefore, once the first phase is completed the researcher should notify the indemnity and ethics committees of their subsequent plans for their study.

Whatever the reasons for making changes, the researcher should write to the chair of both committees describing and justifying the planned changes. In most cases, the chair will write back confirming approval of the proposed changes. It is essential that the researcher follows this procedure rather than just making changes without consultation. To do the latter could mean than when the changes are discovered (and they almost certainly will be at some point), the prior approvals might be withdrawn. More seriously, if an adverse event occurs, the researcher could find themselves without the cover and support provided by the indemnity insurance and ethics committees.

It is not uncommon for researcher to consider the approvals process as being a hurdle to jump over and then forget about. However, it is essential that researchers act in accordance with their professional responsibilities and remain vigilant throughout the conduct of a study to ensure that they, the participants and the organisation are protected and safe from harm.

Website
activity 18.11

SUMMARY

In this chapter we have explored various aspects of research governance. We have considered the origins of ethical research and the ways in which the lessons learned from past events have shaped current practice. We have examined the research governance requirements that a researcher must address before undertaking a health care related study in the UK and we have emphasised that these requirements should be addressed throughout the conduct of a study.

FURTHER READING

Dimond, B. (2015) *Legal Aspects of Nursing* (7th edn). Harlow: Pearson.

This book contains chapters on consent, data protection, confidentiality and consideration of specific client groups such as children, maternity care, the elderly and those with mental health problems or learning disabilities.

Melia, K.M. (2013) *Ethics for Nursing and Healthcare Professionals*. London: Sage Publications.

This text provides a comprehensive overview of factors to consider when undertaking research in health care.

Modi, N., Vohra, J., Preston, J., Elliot, C., Van't Hoff, W., Coad, J., Gibson, F., Partridge, L., Brierley, J., Larcher, V. and Greenhough, A., for a Working Party of the Royal College of Paediatrics and Child Health (2014) Guidance on clinical research involving infants, children and young people: an update for researchers and research ethics committees. *Archives of Disease in Childhood*, 99(10): 887–891.

This paper provides a comprehensive overview of issues to consider when undertaking research involving pregnant women, babies, children and young people including challenging situations such as emergency care and children with life-limiting conditions.

Don't forget to visit https://study.sagepub.com/harveyandland to watch videos, take quizzes and to follow specially designed web activities.

PART IV

DATA ANALYSIS AND EVALUATION

19

QUANTITATIVE DATA ANALYSIS: MEASURES OF CLINICAL EFFECTIVENESS

This chapter will explore how we can measure the effectiveness of treatments and interventions in health care and builds upon Chapter 7. In this chapter we will:

- identify the different measures used to determine the clinical effects of treatment
- examine the difference between traditional medical statistics and measures of clinical effectiveness
- use a worked example to demonstrate how relative risk ratios, absolute risk ratios, odds ratios and number needed to treat are calculated and interpreted
- identify the role of *p*-values and confidence intervals in the analysis of data.

As part of our continuing professional development, we are encouraged to keep up to date with current research, which means that we need to read research articles relating to our area of practice on a regular basis. At the very least we might just skip to the conclusion section and trust the researcher's findings because we perceive that if the research is published in a health journal, then the findings must be accurate. In most cases this is true and the peer review that papers undergo before they appear in print assure us that findings of a study result from appropriate statistical analysis, but sometimes we may come across research that may not be so rigorous. An understanding of data analysis and how findings are produced helps health care professionals to determine whether an intervention is of benefit to their patients and whether it is worth using it in terms of cost or side effects, for example. It is also important that nurses, midwives, allied health professionals and medical practitioners can communicate their views of current research based upon a comprehensive appraisal of the research literature that includes an understanding of the process of data analysis.

The problem with medical statistics is that we need a good grounding and education in the subject to do this effectively but many (although not all) do not find this particularly appealing. Greenhalgh (1997a, 1997b) provides two seminal papers on how to interpret statistics in a randomised controlled trial, including how researchers 'cheat' to produce results that appear significant. These provide a basic but very useful guide for reading research papers where there is limited understanding of statistical analysis.

A different method of analysing data has emerged which is not only more easily calculated but also easier to interpret. See Figure 19.1 and remember this for later in the chapter. Many studies will now use **relative risk** (RR), absolute risk (AR), **odds ratios** (OR) and **number needed to treat** (NNT) to describe the results of a trial instead of traditional methods of analysis using *t* tests, for example. A clue to the difference in the two

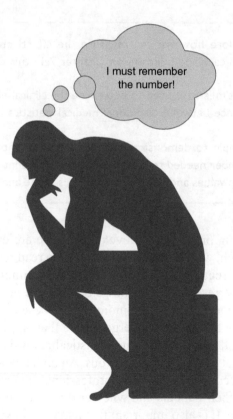

Figure 19.1   Remember

styles of analysis is in their names – one establishes *statistical significance* whereas the other measures *clinical effectiveness*. For example, a researcher could produce a perfect research study and exemplary data analysis to conclude that a new medication reduces a person's diastolic blood pressure by 1 mmHg compared to an existing one, and declare that the result is statistically significant. In the real world we need to consider whether a reduction of 1 mmHg is clinically effective and therefore worth the effort of changing a patient's medication. In this way measures of clinical effectiveness provide an analysis which is directly relevant to a patient's situation.

WHY DO WE NEED STATISTICS ANYWAY?

Almost everyone has a favourite remedy for an ailment and will swear by it. The use of 'special family remedies' for a cold seems to be something widely practised by people all over the world, but how well they work remains anecdotal. It may be that this remedy works on some people or at least the *belief* that it works is sufficient to give the impression that they feel better, but on this basis we wouldn't use this intervention on every person in these countries without establishing that it works by more scientific means.

Statistics is about dealing with uncertainty and variation, and the aim of statistical analysis is to establish that an intervention or medication will work on most of the people

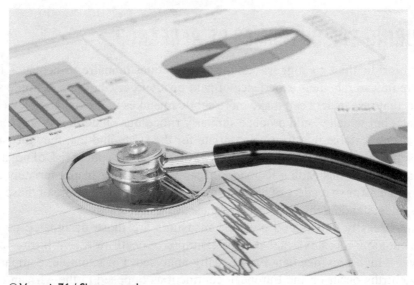

© Voronin76 / Shutterstock

most of the time. Statisticians place a numerical value on the term 'most of the people most of the time' by declaring that an intervention should demonstrate a real effect at least 95 times out of a 100 for it to be beneficial to patients. This is an oversimplification but it is the basis of something called probability and this concept will be revisited later in the chapter.

We know that humans differ in their response to an illness, with some suffering worse with their condition than others, and we also recognise that they will respond differently to the same treatments. For this reason doctors diagnose and treat patients probabilistically, that is, they reason that there is a strong probability that someone has a particular condition and that there is an equally strong probability that a certain treatment will alleviate that condition. Before the widespread use of randomised controlled trials doctors used their experience to determine what would be best for their patients and this sometimes resulted in the use of unusual or bizarre treatments.

A former editor of the *British Medical Journal*, Richard Smith, presented a television programme about evidence-based practice and in the opening scene he is standing by the grave of a woman who had several treatments for her arthritis including being fed raw liver sandwiches, having all her teeth removed as well as taking both steroids and non-steroidal anti-inflammatory medication. He used this example to illustrate that treatments were driven more by fashion than evidence. Much has changed but there are probably still some practitioners who have treatment preferences when there is good evidence that alternative treatments are better. How this is decided depends upon the fundamental question of how we measure the effect of an intervention.

MEASURING THE OUTCOMES OF RESEARCH

It would be ridiculous to suggest administering a questionnaire to neonates in a specialist care unit to rate their experience of pain post-surgery, but this example serves to remind us that researchers can make more subtle mistakes in the method they choose to collect data, but which would produce similarly ridiculous outcomes. It is essential that the data are collectable in a form appropriate for the study and that they measure what they are supposed to measure otherwise the whole research is put at risk of not achieving its aims and worse, misleading its readers. Inappropriate data inappropriately analysed compound the error so readers of health care research need to be aware of these potential errors by understanding the basic rules of measuring outcomes.

The most easily understood outcome measures are those designated as discrete. Discrete outcome measures include, for example, a death or a live birth – a 'yes or no' answer which provides data that is easily analysed. For example, comparing how many live births occur on the European continent as opposed to the African continent per head of population. Two elements of discrete measures need to be considered here, risk and rate. In terms of risk, for example, we might assess the number of people who develop cancer as a result of living near electricity pylons. Rate refers to the actual number of events that occur, for example, the number of deaths that can be directly related to smoking.

The other type of outcome measure is described as continuous and might include a reduction in diastolic blood pressure or pain score or an increase in quality of life. The first of these examples is more easily measured, as we have calibrated instruments to measure it. Measures of quality of life and pain tend to be subjective so we have to be more circumspect about the way in which we collect these data and how they are then analysed. There are a whole host of continuous measures used in health research which require analysis, all of which need to be considered in the context that they are presented.

A FIRST ANALYSIS OF THE DATA

In Chapter 7 we identified that randomisation was needed to makes sure that participants in both the experimental and control arms were equal in terms of baseline equivalence. When we come to the results we need to establish that the participants were indeed equal in the characteristics important to the study. Take for example a study of age related conditions and treatment. We should expect at baseline that both groups would have a similar age range otherwise the direct effects of treatment would not be a fair comparison (refer back to Chapter 7).

AVERAGES, MEAN, MEDIAN AND MODE

It is important to use the right measure to compare the groups and this is often done by comparing the average or mean of the groups in respect of the relevant characteristic. In Figure 19.2 we can see a range of ages of people and by summing their total age (200) then dividing this by the number of people in the group (5), the result is an average age of 40, but looking at the data we can see that actually three of the five people are only 25, so 40 doesn't appear to be representative of the age characteristic of the group because there are two people who are much older. In this case it would be more appropriate to use a median, which is the middle value from the range, which in this case is 25 and is more representative of the group.

The mean cannot be used when instruments are used that provide a score, for example, a Likert type scale (Table 19.1). It is a nonsense to use the mean, if we try $(30 + 32 + 10 + 8 + 20 = 100 \div 5 = 20)$ what does the 20 represent? Agreement or disagreement or something in between?

A third 'average' can be calculated called the mode, which is the value that occurs most often. This can be determined from Figure 19.2 as 25.

Table 19.1   Likert type data

Strongly disagree	Disagree	Don't know	Agree	Strongly agree
30	32	10	8	20

Mean Age 25, 25, 25, 50, 75

$25 + 25 + 25 + 50 + 75 = 200 \div 5 = \underline{40}$

Median 25, 25, <u>25</u>, 50, 75

Mode <u>25, 25, 25</u>, 50, 75 (occurs most often)

Figure 19.2   Determining the mean, median and mode

CALCULATING MEASURES OF EFFECT

The purpose of a randomised controlled trial is to determine whether one treatment or intervention is better than another or better than nothing at all. This can be done by constructing a 2×2 table (Table 19.2). Using this table we can enter the results of a trial and calculate relative and absolute risk ratios, odds ratios and number needed to treat or **number needed to harm** (NNH).

CLINICAL SCENARIO

The principles of evidence-based practice demand that the research process begins and ends in clinical practice and so we will use a scenario to demonstrate the calculation and interpretation of specific effect measures.

Imagine there is a threat of a swine flu epidemic and that there is a vaccination currently available, but there is a need for a more effective vaccine to protect people, particularly the vulnerable, and it has become an urgent public health issue. Scientists have developed a new vaccine which they have trialled in accordance with the conventions outlined in Chapter 7 and we need to assess whether it is better than the existing one.

Table 19.2   Calculating effect measures

	Disease		
Exposure	Yes	No	
Yes	a	b	a + b
No	c	d	c + d
	a + c	b + d	

THE CLINICAL BOTTOM LINE: IS THE NEW VACCINE BETTER THAN THE OLD ONE?

The results of this trial are recorded in Table 19.3. You can see from this table, for example, that 43 people who received the new vaccine got swine flu, whilst 52 who had the old vaccine got swine flu. On the face of it there doesn't seem to be much difference between the two vaccines but if we do some relatively simple calculations we can make an informed decision about which is better. Don't be put off by the formulae used in these calculations, there is no need to memorise them and all can be performed by using the calculator on your cell phone.

Table 19.3 Results from the trial of two vaccines for swine flu

	Swine flu		
Exposure	Had swine flu	Did not get swine flu	Total
Experimental group (new vaccine)	43	237	280
Control group (old vaccine)	52	198	250
Total	95	435	

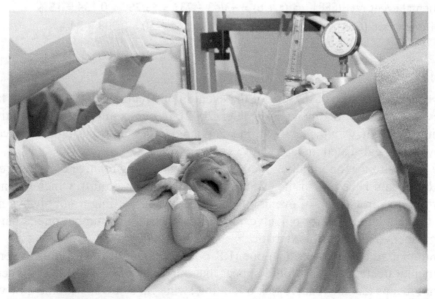

© nattanan726 / iStock

RISK

The first piece of information we can retrieve is to determine what risk the control group has of getting swine flu using the old vaccine and similarly what risk the experimental group are at by using the new vaccine (Table 19.4). If we call getting the flu despite vaccination an event, we can compare the number of events in each group; that is, if swine flu occurs in the group taking the new (experimental) vaccine we have an **experimental event rate** (EER). Similarly if we count the number of people getting swine flu in the old (control) vaccine we have a **control event rate** (CER). If we convert the formula to numbers extracted from Table 19.4 you can see that if people use the new vaccine they are at 15% risk of getting flu, whereas if people use the old vaccine they are at 21% risk of getting flu. It appears now that we may have a clearer picture of which vaccine is most effective. We do need to go further, however, as a more reliable calculation can be performed and one which is often used in the analysis of clinical trials.

Table 19.4   Event rates

Exposure		Swine flu		
		Had swine flu	Did not get swine flu	Total
Experimental group (new vaccine)	Yes	43	237	280
Control group (old vaccine)	No	52	198	250
Total		95	435	

Experimental event rate (EER) = a/(a + b) = 43/43 + 237 = 43/280 = 0.154 = **15%**
Control event rate (CER) = c/(c + d) = 52/52 + 198 = 52 /250 = 0.208 = **21%**

RELATIVE RISK

Relative risk is the ratio of the risk of the event in one regimen compared with the risk of an event in another regimen (Earl-Slater, 2002). In our example it is the relative risk of getting swine flu with the new vaccine compared to getting flu using the old vaccine. See how this is calculated in Table 19.5.

The number one is an important number in understanding relative risk (Figure 19.1). If the RR equals 1 the risk of the event is the same in both groups, which means there is *no difference* in the risk of events of both treatments. We might not always need to calculate the relative risk for ourselves, but remembering the number one is handy for reading papers that report this statistic.

If the relative risk is lower than one (RR = <1), the risk of the event is lower in the experimental treatment, so it would appear that our value of 0.74 (which is indeed less than one) means that the relative risk of getting swine flu is lower with the new vaccine compared to the old one.

Table 19.5   Calculating the relative risk ratio

Exposure		Swine flu		
		Had swine flu	**Did not get swine flu**	**Total**
Experimental group (new vaccine)	Yes	43	237	280
Control group (old vaccine)	No	52	198	250
Total		95	435	
Relative risk (RR) EER/CER = a/(a + b) / c/(c + d) = 0.154/0.208 = **0.74**				

If the relative risk is above one (RR > 1), the risk of the event is higher in the experimental treatment, therefore had the result been higher than the number one, the risk of getting swine flu would have been higher with the new vaccine. On first appearance it may seem that these are complex calculations, but in fact they are relatively quick and simple.

ODDS RATIO

The odds ratio is a measure of treatment effectiveness; it is the ratio of two odds (Earl-Slater, 2002). This is even simpler to calculate (see Table 19.6) and in our example produces the value 0.69. Using the number one as our reference point we can apply the same principle to understand that if the OR equals one the odds are the same in both groups (equivalent) and therefore there is no difference in the effect of either treatment.

If the OR is lower (OR < 1), the odds of the event are lower and the treatment effect is better in the experimental group. That is, the experimental swine flu vaccine is better. Since 0.69 is lower than one, we can make this conclusion.

If the OR is higher than one (OR > 1), the odds of the event are higher, which means the control groups has the better treatment effect and means in our example that the old vaccine has a better treatment effect.

Table 19.6   Calculation of the odds ratio

Exposure		Swine flu		
		Had swine flu	**Did not get swine flu**	**Total**
Experimental group (new vaccine)	Yes	43	237	280
Control group (old vaccine)	No	52	198	250
Total		95	435	
Odds ratio (OR) = (a/b)/(c/d) = 43/237/52/198 = 0.19/0.26 = **0.69**				

To make it even simpler, we could represent the OR visually (see Figure 19.3). This is called a forest plot and although this figure is a very simplified one the results of the swine flu trial can be visualised easily. The 'line of 1' is seen here as the vertical line and the horizontal line provides us with an axis along which we can plot our result.

In summary, the use of risk and odds ratios can tell use a great deal. Relative risk ratios might help to put a numerical value about the risk of having a live birth in Europe compared to Africa and an odds ratio might help us interpret how clinically effective a reduction of 1 mmHg in diastolic blood pressure actually is.

Website
activity 19.1

NUMBER NEEDED TO TREAT

The number needed to treat represents the number of patients who must be treated in order to achieve a result. In our example we could find out how many people we need to give the new vaccine in order to prevent one person from getting swine flu. It can be used as a measure of treatment effect, although it needs to be regarded in the context of the treatment it provides. The calculation for this is slightly more convoluted because it involves more than one step, although the sums themselves are not particularly challenging. To arrive at an NNT we first need to calculate the absolute risk reduction, which is the absolute arithmetic difference between the control event rate and the experimental event rate. See the rough calculation in Figure 19.4 and refer back to Table 19.5 as a reminder of how experimental event rates and control event rates are calculated. The absolute risk reduction is 6%. This can also be visualised in Figure 19.4.

To ascertain the number needed to treat using our rough measurements we produce a number needed to treat of 14 (Figure 19.4). This means that for every 14 people treated with the new vaccine one additional person would be protected compared to the control group. If this seems difficult to grasp it makes more sense if we think about the real-world need for mass vaccination (see Table 19.7). In this way you can see that the additional protection is considerable given that vaccination programmes are generally very large.

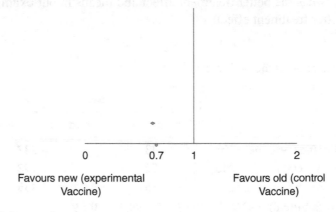

Figure 19.3   A forest plot

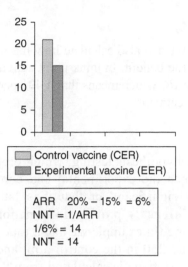

ARR   20% − 15% = 6%
NNT = 1/ARR
1/6% = 14
NNT = 14

Figure 19.4 Absolute risk reduction

Table 19.7 Calculating the absolute risk reduction

Number of people given a vaccine	Number likely to be protected using new vaccine	Number likely to be protected using old vaccine
98	105	98
980	1050	980
9,800	10,500	9,800
98,000	105,000	98,000
980,000	105,0000	980,000
9,800,000	10,500,000	9,800,000
Additional number protected	700,000	

THINK POINT ACTIVITY   19.1

It is estimated that 735,000 Americans die from a heart attack every year (Center for Disease Control Atlanta). The ISIS2 Trial demonstrated that the NNT (lives saved) for those receiving aspirin for a suspected heart attack is 42. Calculate how many additional lives would be saved if this treatment was given to all of these people.

NUMBER NEEDED TO HARM

Using the same calculation we can also calculate how harmful a treatment might be and whether the risks outweigh the benefit. In think point activity 19.2 the NNH is 167 with regard to *non-dangerous bleeds,* which means that 4,401 people may have a non-dangerous bleed as a result of the treatment.

CONFIDENCE INTERVALS

In Chapter 7 we looked at hypothesis testing, which produces a decision about any observed difference between the experimental and control group, either that this difference is 'statistically significant' or that it is 'statistically non-significant'. In contrast, **confidence intervals** provide information about the range of the observed effect. In our swine flu example we had a total sample of 530 people, 280 in the experimental arm and 250 in the control arm, and when a sample of data is taken from a process, and a statistic is calculated from that sample of data, we have to remember that the statistic doesn't necessarily represent the entire population, it's just a sample! If the flu vaccine trial were repeated again and again on different people, even if they had similar characteristics it is possible that we might produce a different answer.

So, because sample statistics don't necessarily reflect the true process, we place an interval around each statistic, and say that we are confident that the true process statistics fall within those intervals. Those intervals are known as confidence intervals.

AN EXAMPLE

We could estimate some characteristic of a population, for example, the average length of a newborn baby by measuring the length of every newborn baby born during a specified time on one designated maternity unit. That is, we ask all the mothers (this may number a couple of dozen) if we could measure their babies. We then calculate the average length of these babies, and presume this average to be the same as that of all newborn babies.

Unfortunately, we know that's not completely accurate. In fact, if we were to sample again, we'd likely find a somewhat different average. A third would likely produce yet another. Occasionally, we'd even find a baby who was much longer and get a really bizarre result.

So a confidence interval is just a range that we believe will include the true population parameter 'most of the time' – that is, to some level of confidence. When we say that we are 95% confident that the average length of a newborn baby is between 46 cm (18 inches) and 56 cm (22 inches), we mean that if we repeated our sampling procedure say, 1,000 times, 95% of the time (950 out of 1,000) the calculated interval would include the true mean length of a newborn baby.

In addition to calculating the risk or odds ratio and the confidence intervals, a third piece of information is required to estimate the significance of the result, which we call statistical significance. In Chapter 7 we looked at the role of statistical significance in determining whether there was a real difference in treatments that were unlikely to have occurred by chance. There was a note of caution to this explanation, which identified the difference between statistical significance and clinical significance by using an example (refer back to Chapter 7). When using measures of clinical effectiveness we still need an idea of whether the probability that the odds ratio calculated in this chapter for the new influenza vaccine represents a clinical or practical significance. Confidence intervals help here because they place a parameter around where the true value is said to lie, but it is also usual to calculate the statistical significance, which involves the production of a p-value.

P is short for probability and a p-value is a number between 0 and 1 and is interpreted in the following way:

- A small p-value (typically ≤ 0.05) indicates strong evidence against the null hypothesis, so you reject the null hypothesis. (See Chapter 7 for an explanation of the null hypothesis.)
- A large p-value (> 0.05) indicates weak evidence against the null hypothesis, so you fail to reject the null hypothesis.
- p-values very close to the cutoff (0.05) are considered to be marginal (could go either way).

For example, suppose an out-patient department claims their waiting times for an appointment are 30 minutes or less on average but you think they are more than that. You conduct a hypothesis test because you believe the null hypothesis (H_0), that the mean delivery time is 30 minutes max, is incorrect. Your alternative hypothesis (H_1) is that the mean time is greater than 30 minutes. You randomly sample some out-patient waiting time records and analyse the data, and your p-value turns out to be 0.001. In real terms, this means that there is a probability that there is a 1 in 1,000 chance you will mistakenly reject the out-patient department's claim that all patients are seen within 30 minutes of their appointment time. Since typically we are willing to reject the null hypothesis when this probability is less than 0.05, you can conclude that the out-patient data do not support their claim and waiting times are in fact more than 30 minutes on average. See further reading for additional information.

SUMMARY

In this chapter we have learned how several measures of clinical effectiveness can be calculated. In normal day-to-day practice, health professionals would not need to perform these calculations but some understanding of how we arrive at the measures is important in the critical evaluation of papers we need to read.

FURTHER READING

Davies, H.T.O. and Crombie, I.K. (2009) What are confidence intervals and p-values? www.medicine.ox.ac.uk/bandolier/painres/download/whatis/what_are_conf_inter.pdf (last accessed 7 June 2016).

A useful PDF exploring one of the key questions in health statistics.

Kent, R.A. (2014) *Analysing Quantitative Data*. London: Sage Publications.

A good overview of research using quantitative data, this book includes case-based methods as well as variable-based methods. It uses multidisciplinary non-experimental data-sets, including one big case study about alcohol consumption in Scotland.

Salkind, N.J. (2016) *Statistics for People Who (Think They) Hate Statistics* (6th edn). London: Sage Publications.

A very accessible introduction that can help you get to grips with statistics and to understand how analysing numbers fits into your broader research.

Don't forget to visit https://study.sagepub.com/harveyandland to watch videos, take quizzes and to follow specially designed web activities.

20

MANAGING AND ANALYSING QUALITATIVE DATA

In this chapter, we will explore qualitative data analysis in depth and in doing so we will:

- explore issues surrounding the transcription of data recordings or field notes
- explore the principles of qualitative data analysis
- consider the most commonly utilised methods of qualitative data analysis: thematic analysis, conversation analysis and interpretative phenomenological analysis
- explore factors that the researcher should consider when undertaking qualitative data analysis; this will include consideration of ethical, moral, legal and professional responsibilities.

In the previous chapter we explored quantitative data analysis. It is now time for the analysis of qualitative data to take centre stage. Some would-be researchers, particularly perhaps those who are not enthusiastic about mathematics, tend to assume that qualitative analysis is easier and more straightforward than quantitative data analysis. However, the analysis of qualitative data can present challenges for the researcher and we will explore some of these in this chapter.

As we have identified in earlier chapters qualitative data can be generated in a number of ways (see Chapters 8 and 17). The first challenge for the researcher is to turn these data into a usable format for data analysis. In most cases this requires the data to be in text format (Miles et al., 2014). Some data collection methods, such as written diaries and the responses to open questions on a questionnaire, will already be in the form of words. However, others, such as audio-recordings from interviews and focus groups will need to be turned into text and artwork will need to be described and summarised.

TRANSCRIPTION OF DATA RECORDINGS

The transcription of audio- and video-recordings is an integral, but often overlooked part of the data analysis process (Bird, 2005). Although voice recognition software is currently being developed and refined at a rapid pace, audio-recordings usually need to be transcribed into a word-processing document. The researcher will firstly have to decide who carries out the transcription. A number of factors will influence their decision:

- time
- cost
- resources and skills available
- data security
- maintaining confidentiality
- the nature of the recordings
- potential impact on the transcriber
- impact on the data analysis process.

There are varying opinions about whether or not the researcher should carry out the transcription. A strong argument for the researcher doing this is that doing the transcription becomes the first phase of the data analysis process. As the researcher listens to the recordings and types the text, he or she will be thinking about the data. Even at this very early stage the researcher will begin to notice similarities and differences, aspects of the data that are unusual or surprising and connections in the data. Another reason why researchers often transcribe their data is cost. It may simply be too expensive to pay someone else to do this. However, transcription is time consuming. Estimates vary and the length of time will depend on the typing skills of the transcriber, the quality of the recording and the nature of the discussion. However, it is suggested that a one-hour recording can take five to eight hours to transcribe (Smith and Osborn, 2008). If more than one participant is speaking, as in a focus group, the process will take longer.

If the researcher transcribes the data, he or she will need to do this in an appropriate environment. They will need a quiet, private location where the data can be securely stored. If someone else is transcribing the data, this may be someone doing this as a favour for the researcher or as casual work. Whilst it is understandable that these sorts of arrangements might be made, the researcher needs to be very careful that data are stored securely and that any other research governance requirements (see Chapter 18) and employment arrangements are not breached. There are a number of professional organisations who will transcribe data. Whilst these might be more costly, the turnaround is usually very quick and they should have established strategies in place for the secure transfer and storage of data and agreements about maintaining confidentiality.

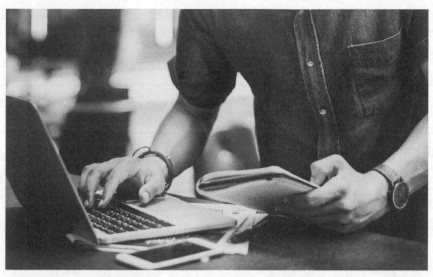

© Rawpixel.com / Shutterstock

The nature of the recording should also influence the researcher's decision about who transcribes the data. Recordings that involve complex terms may be a challenge and more time consuming for those who are unfamiliar with the terminology. The researcher should also consider the potential impact on the transcriber (Rager, 2005; Wilkes et al., 2015) because the content of recordings can sometimes be distressing. The researcher may need to carefully select which tapes someone other than themselves transcribes. Recordings involving highly emotional incidents and/or when participants became distressed should probably not be included for external transcription.

The researcher will need to decide if all or just part of the recording should be transcribed. One of the risks of partial transcription is that important or significant data may be overlooked (Alcock and Iphofen, 2007). Similarly, digressions or seemingly irrelevant data may become important during data analysis (Richards, 2009). Whilst it may not be necessary to transcribe the researcher's questions verbatim (word for word), summarising these will only make a small reduction in the overall transcription process.

There are no standard rules regarding the format for transcription. For example, some researchers advocate that every line is numbered, whilst others find this distracting and unnecessary. Nevertheless, there are practical issues to be addressed. The researcher should decide which conventions should be used before the process commences (Bird, 2005; Brinkmann and Kvale, 2015). For example, should intonations and emotional expressions such as laughter be included and should the length of pauses be timed? To some extent, the format of the transcription will be determined by the type of data

Website
activity 20.1

analysis to be conducted (see below). In most cases, however, the recordings should be transcribed verbatim and therefore pauses, intonations, emotional expressions, incomplete words and overlapping speech should be transcribed (see Box 20.1).

BOX 20.1   SUGGESTED TRANSCRIPTION CONVENTIONS

UPPER CASE	Speaking loudly
Italics	Stressing or emphasising a point
(0.5)	Pauses in tenths of a second
((...))	Explanation of additional information
-	Incomplete word, either cut off or self-terminated
(inaudible)	Words that cannot be identified
[....]	Overlapping speech

Taken in part from Gibson and Brown (2009: 120–121)

EXAMPLE

Participant:	So I said to her, the nurse at X ((hospital)), HOW DARE YOU, I mean (0.3), she was, you know, really rude to me.
Researcher:	And how did that-
Participant:	Well, I thought, I'm not coming here again ((laughs)).

ANALYSING THE DATA

Having converted all of the data to words, the researcher now needs to decide what to do with them. The purpose of qualitative data analysis is to understand meaning and to provide an accurate portrayal of that meaning for others (Robson, 2011). Qualitative researchers also endeavour to determine individual interpretations of phenomena and the impact of the context (Yardley, 2008). Although a number of strategies and frameworks for qualitative data analysis exist, there is no definitive method for this process in the way that there is for quantitative data analysis (Jacelon and O'Dell, 2005; Braun and Clarke, 2006). In addition, some frameworks have been criticised for being too restrictive (Van der Zalm and Bergum, 2000).

However, whichever method of qualitative data analysis is used, the fundamental principles are the same. Qualitative data analysis is an iterative process (Robson, 2011). This means that the researcher engages in a 'conversation' with the data in order to facilitate their understanding and interpretation. To do this, the researcher must be open and curious (Johnson, 2000; Jacelon and O'Dell, 2005). A phrase that is often used to describe the perspective that the researcher must take is 'standing in the shoes of the participants'. In their interpretation, the researcher will draw on their personal experiences whether intentionally or otherwise (Birks et al., 2008; Richards, 2009). Qualitative methods can therefore be referred to as being dialectical; whereby the researcher is affected by the phenomena they seek to understand and in turn affects the phenomena themselves (Coyle, 2007; Birks et al., 2008). As a consequence the researcher should reflect throughout the study on their preconceived ideas and the impact of these on their interpretation of the findings (Yardley, 2008) (see Chapter 21).

The ultimate aim of qualitative data analysis is to make sense of the data and present the researcher's interpretation without losing the essence of the data or contrasting views. Therefore the richness and nuances within the data must be retained. Doing qualitative data analysis is rather like doing a jigsaw without the picture, whereby the researcher sifts through the pieces (the data) and makes a picture. However, unlike a jigsaw puzzle, when doing qualitative analysis, more than one picture could be produced. This is because the idiosyncratic nature of qualitative research means that it is likely that two researchers analysing the same data would generate similar but in some ways different findings. However, rather than seeing this as a flaw, proponents of qualitative research believe that this potential for individual interpretation is the strength of the research (Rolfe, 2006).

PRINCIPLES OF QUALITATIVE DATA ANALYSIS

Whilst a number of methods of qualitative data analysis exist (see below), the fundamental principles are the same. Therefore the following overview applies whichever specific method is used. In terms of the actual process, the key features are generally the same and include the following phases:

- breaking down the data into manageable pieces
- reviewing and organising the data
- building the data into manageable portions so the findings can be reported. (adapted from Miles et al., 2014)

When exactly does qualitative data analysis begin? Some might argue that it begins during the collection of the very first data for the study, for example, during the first interview or focus group. The researcher will be thinking about the key issues arising from the participant's responses, actions or comments during the data collection process. Even if this view is not supported, qualitative data analysis usually begins early on in a study. This is because, irrespective of the specific research method used, the initial analysis is likely to be used to inform subsequent data collection as the two processes usually occur concurrently (Miles et al., 2014; Polit and Beck, 2014).

The researcher should keep an audit trail which documents the data collection and analysis processes from beginning to end. This is usually done by keeping a research diary. In this, the researcher reflects on the data and their actions and decisions as they collect and analyse them. This audit trail will be invaluable when the researcher writes up the study and can also be a powerful tool in the facilitation of rigour within the study (see Chapter 21). Each episode of data collection and analysis should be reflected on either during, or as soon as possible after, the event to ensure accurate recall.

If transcription has taken place, the transcripts must be checked against the recordings. Any transcription errors should be corrected. These usually occur because the recording has been misheard rather than any malicious intent. Nevertheless, inaccurate transcription can change the meaning of the data so the researcher should ensure the transcripts are as accurate as possible.

The researcher should then read and re-read the data. The phrase that is commonly used in relation to this phase is that the researcher becomes 'immersed' in the data.

THINK POINT ACTIVITY   20.1

Think about the statement that the researcher becomes immersed in the data. What do you think this means? To help you, think about the meaning of the word 'immerse'.

As they read through the data, the key questions the researcher should ask are:

- What stands out here?
- What are my initial thoughts about this?
- What surprises me about this?
- What is unexpected about this?
- What about this is as I would have expected?

It may be helpful at this stage to draw a mind-map that illustrates these initial thoughts (see Figure 20.1).

Although qualitative methods generally involve small samples, they usually generate vast quantities of data and this can be overwhelming. The researcher therefore needs to decide how the data will be organised and managed. In the past, researchers used what is

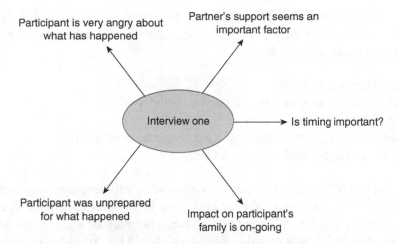

Figure 20.1   Example of a mind-map illustrating a researcher's initial thoughts following an interview

sometimes called the 'long table approach'. As the name suggests this involves laying out the data, for example, a focus group transcript or field notes from an observation, on a long table or perhaps the floor. In this way all the data from one episode of data collection can be seen at the same time. Using highlighter pens, Post-it notes and annotations the researcher then codes the text from start to finish. To do this, codes are assigned to portions of the text. The researcher gives a name or a label to the code which captures the essence of or summarises the data. Codes may be descriptive (factual) such as 'antenatal care' or 'wound treatment', or they may be interpretative (analytical) such as 'anger' or 'isolation'.

As an alternative to the process described above, a paper copy of the data-set can be cut into sections of text, each of which represents a code. Note that if using this strategy the researcher will need lots of copies of each transcript, otherwise they will lose the perspective of the bigger picture and also risk losing important data.

In contrast to the manual approach, software packages such as NVivo or NUDIST can be used (Noble and Smith, 2014). These facilitate the management and organisation of data in a way that can be difficult to replicate manually (Jacelon and O'Dell, 2005; Plummer-D'Amato, 2008). Software packages enable the researcher to sort the data in one place and see them more clearly. However, the researcher still needs to do the thinking because the package does not create or assign codes to the text. This needs to be done by the researcher, whereby codes are created and sections of data are cut and pasted into the relevant code(s). The novice researcher will almost certainly need some training to use the software (O'Leary, 2014) and it must be acknowledged that some researchers ultimately find these packages more of a hindrance than a help (Noble and Smith, 2014).

Whether done manually or using a software package, coding can be a challenge, particularly for novice researchers. A useful strategy for the researcher is to constantly ask questions when looking at the data:

- What is happening here?
- What is the meaning of this comment or behaviour?
- Have I heard or seen this before?
- Is this something new, surprising, unexpected or contrasting?
- Why is this happening?

During the analysis of the first set of data the researcher will develop many, perhaps hundreds of codes. Some sections of the data may also be in several different codes simply because it covers a number of issues or the researcher may be unsure into which code it should go. Having initially coded a data-set, it should be reviewed for coding errors. When doing this, the researcher may find that several codes have been created for the same or similar feelings, behaviours or comments (see Box 20.2).

Website activity 20.2

BOX 20.2   EXAMPLE ILLUSTRATING THE GENERATION OF CODES

Simon has coded the first interview transcript from a study of mothers caring for a chronically ill child. Simon has created separate codes for text in which the participant talked about feeling isolated, lonely, abandoned, cut off and ignored by friends and family.

As part of the review, codes may be amended, amalgamated or perhaps separated. The researcher should also look for relationships, contrasts, associations and links between the codes. The use of memos and the researcher's reflective diary can help with this process by facilitating engagement with and exploration of the data (Birks et al., 2008; Charmaz, 2008). The second and subsequent sets of data are then coded following the same process. As the coding continues, the researcher will probably spend time amending the codes, perhaps renaming them, merging them together or creating new ones. This process continues until a final coding framework is produced.

It is quite likely that another person would code the data in a different way (Noble and Smith, 2014). Different names may be given to codes and there may be differences in interpretation. Therefore, whilst there will be many similarities, there may also be some differences. Neither approach to the coding will be wrong. The fundamental principle of qualitative data analysis is the researcher's interpretation of the data.

THINK POINT ACTIVITY   20.2

Think about a time when you have discussed a film or book with a group of friends. You will all have had slightly different interpretations of what you have seen or read. There may be commonalities in your interpretation of the film/book but it is also quite likely that at least one person will have interpreted some aspect of it in a different way.

Nevertheless, novice researchers and particularly those undertaking research as academic work may discuss their coding with a colleague or supervisor. This can be useful, because explaining what they have coded and why, means that the researcher must justify the decisions they have made. It may be that this discussion reveals to the researcher that there are gaps or duplications in their coding. In addition, if the researcher cannot explain their actions, the coding may need to be amended or their rationale strengthened.

In large qualitative studies, more than one person may be involved in the analysis of the data. Achieving consistency between data analysts (**inter-rater reliability**) can be a way of minimising coding errors or misunderstandings. However, involving more than one person can also present challenges and difficulties. This is because in many ways the ethos of qualitative data analysis is an individual's interpretation of the data (Grubs and Piantanida, 2010). Having more than one person involved may mean that compromises have to be made in order to reach some form of agreement.

Another way of checking for coding errors is to ask the participant to check the coded transcript. Whilst this process has been recommended (Polit and Beck, 2014), its usefulness has been questioned (Tuckett, 2005). Use of this strategy appears to support the notion of a fixed truth, yet this is counter to the underpinning philosophy of qualitative research. In addition, the accounts or behaviours of participants are context-bound (Angen, 2000). They may also forget what they meant, change their point of view, be unable to explain their actions or feel obliged to agree with or contradict the coding. Consequently, participant checking can lead to confusion rather than confirmation (Angen, 2000).

Website activity 20.3

The final phase of data analysis usually occurs when the researcher writes up the findings. The research report should clearly describe the data analysis process and quotes or excerpts from the data should be used to illustrate the codes. At this point, it is not unusual for the researcher to see connections and contradictions between the codes that they had not noticed before. Therefore, there may be some further adjustment to the coding framework. The researcher should avoid the temptation to use numerical values, such as percentages, to describe a code. Whilst the sample may reflect the population, it is unlikely to be numerically representative. It is therefore risky to use numerical values as others may use the information to inaccurately generalise the findings. When describing the data analysis process, the researcher should acknowledge the ways in which their prior knowledge and experiences may have unduly influenced data interpretation. Including all of this information means that the data analysis and findings section of a qualitative study are often quite lengthy.

METHODS OF QUALITATIVE DATA ANALYSIS

There are numerous specific ways in which qualitative data can be analysed and there are frameworks to support the process. The most commonly used qualitative data analysis methods are thematic analysis, **interpretative phenomenological analysis, conversation analysis, discourse analysis** and **content analysis**. However, it is important to note that a researcher need not necessarily be limited to using just one strategy in a study.

THEMATIC ANALYSIS

Website activity 20.4

This is the most commonly used method to analyse qualitative data. Using this method, text is coded into broad or key themes (or categories) and sub-themes. The process begins in the way previously described with the researcher reading and then re-reading the first transcript in order to become familiar with the data and to begin to develop an understanding. The transcript is then coded from start to finish. As the second and subsequent sets of data are coded the researcher begins to form these codes into themes with each theme capturing the essence of the data it contains. Gradually, as the researcher begins to make sense of the similarities, differences, links, patterns and contradictions between the themes, a framework or hierarchy evolves which consists of broad themes each of which incorporates a number of sub-themes. This thematic framework or hierarchy is like a large filing system which contains the data (see Box 20.3).

BOX 20.3   EXAMPLE ILLUSTRATING THE DEVELOPMENT OF A CODING FRAMEWORK

Imagine you are filing the notes that you have made during your nurse or midwifery training. One option would be to have different folders for different subject areas. For example, you may have individual folders for anatomy and physiology, psychology and pharmacology. In each folder, you will divide the notes into sections, for example, in your anatomy and physiology folder you might have a section for the circulatory system and one for the nervous system. Developing this filing system is the same approach that a researcher takes when using thematic analysis to develop a framework or hierarchy. The researcher designs the system and decides what goes where.

The key principle of thematic analysis is the *analysis* of the data. In the same way that you would critically analyse a paper used in an assignment, in thematic analysis the researcher must demonstrate that they have analysed the data rather than just para-phrasing or describing it.

BOX 20.4   EXAMPLE ILLUSTRATING A BROAD THEME AND SUB-THEMES

In Simon's study of mothers' experiences of caring for a chronically ill child, he has identified a broad theme, which he has called 'I travel this journey alone'. This broad theme incorpo-rates a number of sub-themes, which include mothers talking about feeling unsupported by the health services and abandoned by family and friends.

As the analysis continues, the researcher will probably spend time amending the themes and sub-themes, perhaps renaming them, merging them or creating new themes and sub-themes (see Box 20.4). The process continues until all transcripts have been coded. At this point, the researcher reviews the entire framework and may make some final adjustments. Usually the researcher will have developed between four and six broad themes, each of which may incorporate a number of sub-themes. It is likely that some portions of text will appear in more than one sub-theme. It is also possible that some sub-themes will only contain data relating to one participant whilst others will contain data pertaining to almost all of them (Daly et al., 2007). This is to be expected, because the whole data-set should reflect a range of views, expe-riences and responses, and the contradictions are as important as the similarities. It should also be noted that a counter or contradictory theme also indirectly supports the opposing theme.

It is often stated that during thematic analysis the themes 'emerge' from the data. However, this notion is inaccurate because the researcher plays an active and integral part in the process of discovering and describing themes which are therefore both con-text- and researcher-related (Richards, 2009). To facilitate effective thematic analysis, a checklist devised by Braun and Clarke (2006: 96) can be utilised (see Table 20.1). Some of these issues will be explored in more depth in Chapter 21.

When the researcher writes up the findings of the thematic analysis, each theme and sub-theme should be described with excerpts of the data used as illustrations. A mind-map may be a helpful way of explaining the relationships between themes and sub-themes (see Figure 20.2). In writing up the analysis, the researcher may see

Table 20.1   Checklist to facilitate effective thematic analysis

Process	Criteria
Transcription	Data transcribed to an appropriate level of detail.
	Transcripts checked for accuracy.
Coding	Each data item given equal attention in coding process.
	Coding process thorough, inclusive and comprehensive.
	All relevant extracts for all themes collated.
	Themes checked against each other and original data-set.
	Themes coherent, consistent and distinctive.
Analysis	Data have been analysed rather than paraphrased or described.
	Extracts illustrate analysis.
	Analysis presents a convincing and well-organised argument.
	Enough time allocated to adequately complete the analysis.
Writing report	Assumptions about and specific approach to analysis clearly explicated.
	Described method and reported analysis are consistent.
	Language and concepts used are consistent with epistemological position of analysis.
	Researcher active in the process, themes have not just emerged.

Source: adapted from Braun and Clarke (2006: 96)

connections and contradictions between the themes and sub-themes that they had not noticed previously. Writing the research report therefore becomes the final stage of the thematic analysis process.

INTERPRETATIVE PHENOMENOLOGICAL ANALYSIS (IPA)

This has many similarities to thematic analysis as previously described. It is an approach to analyse data commonly used in phenomenological studies. Using this approach the researcher actively draws on their prior knowledge and experiences when interpreting data. The phrase that is often used when referring to IPA is analytical induction, whereby the analysis or the findings come from the data.

In terms of the actual process, IPA researchers usually print off the data (e.g. an interview transcript). Annotations in the left hand margin identify codes whilst the researcher uses the right hand margin to make annotations about their analysis. Eventually the annotations on the right hand side become themes and sub-themes.

Website activity 20.5

CONVERSATION ANALYSIS

This method of qualitative data analysis is usually used to analyse naturally occurring everyday conversation between individuals rather than more formal interviews and

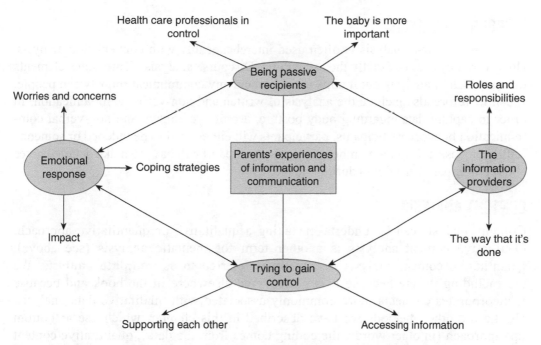

Figure 20.2 Mind-map of themes and sub-themes (Harvey et al., 2013: 362)

focus groups. Again, the general principles of conducting qualitative data analysis apply but in conversation analysis, the researcher is not only interested in *what* the participant says but also *how* they say it (O'Leary, 2014). The researcher therefore will analyse:

- the overall structure of the dialogue
- language and terminology used
- intonations and emphasis
- emotional expressions
- pauses and gaps
- repetition
- echoing
- turn taking
- the way in which new topics are introduced or terminated
- interruptions and overlapping speech
- metaphors and euphemisms used.

Website
activity 20.6

In order to ensure conversation analysis is undertaken correctly, detailed and accurate transcription is essential. The transcriptions will need to be carefully checked against the recordings before analysis can begin.

Website
activity 20.7

DISCOURSE ANALYSIS

The term discourse analysis is often used interchangeably with conversation analysis. However, they are not exactly the same thing. Discourse analysis incorporates elements of conversation analysis but it aims to understand any communication between people. It can therefore also include the analysis of written and non-verbal communication. In order to capture data regarding body posture, use of eye-contact and non-verbal communication between participants, participants will either need to be videoed or someone (either the researcher or a member of the research team) will have to make detailed notes about participant behaviours during the interaction.

Website activity 20.8

CONTENT ANALYSIS

Content analysis can be undertaken taking a qualitative or quantitative approach. Qualitative content analysis is another term for thematic analysis (see above). Quantitative content analysis is sometimes referred to as **template analysis**. We are including it here because it is not covered elsewhere in the book and because it incorporates elements more commonly associated with qualitative data analysis. Unlike the other methods we have described in this chapter, which use a 'bottom up' approach (in other words, the coding comes from the data), quantitative content analysis uses a 'top down' approach. This means that a coding framework is devised before data analysis begins. The researcher decides in advance what they are going to look for in the data and develops a list of codes or categories. In a similar way the questions from a structured questionnaire could be used as the coding framework. The researcher then reads through the data and counts the number of cases within that category (O'Leary, 2014). An advantage of this approach is that different coders should obtain the same results so long as the codes are clear and unambiguous. Content analysis can also be a useful way of analysing written material such as news reports or journal articles.

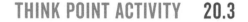

THINK POINT ACTIVITY   20.3

Website activity 20.9

Do you think content analysis, as described in this section, should be regarded as being a quantitative or qualitative method of data analysis? Give a rationale for your decision.

WHICH METHOD OF QUALITATIVE DATA ANALYSIS SHOULD I USE?

When it comes to choosing which method to use, a key factor for the researcher to consider is whether they should take a 'top down' approach or a 'bottom up' approach.

The choice of specific method should be determined by the research question and the research method used. However, as we have previously identified, thematic analysis is most commonly used.

CHALLENGES OF QUALITATIVE DATA ANALYSIS

THINK POINT ACTIVITY   20.4

Make a list of the challenges the researcher may face when undertaking qualitative data analysis.

As we identified at the beginning of this chapter, qualitative data analysis is not as straightforward as might be supposed. The researcher will encounter a number of challenges and these might include:

- Choosing which approach to use. Unlike quantitative data analysis there are no agreed 'rules' on how the process should be undertaken.
- The researcher may face criticism, particularly from proponents of quantitative research. They have to justify the approach they have taken and counter the view that subjectivity and bias are the same thing (see Chapters 5 and 21).
- For most of the methods we have described the researcher must allow the codes or themes and the subsequent framework or hierarchy to come from the data. This process should not be rushed. Qualitative data analysis requires a lot of thinking time and it can therefore be a lengthy, time consuming and consequently costly process.
- To undertake qualitative data analysis the researcher must be creative and thoughtful. The researcher also needs to be able to 'think outside the box'.
- Unlike quantitative data analysis, which usually has only one 'answer', qualitative data analysis lends itself to multiple interpretations. Whilst advocates of qualitative research regard this as a strength, some can find the concept difficult to grasp.
- Keeping qualitative data analysis meaningful can be problematic as the researcher must ensure the subtleties, nuances and extremes are retained.

Website activity 20.10

SUMMARY

In this chapter we have explored qualitative data analysis. We have reviewed factors surrounding data transcription that the researcher should consider. We have explored the principles of qualitative data analysis and have reviewed the most commonly utilised methods of qualitative data analysis. We have also acknowledged the challenges that the researcher may face when undertaking qualitative data analysis.

FURTHER READING

Bazeley, P. (2013) *Qualitative Data Analysis: Practical Strategies*. London: Sage Publications.

This book provides a more detailed consideration of doing qualitative data analysis in the real world. It is very strong on the software you can use as well as providing practical tips and advice.

Grubs, R.E. and Piantanida, M. (2010) Grounded theory in genetic counseling research: an interpretive perspective. *Journal of Genetic Counseling*, 19(2): 99–111.

This paper includes discussion about constant comparison data analysis and provides examples of coding.

O'Leary, Z. (2014) *The Essential Guide to Doing Your Research Project* (2nd edn). London: Sage Publications.

See Chapter 14, 'Analysing qualitative data', a no-nonsense guide to incorporating qualitative data into your research project.

> Don't forget to visit https://study.sagepub.com/harveyandland to watch videos, take quizzes and to follow specially designed web activities.

21
RIGOUR

In this chapter, we will explore strategies that researchers can use to ensure their research is rigorous. In doing this we will:

- clarify definitions that are commonly used when describing strategies to ensure the production of good quality research, these terms will include validity, reliability, generalisability, trustworthiness and rigour
- consider the ways in which researchers can strengthen the rigour of quantitative research, this will include the use of pilot studies
- explore fidelity assessment of quantitative research
- consider the ways in which researchers can strengthen the rigour of qualitative and mixed methods research, this will include the use of Yardley's (2008) framework
- explore the concept of triangulation.

Throughout this book we have emphasised the importance of researchers ensuring that their research is robust, in other words is of good quality. In this chapter we will explore the strategies researchers can use to facilitate the production of good quality research. These strategies can also be used to effectively evaluate a research study (see Chapters 10, 14 and 22).

CLARIFYING TERMINOLOGY

THINK POINT ACTIVITY   21.1

We have previously referred to terms that are often used when discussing the production of good quality research earlier in the book. Try to give a definition for the following terms: validity, reliability, generalisability, trustworthiness and rigour.

Validity means 'truth'. In the context of research it refers to the extent to which what was intended to be measured, actually has been and that the findings are therefore accurate. There are several different types of validity:

- **Construct validity**: the outcome measure of the current study which has previously been confirmed or established in another study.
- **Content validity**: the extent to which a data collection tool encompasses all aspects of the variables being measured.
- **Face validity**: the extent to which a data collection tool appears to measure what is intended.
- **Internal validity**: the extent to which other possible explanations of the findings can be excluded.
- **External validity**: the extent to which the findings can be generalised to the total population and other settings.
- **Reliability**: this relates to the uniformity and accuracy of the data collection tool used and the researcher using it.

BOX 21.1   EXAMPLE OF A STRATEGY TO ENHANCE RELIABILITY

A study is being carried out to investigate the short term effect of a drug on blood pressure. The same piece of equipment is used by the same nurse (Sally) to measure all participants' blood pressure throughout the whole study. This is likely to be more reliable than the blood pressure being measured by ten nurses using ten different pieces of equipment.

Validity and reliability go hand-in-hand. In order for valid data to be collected the process for doing this must be reliable (see Box 21.1). However, reliability does not guarantee validity (see Box 21.2).

Website activity 21.1

BOX 21.2   EXAMPLE ILLUSTRATING LACK OF VALIDITY

In the scenario given above, at the end of the study it is discovered that Sally has been using a faulty piece of equipment. Therefore, whilst the data collection process has been reliable (i.e. done is a consistent way, by the same person) the data are not valid because the blood pressure readings are inaccurate.

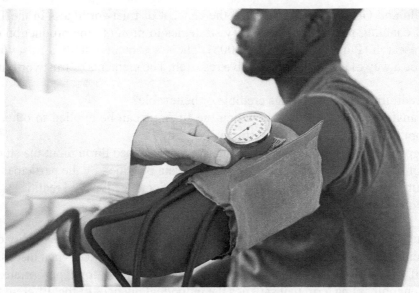

© annebaek / iStock

Generalisability is a term closely associated with quantitative research. It is the extent to which the findings of a study can be applied to the wider population. In order for this to be possible, the study sample must be representative of the wider or total population. Representativeness and generalisability therefore go hand-in-hand (see Chapter 15).

Whilst the terms validity, reliability and generalisability have become synonymous with quantitative research they have been deemed inappropriate in the context of qualitative research and the qualitative aspects of mixed methods studies (Gibson and Brown, 2009; Silverman, 2015). However, in order for their work to be universally accepted, some qualitative researchers use quantitative criteria when advocating the quality of their study (Yardley, 2008). This has been particularly apparent in nursing and midwifery research, in an attempt to attain 'scientific' acceptance (Rolfe, 2006). Differing views over the use of 'quantitative' terminology will be determined by an individual's beliefs and assumptions and the extent to which they uphold the ontological and epistemological suppositions upon which positivistic (quantitative) research is based (Angen, 2000). Nevertheless, rejection of the terms validity, reliability and generalisability does not mean that the quality of qualitative and mixed methods research is unimportant. The need for academic authenticity has led researchers, and those working in health care in particular, to finding other ways in which to determine the quality and legitimise their work (Angen, 2000; Thorne, 2008). Probably the most commonly used is the criteria devised by Lincoln and Guba (Houghton et al., 2013).

Lincoln and Guba (1985) introduced the concept of trustworthiness in the 1980s as a way of enabling researchers to identify strategies to promote the production of good quality research (Plummer-D'Amato, 2008). The assessment a study's trustworthiness can also be a way of evaluating qualitative research. The elements of trustworthiness are:

- Credibility: are the findings credible or believable?
- Transferability: the extent to which the findings can be applied to other similar populations in other similar settings.
- Dependability: the consistency of the approaches used throughout the study.
- Confirmability: do the findings reflect the data provided by the participants?
- Authenticity: do the findings portray a range of perspectives and realities? (Lincoln and Guba, 1985; Guba and Lincoln, 1994)

Given the polarisation of the specific terminology used in relation to the quality of quantitative and qualitative research (see Figure 21.1), we advocate that when discussing the quality of research in a more general way the term 'rigour' is more appropriate. Rigour is an all-encompassing term that satisfies the individual nuances of the different types of research. In the context of research, rigour means that the study has been conducted in a thorough, consistent and meticulous way, in accordance with the principles of the particular method and design used. A study conducted in a rigorous way will also generate accurate and believable findings.

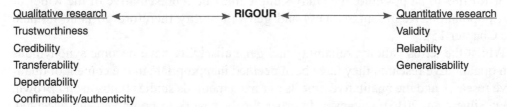

Figure 21.1 Strategies to promote and evaluate the quality of research

PROMOTING RIGOUR IN QUANTITATIVE RESEARCH

THINK POINT ACTIVITY   21.2

List the strategies a researcher could use to enhance the rigour of a quantitative study.

There are a number of ways in which a researcher can promote the rigour of a quantitative study and the quantitative aspects of a mixed methods study. If these strategies are adopted the research is more likely to be deemed valid and reliable and the data generalisable. Not all of the following strategies may apply to a particular study, but they could include:

- Addressing the research hypothesis, aim(s) and answering the research question(s). In other words the research has achieved what the researcher intended.
- Conducting a pilot study and assessing a study's **fidelity** (see below).
- Ensuring appropriate training for all the researchers involved in participant recruitment, data collection and data analysis to facilitate a consistent approach in accordance with the research proposal.
- Giving a detailed account of the way in which the research was conducted along with acknowledgement of any potential bias or limitations (Robson, 2011; Creswell, 2014; Silverman, 2015) (see Chapters 5 and 8).
- Considering the timing of the research, for example, are there any seasonal factors which may inadvertently influence the findings?
- Using an appropriate sampling strategy and having clearly defined inclusion and exclusion criteria (see Chapter 15).
- Establishing the content and face validity of the data collection tool by having it scrutinised by experts in the field, the research supervisor, colleagues, peers or people with the same characteristics as the participants in the proposed study (Dunne et al., 2014).
- Using previously validated data collection tools. However, the researcher should note that payment to the creator may be required.
- Ensuring that data collection tools to be completed by participants include clear and comprehensive instructions about when and how they should be completed and when and how they should be returned to the researcher. The need for accuracy should be highlighted.
- Using strategies that will promote validity and reliability of questionnaires identified in Chapter 16.
- Providing statistical assessment of the reliability of the data collection tool (see Chapter 19).
- Facilitating the return of the data collection tool: where appropriate a stamped address envelope should be provided with follow-up reminders as required.
- Minimising participant drop-out by maintaining contact with participants. The use of incentives may also be appropriate (see Chapter 18).
- Explaining strategies used to minimise the Hawthorne effect (see Chapter 7).
- Assessing intra- and inter-observer reliability when observations have been undertaken. This means ensuring there is consistency in the way that observation data are recorded over time. This can be easily done if the observations have been video-recorded. When two more researchers have been involved, inter-observer reliability can be assessed by checking whether they have documented the same information and in the same way. When only one researcher has been involved intra-observer reliability is more likely, but it should nevertheless be established.

PILOT STUDIES IN QUANTITATIVE RESEARCH

Website
activity 21.2

The use of a pilot study is a specific way in which the researcher can promote the validity, reliability and generalisability of a study (see Box 21.3). A preliminary pilot study is commonly used in larger-scale quantitative studies. A pilot study is a small-scale study which is carried out in exactly the same way, using the same methods of participant recruitment, data collection and data analysis that the researcher plans to use in the larger or main study. In other words, the pilot study is an exact replica of the proposed main study. A pilot study may sometimes be referred to as a **feasibility study**. This is because the purpose of this small-scale study is to determine the feasibility of the main study. A pilot study should not therefore be confused with a pre-test, which is the collection of data before manipulation of the independent variable in experimental research (see Chapters 4, 7 and 11).

BOX 21.3   EXAMPLE ILLUSTRATING THE VALUE OF CONDUCTING A PILOT STUDY

Despite careful planning of participant recruitment strategies, a pilot study may indicate that the main study is unlikely to recruit the required number of participants in the time available. Alternatively a pilot study may demonstrate that participants misunderstand the wording of a number of questions on a questionnaire.

As the examples above suggest, one of the advantages of doing a pilot study can be that they save time and money in the long run. Finding out from a pilot study that a questionnaire needs further development will reduce the likelihood that the researcher collects a large amount of unusable data in the main study. Collecting unusable data wastes the researcher's and participants' time, it has implications for the funders and indeed is unethical. It may therefore be assumed that all quantitative studies will involve a preliminary pilot study, but this is not always the case. This is usually because of time and financial pressures, particularly in smaller studies. However, as we have indicated, this may be a false economy in the long run.

If a pilot study has been undertaken there may be a number of issues that the researcher should consider. If it is identified that aspects of the research require change, for example, the strategy for recruiting participants or the design of the data collection tool, the resigned study should, in principle, be re-piloted before the main study is undertaken. However, time and financial pressures may prevent this from happening. Also, the researcher should consider whether the data from the pilot study should be added to the main study data for analysis. This might be feasible if the pilot and main study have been conducted in exactly the same way but the general view is that pilot and main study data should be kept separate (Peat, 2002). To illustrate this point, an increasing number of pilot studies have been published over recent years (Anderson et al., 2014; Booth, 2014).

ASSESSING THE FIDELITY OF QUANTITATIVE RESEARCH

Fidelity assessments are being increasingly undertaken (Teague et al., 2012; Dyas et al., 2014), particularly in large scale randomised controlled trials (Farchaus Stein et al., 2007; Lawton et al., 2011). Fidelity assessment involves evaluation of the way in which the study was conducted to determine the validity, reliability and generalisability of the findings. In order to undertake the assessment, two approaches are commonly taken. Firstly, aspects of the research process are evaluated in a quantitative way in relation to the study protocol or **standard operating procedures** (SOPs). The SOPs explain in detail each aspect of the research so that in effect they become the 'operation manual'. Fidelity assessment therefore determines whether the study has been conducted in the way it was intended. Aspects of the fidelity assessment may include determining whether:

- members of the research team were adequately prepared (did they attend the required training sessions before the study commenced?)
- researchers adhered to the study protocol/SOPs in all aspects of the research process
- participants were recruited in accordance with the study protocol/SOP
- participants receive the allocated treatment/intervention (experimental or control)
- data collection tools were completed within the required timeframe
- the documentation devised for use in the study was user-friendly and fit for purpose.

Fidelity assessment may also include a more qualitative approach whereby the views and insights of participants and researchers are obtained (Dyas et al., 2014). This type of evaluation of a study's fidelity may therefore discover what participants think about the study, why they agreed to participate, if they found the intervention/treatment acceptable and whether they were able to comply with the requirements of the study.

Website activity 21.3

Ideally the fidelity assessment will clearly demonstrate that all aspects of the research were conducted in accordance with the study protocol and SOPs and that all participants endorsed the research. If this is the case, the researchers can claim the study's validity and reliability have been demonstrated and that the findings are generalisable. If, however, the fidelity assessment is more negative, this may be an uncomfortable truth for the research team.

Website activity 21.4

PROMOTING RIGOUR IN QUALITATIVE RESEARCH

THINK POINT ACTIVITY   21.3

List the strategies that a researcher could use to enhance the rigour of a qualitative study.

In order to promote the rigour of a qualitative study or the qualitative aspects of a mixed methods study, the researcher can use a number of strategies. If these strategies are adopted qualitative research can be both systematic and rigorous. Not all of the following may apply to a particular study, but strategies could include:

- Achieving the research aim(s) and answering the research question(s), in other words the researcher achieves what they set out to do.
- Considering the timing of the research, for example, are there any seasonal factors which may inadvertently influence the findings?
- Using an audit trail. This should document all decisions made by the researcher during the research process. It therefore should enable others to track all research activity and verify the researcher's final interpretation of the data (Birks et al., 2008; Yardley, 2008).
- Being reflexive by reflecting throughout the study (Darawsheh, 2014). This can be facilitated by using a contemporaneously recorded reflective diary. In this the researcher should consider each aspect of the research process, their decision making and their interpretations (Gardner, 2008). The reflective diary also provides a means by which the researcher can consider the impact and repercussions of any sensitive or emotionally difficult issues (Rager, 2005; Darawsheh, 2014).
- Providing a detailed account of the research process along with acknowledgement of any potential researcher bias (Robson, 2011; Creswell, 2014; Silverman, 2015) (see Chapters 5 and 8).
- Using an appropriate sampling strategy and having clearly defined inclusion and exclusion criteria (see Chapter 15).
- Recruiting participants and collecting data until data saturation is achieved.
- Giving a detailed description of the context of a study and the participants. This is sometimes referred to as thick description (Richards, 2009).
- Scrutiny of the proposed data collection tool by experts in the field, the research supervisor, colleagues or peers.
- Promoting consistency by minimising the number of researchers involved in participant recruitment, data collection and data analysis.

- Ensuring appropriate training for all the researchers involved in participant recruitment, data collection and data analysis to facilitate a consistent approach in accordance with the research proposal.
- Involving participants in checking the analysed data. Note that opinions vary regarding the usefulness of this approach (see Chapter 20).
- Standardising the transcription process.
- Auditing interviews transcribed by a third party to confirm accuracy.
- Using verbatim quotes or excerpts from field notes to illustrate data analysis.
- Ensuring the data involving all participants are included in the data analysis and examples involving all participants are presented in the research report.
- Ensuring contradictory themes or findings are reported (Endacott, 2005; Yardley, 2008).
- Providing evidence to support claims of data saturation.
- Discussing the data analysis with a supervisor, colleague or peers to refine the researcher's thinking, facilitate accuracy and defend their interpretation.
- Providing evidence of inductive reasoning; in other words reasoning from a case or cases to a more general theory or conclusion.

Website activity 21.5

It will be recalled that the findings of a qualitative study are not generalisable and causal relationships cannot be established (see Chapters 8 and 20). However, findings can be substantiated by similar studies or corroborated by people who have had similar experiences (Angen, 2000; Yardley, 2008). Whilst the findings are time- and context-bound, they should appear plausible and may resonate with other similar populations and settings (Baker, 2006).

To support the evaluation of the rigour of qualitative research, a number of frameworks have been devised. Whilst rigid checklists can be counter-productive, Yardley's (2008) framework provides a versatile and thorough means by which the rigour of a study can be evaluated (see Table 21.1). The framework was first published in 2000 and is based on earlier work (Yardley, 1997; 2008). The framework consists of four core principles: 'sensitivity to context', 'commitment and rigour', 'coherence and transparency' and 'impact and importance' (Yardley 2008: 243–244). A criticism of many other frameworks is that criteria cannot always be applied to a diverse range of approaches (Braun and Clarke, 2006). However, Yardley's framework can be used with a variety of qualitative methods (Yardley, 2008) and therefore provides a means by which the rigour of any qualitative study can be assessed.

DEMONSTRATING SENSITIVITY TO CONTEXT

This can be achieved by drawing on literature from a range of disciplines as appropriate. This literature should be used: to provide the foundation for the study, in the literature review, to support the data analysis and in the discussion of the findings. The researcher

Table 21.1 Yardley's (2008) framework

Core principles	Key features
Sensitivity to context	Use of relevant theoretical literature
	Sensitive to socio-cultural setting and participants' perspectives
	Ethical issues identified and addressed
	Generation of empirical data
Commitment and rigour	Thorough data collection
	Depth and breadth of analysis
	Methodological competence and skill
	In-depth engagement with topic
Coherence and transparency	Clarity and power of argument
	Fit between theory and method
	Transparent methods and data presentation
	Reflexivity
Impact and importance	Practical and applied
	Theoretical
	Socio-cultural

Source: adapted from Yardley (2008: 243–246)

should also try to ensure they remain sensitive to and respectful of both the participants and the study setting. This can be demonstrated in the participant recruitment and data collection processes. Whilst in most qualitative studies there is a risk that the researcher's prior knowledge and preconceived ideas will be superimposed on the analysis of the data, strategies can be put in place to minimise the chances of this occurring (see Chapter 20). Counter themes and inconsistencies should also be acknowledged. Although ethics committee and indemnity insurance approvals are required before a study can be undertaken in a health care setting (see Chapter 18), it is essential that ethical issues are constantly monitored and addressed throughout the study (Yardley, 2008).

DEMONSTRATING COMMITMENT AND RIGOUR

Evidence of this can be provided through use of an appropriate sampling strategy, extensive data collection and detailed data analysis. These should all demonstrate that the researcher understands the methodological processes. Support from and the involvement of others, including the participants, funding bodies, user groups, gate-keepers and supervisors also provides evidence of commitment to the research. In recognition and appreciation of this sort of commitment, it is essential that the researcher ensures they have the research skills required to ensure successful completion of the study (Angen, 2000; Baker, 2006).

DEMONSTRATING COHERENCE AND TRANSPARENCY

This can be achieved in a number of ways. Whilst the researcher's clarity of expression and the power of their argument are for others to judge, they should ensure sufficient detail is provided of the research processes, in particular regarding data analysis. A contemporaneous reflective diary and a detailed audit trail can provide additional evidence (Darawsheh, 2014; Engward and Davis, 2015). The methods and approaches used should reflect the theoretical background of the study. An extensive range of data should be presented and the researcher should not generalise the findings to the wider population. However, ways in which the findings may be applied in a wider context should be indicated.

DEMONSTRATING IMPACT AND IMPORTANCE

The extent to which the study provides a better understanding of the phenomena under investigation should be made explicit. Implications for practice should also be apparent. Many studies can be the catalyst for change, and recommendations for future practice should be made. The findings of the study may also indicate the need for further research and this should be articulated.

TRIANGULATION

A further way of strengthening the rigour or quality of a research study is through triangulation. Triangulation is most commonly associated with the use of more than one research method, types of data or theoretical perspectives in a study. Triangulation is a key feature of mixed methods research (see Chapter 6) and this probably explains the increased use of this research approach in recent years. Triangulation can also be achieved by repeatedly collecting the same data from the same participants at different time points or collecting the same data from similar participants in different settings at the same time (Polit and Beck, 2014).

Combining methods, data and theoretical underpinnings and the corroboration of findings has the potential to strengthen the overall study through the verification or confirmation of the findings (Creswell and Plano Clark, 2011; Houghton et al., 2013). Triangulation also provides the researcher with a deeper understanding of the phenomena under investigation (Gibson and Brown, 2009).

Website activity 21.6

SUMMARY

In this chapter we have clarified definitions commonly used when discussing the strategies used to facilitate the production of good quality research. We have explored the strategies available to researchers to enhance the rigour of their research and discussed the effective use of triangulation.

FURTHER READING

Holloway, I. and Wheeler, S. (2013) *Qualitative Research in Nursing and Health* (3rd edn). Chichester: Wiley-Blackwell.

Chapter 18, 'Establishing quality: trustworthiness or validity', provides more detailed discussion on the strategies to facilitate rigour in qualitative and quantitative research.

LoBiondo-Wood, G. and Haber, J. (2014) *Nursing Research: Methods and Critical Appraisal for Evidence-based Practice* (8th edn). St Louis: Elsevier Mosby.

Chapter 15, 'Reliability and validity', provides more detailed discussion on the strategies to facilitate rigour in quantitative research.

Polit, D.F. and Beck, C.T. (2014) *Essentials of Nursing Research* (8th edn). Philadelphia: Wolters Kluwer Health, Lippincott Williams & Wilkins.

Chapter 17, 'Trustworthiness and integrity in qualitative research', provides more detailed discussion on the strategies to facilitate rigour in qualitative research.

Don't forget to visit https://study.sagepub.com/harveyandland to watch videos, take quizzes and to follow specially designed web activities.

22
EVALUATING RESEARCH

In this chapter we will focus on reading and appraising research rather than doing it. We will build upon earlier content in the book and in this chapter we will:

- clarify what the term 'critical appraisal' means when evaluating research
- reiterate why critical appraisal of research is important
- identify strategies to develop critical appraisal skills
- examine the range of frameworks available to facilitate critical appraisal
- establish the key elements to be considered when critically appraising a research study.

In previous chapters we have considered a variety of topics, such as searching the literature, aspects of the research process and the different ways in which research can be conducted. This earlier content provides the foundation for the evaluation or critical appraisal of research, and this is what we will explore in this chapter. We will begin by clarifying what the term critical appraisal means, what it involves when evaluating research and why it is important. Strategies that can be used to critically appraise research effectively will then be examined. This will include avoiding unnecessary reading and the use of frameworks such as tools, checklists or key questions to ask, which can facilitate the process. This will culminate in the identification of the key elements that should be considered when critically appraising a research study.

WHAT IS CRITICAL APPRAISAL OF RESEARCH AND WHAT DOES IT INVOLVE?

As we have seen in earlier chapters, unfortunately not all research that is published is sound (Andrews, 2006). Readers of published research therefore need to be able to discriminate between studies that have been undertaken appropriately and those that are seriously flawed. In the context of research, evaluating, critiquing or critically appraising a study all mean the same thing (Coughlan et al., 2007; Baker, 2014).

THINK POINT ACTIVITY   22.1

Think about what the term 'critical appraisal' means in the context of research. How would you explain critical appraisal to someone else? To complete this task, it may help you to make a list of the key features of the critical appraisal of research.

When evaluating research, **critical appraisal** means:

- identifying the study's strengths, weaknesses and limitations
- challenging the approach taken and suggesting alternative approaches
- evaluating whether the findings should be applied to local clinical settings
- identifying whether the study is valid and reliable or trustworthy
- comparing the findings with the current body of knowledge
- being objective and taking a balanced view.

Critical appraisal means not taking a published study at face value, but having read a research paper, making an informed judgement about it (Fothergill and Lipp, 2014). In order to do this, the process of critical appraisal involves making decisions about the study's strengths, weaknesses and limitations. Doing this will enable the reader to decide whether or not the study findings should be used to inform their practice. In order to carry out an effective critical appraisal of a study, nurses and midwives must therefore have a sound knowledge base regarding research methods and the research process.

For some people, the term 'critical' when used in relation to the appraisal of research has negative connotations. They therefore assume that critical appraisal only involves identifying a study's flaws or negative aspects. However, critical appraisal should also include identifying and acknowledging a study's strengths because this adds weight to the assessment of whether or not the study is robust and ultimately whether the findings should be used to inform practice (Morse, 2006). For example, if the weaknesses and limitations outweigh the strengths, the reader may decide on balance that the findings should not be implemented. However, following the critical appraisal of another study the reader may conclude that the strengths outweigh some minor weaknesses and that therefore the findings should be used to inform their practice.

As has been alluded to in earlier chapters, there is no such thing as the perfect study; particularly when the research is undertaken in health care settings and involves human beings. In the conduct of research, compromises often have to be made at some point. In addition, all research methods have weaknesses or limitations to some extent. However, researchers can put strategies in place to minimise the effects of these weaknesses and limitations. A key part of the critical appraisal process therefore also involves establishing

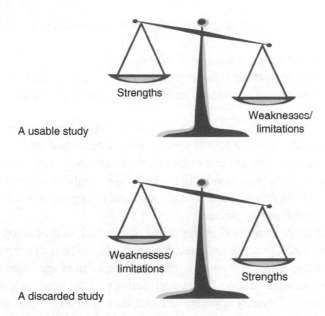

Figure 22.1 Balancing the strengths and weaknesses of a study to make decisions about the use of the findings to inform practice

whether the researcher has identified their study's potential weaknesses and limitations and the extent to which they have tried to minimise the effect of these.

WHY SHOULD NURSES AND MIDWIVES CRITICALLY APPRAISE RESEARCH?

THINK POINT ACTIVITY   22.2

Make a list of the reasons why nurses and midwives should critically appraise research. You may wish to revisit Chapter 1.

Nurses and midwives should critically appraise research for a number of reasons, these include:

- to distinguish between robust and flawed research; not all published research is sound
- to inform clinical practice
- to facilitate practice change

- to adhere to professional responsibilities to ensure practice is evidence-based
- to aid the literature review process
- to provide a rationale for a research proposal
- as an academic assignment; the critical appraisal of a research study is a common method of assessment in nursing and midwifery undergraduate programmes.

The critical appraisal of a study is not a one-off activity. This is because a study that was previously considered to be robust may no longer be considered to be so in the light of new knowledge, a greater understanding of research processes or clarification about the way in which a study was conducted. The MMR study is a good example of this (Wakefield et al., 1998). Consequently evidence used to support clinical practice should be constantly reviewed and appraised.

As we become more immersed in the world of research and develop a deeper understanding of the research process and research methods, critical appraisal skills become more refined. It is also important to remember that the critical appraisal of research does not only occur in relation to a specific research activity or the academic study of research modules. The ability to critically appraise research should be an integral activity for nurses and midwives in many other contexts, such as providing a rationale or justification for care, writing a business, funding or job application, the preparation of teaching or health education materials or the development of assignments on topics for modules that are not specifically research-focused. The critical appraisal of research demonstrates depth and breadth of reading and that the key concepts are understood. The principles are the same regardless of the purpose of the appraisal. The ability to evaluate research is therefore an on-going process and a skill to be utilised by nurses and midwives throughout their professional practice (Fothergill and Lipp, 2014).

STRATEGIES TO DEVELOP CRITICAL APPRAISAL SKILLS

Much of our guidance about developing the skills to critically appraise research will apply to developing critical appraisal skills more generally. Therefore, some of our suggestions may already be familiar to you. Undoubtedly, the first step is reading papers about research studies. If you are undertaking academic study remember that in addition to attaining a professional qualification or academic credits you are also *reading* for a degree whether it be at graduate, Master's or PhD level. Through reading as much relevant literature as you can, you will develop a deeper understanding of the research process and research methods. You will begin to notice the different strategies researchers put in place to enhance their study's strengths and minimise the limitations and weaknesses. You will also begin to identify approaches researchers should have taken, but did not.

Whilst reading as much as you can is important, the key thing is to ensure that what you are reading is relevant. In order to do this, you will need to develop 'filter reading' skills to ensure that you avoid unnecessary reading. It is essential therefore that you read the right studies. The definition of 'right' will vary but in addition to the right topic, this may include the right research method, research design, participant group, geographical location and/or method of data collection. The way to maximise the likelihood that you select the right research paper to read, is by ensuring that your literature search question and search strategy will lead you to the sort of research that you need to be reading (Chapter 13). Having found a paper that appears to be appropriate, the title and abstract should confirm whether this is the case. If you are still uncertain, it may be helpful to read specific sections of the paper such as information about the sample or the findings to help you make your final decision. You will, however, have to read the whole paper at some point. To skim read or focus only on specific sections of a paper may mean that you miss important details that you should consider in the critical appraisal of the study. It is important to note that your reading skills will develop over time, the more you read, the more fine-tuned your skills will become.

Frameworks are available to support the critical appraisal process and we will review some of these later in the chapter. In terms of developing your own critical appraisal skills, a useful approach when having read the paper through once is to ask yourself, what is my *gut* feeling about the study? As you read more and more research, your instincts will become more finely tuned. As you read the paper you should clarify any terminology or aspects of the research process/method that you are unfamiliar with. This will strengthen your understanding and thereby your critical appraisal skills.

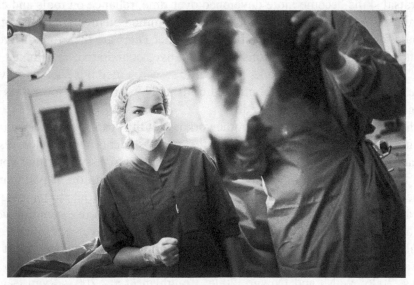

© knape / iStock

Some journals such as the *MIDIRS Midwifery Digest* regularly publish **critiques** of research studies, for example, the review undertaken by Evans et al. (2014) of the study by Shirvani and Ganji (2014). These critiques provide an insight into the critical appraisal process and help readers to identify factors to consider when reviewing a study. In addition, these and other journals often provide opportunities for new reviewers to become involved in the critical appraisal of research papers and other resources such as books and teaching packages (Chapter 26). Involvement in these peer review activities will help to develop your critical appraisal skills. Participation in peer review will also support the development of a researcher's writing skills because he or she will gain a greater awareness of the sorts of things peer reviewers and editors are looking for and the pitfalls that writers sometimes fall into.

Website activity 22.1

FRAMEWORKS FOR CRITICAL APPRAISAL

As we have previously identified, critical appraisal of a research study is a common method of assessment in nursing and midwifery undergraduate programmes. Nurses and midwives in this situation may find that their academic institution expects them to use a particular framework such as a critical appraisal tool, checklist or list of questions. Similarly, if you are undertaking a literature or systematic review as part of an academic assessment you should follow your institution's guidelines regarding which framework to use.

The advantage of using a framework is that it provides structure to the appraisal process and reduces the likelihood that important elements are overlooked (Andrews, 2006). Students and novice researchers therefore find them particularly useful. As critical appraisal skills become more developed over time, reliance on tools and checklists may diminish. Whilst all frameworks will have common elements, finding one that is appropriate for all types of study can be problematic. There are therefore different tools, checklists and lists of key questions for qualitative, quantitative and mixed methods research. There are also frameworks for specific research methods such as surveys, historical research and randomised controlled trials and systematic reviews. It is essential that the correct framework is selected.

Another disadvantage of using a framework is that they can sometimes be unwieldy, over-complicated and lengthy. Consequently, some students and novice researchers rather than finding them helpful, feel they are intimidating. Assuming that you are not required to use a specific framework by your academic institution, it is important that you select one that you are comfortable with and that is appropriate to the type of study you are appraising. For example, it would be inappropriate to use quantitative parameters to make judgements about qualitative research and vice versa. Probably the most commonly used tools are the CASP tools (www.casp-uk.net). However, most research textbooks also include tools, checklists and key questions for the reviewer to consider (Andrews, 2006; Walsh and Downe, 2006; Coughlan et al., 2007; Ryan et al., 2007;

Aveyard, 2014; Fothergill and Lipp, 2014; Kelly and Watson, 2014; Polit and Beck, 2014; Lipp and Fothergill, 2015; Rees et al., 2015). You may, however, prefer to develop your own checklist, tool or list of key questions.

**Website
activity 22.2**

KEY ELEMENTS OF CRITICAL APPRAISAL

We have devised Table 22.1 to assist the evaluation of research. In an attempt not to over-complicate the process, the table consists of core or key elements that would be relevant to any type of research. The table also includes components specific to qualitative and quantitative research. If you are appraising a mixed methods study both qualitative and quantitative elements of the table should be used.

Table 22.1 Issues to be considered when critically appraising a research study

Qualitative	Quantitative
How was the sample size determined? Is data saturation discussed? Do participants reflect the wider population?	How was the sample size determined? Was a power calculation undertaken? Are participants representative of the wider population?
Are all participants accounted for? Was the response/recruitment rate acceptable? Was there a high participant drop out rate?	
Are data collection methods appropriate and justified? Were previously validated tools used? Who carried out the data collection?	
Qualitative Were experts involved in the review of aspects of the proposed study, such as the data collection tools?	**Quantitative** Was a pilot study conducted? Were any changes made following the pilot study?
Are data analysis processes adequately explained? Who carried out the data analysis?	
Qualitative Were appropriate qualitative data analysis strategies used? Were participants involved in confirmation of the data analysis? Does the findings section include direct quotes or excerpts from the researcher's field notes?	**Quantitative** Were the correct/appropriate statistical tests used? Do data in the tables and charts match information provided in the text? Are all participants accounted for in the findings?

(Continued)

Table 22.1   (Continued)

Has the potential impact of co-founding factors such as culture, location, time of year, time of day been taken into consideration?
Is there evidence of triangulation? Are the findings corroborated by other literature?
Do the conclusions relate to the findings? Are unsubstantiated conclusions made?
Were there any conflicts of interest for the funder, research setting or members of the research team?
Were research governance requirements adhered to?
Have ethical issues been identified and addressed?
Were service users involved in the design and conduct of the research?
Was the study conducted in the way initially described? Was justification given for any changes made?
Is the study adequately described? Do you have a clear picture of what happened?

Qualitative	Quantitative
What, if any, strategies were put in place to facilitate trustworthiness? Have the research question/aims/objectives been addressed? If not, why not?	What, if any, strategies were put in place to facilitate validity and reliability? Have the hypothesis/research question/aims/objectives been addressed? If not, why not?

What are the study's key strengths, weaknesses and limitations?
Do the researchers acknowledge the study limitations and weaknesses? What did they do to minimise the effect of these?
What relevance are the findings to clinical practice generally?
What relevance are the findings to your practice specifically? Does the country of origin or date of the study have implications for your practice?
Is the study published in a reputable, peer reviewed journal?
Is there anything else about the study that concerns you?

If you require clarification on points identified in Table 22.1, for example, strategies to promote trustworthiness or research governance requirements, you should refer to the relevant sections earlier in this book. You will notice that the last section of Table 22.1 asks if there is anything else about the study that concerns you. This could be something unusual that you have noted such as a 100% response rate or no negative cases in a qualitative data analysis.

CRITICAL APPRAISAL IN ACADEMIC ASSESSMENTS

We will assume in this section that you are undertaking the critical appraisal as part of an academic assignment. The first thing to be clear about is whether you are appraising the study, a paper (for example a journal article) about a study or both. This is because there may be some aspects of a publication that you may appraise such as the way the paper is written, which may not be relevant if you are only appraising the study per se. If you are uncertain about this, your assignment brief and criteria and module leader(s) should clarify the situation. You also should establish whether you are required to use a particular framework to facilitate the appraisal.

When reading a research paper, you should try to set out with an open mind about it, expecting to find neither negative nor positive elements (Coughlan et al., 2007). You should therefore aim to take a balanced and constructive view of the study. Critical appraisal should be done in a structured and objective way, whereby having read the paper, you weigh up the study's pros and cons (Lipp and Fothergill, 2015). Remember critical appraisal is not only about being negative. It also involves commending the positive elements of a study.

Having read the paper through once, you then need to go back and read it again, perhaps this time more slowly (Baker, 2014). You may find it helpful to annotate the paper, highlighting the strengths, weaknesses and limitations as you read. Using different colour highlighter pens can help to identify the different sections, for example, blue for sampling and red for data collection. This can be useful because sometimes authors discuss different aspects of the research process in several places in the paper. At this second reading you should clarify any terminology or aspects of the research process/ method that you are unfamiliar with. It is at this stage that referral to a tool or checklist may be useful.

As you then begin to construct your assignment, follow the structure of the framework that you are using or the research process. Remember that the purpose of the appraisal is to analyse the paper and not to rewrite it. You should therefore use supporting evidence to substantiate each point that you make about the study's strengths, weaknesses and limitations or suggestions that you make about alternative approaches (Coughlan et al., 2007). For example, you may wish to make a comment that the sampling strategy was inappropriate for that particular type of study or that an alternative research method would have been more effective. You should support these statements with a reference from an appropriate source such as a research textbook or a journal article.

Depending on the word limit of your assignment, you may not be able to address all of the elements of the framework. You should therefore acknowledge this in your assignment and focus on the elements that you think are most important. Essentially, your assignment should show that you have read the whole paper, that you have tried to understand it and that you can demonstrate critical appraisal skills. One of the issues students sometimes struggle with is when a framework directs them to comment on particular information that cannot be located in the paper, for example, how the researchers calculated the required sample size. Being unable to find such information it is not necessarily the reviewer's fault. If the information is not there, you should ask yourself why the information is missing. If the information is there but it is not clearly expressed, you should also comment on this. In terms of the latter, you should take into account the target audience of the journal before stating that this is a weakness. Ultimately, you should decide whether the missing or unclear information weakens the study. You should always comment on missing or unclear information in your assignment, because this demonstrates to the assessor that you attempted to look for the information. To omit making a comment about this may mean that the assessor will assume that you have not looked for the information yourself. There may be some instances where the information you are looking for is not provided in a direct way, for example, the study aims are not specifically stated, but they can be deduced on reading the paper. This and confirming whether or not important information has been included, can only be established by reading the whole paper.

The points that you make throughout the appraisal should lead to an overall judgement about the study; whether the strengths outweigh any weaknesses or limitations, or vice versa. This judgement should in turn inform your decision about the implementation of the study findings in practice and the ways in which the findings compare to the findings of other similar studies.

Website activity 22.3

If, rather than appraising one study for an academic assignment, you are evaluating a study as part of a larger literature review or discussion, you will be unable to comment on all aspects of the study as identified by a framework. You should, however, try to comment on at least one aspect (either positive or negative) to demonstrate that you have read the paper and to support your claim that it is either robust or flawed.

SUMMARY

Within this chapter we have clarified that in the context of research, the critical appraisal, evaluation or critique of a study means the same thing; making an informed, balanced and objective judgement about it, in order to determine whether the study is robust or flawed. We have established why the critical appraisal of research is an essential 'skill for life' for nurses and midwives. We have also identified strategies that can be used to critically appraise research including avoiding unnecessary reading and the use of frameworks to facilitate the process. The chapter concluded with the identification of the key elements that should be considered when critically appraising a research study.

FURTHER READING

Fothergill, A. and Lipp, A. (2014) A guide to critiquing a research paper on clinical supervision: enhancing skills for practice. *Journal of Psychiatric and Mental Health Nursing*, 219: 834–840.

This paper guides the readers on how to critically appraise a quantitative study using a published paper.

Fox, C., Grimm, R. and Caldeira, R. (2016) *An Introduction to Evaluation*. London: Sage Publications.

This book provides an introduction to evaluation and includes material on both academic and policy-based research.

Lipp, A. and Fothergill, A. (2015) A guide to critiquing a research paper. methodological appraisal of a paper on nurses in abortion care. *Nurse Education Today*, 35: e14–e17.

This paper guides the readers how to critically appraise a qualitative study using a published paper.

Maltby, J., Williams, G., McGarry, J. and Day, L. (2010) *Research Methods for Nursing and Healthcare*. Harlow: Pearson.

This digital source includes a chapter on the critical appraisal of quantitative and qualitative research.

Don't forget to visit https://study.sagepub.com/harveyandland to watch videos, take quizzes and to follow specially designed web activities.

PART V

RESEARCH IN ACTION: DISSEMINATION AND APPLICATION

23

WRITING UP AND DISSEMINATING YOUR RESEARCH

In this chapter, we will explore strategies that can facilitate the process of writing up research and disseminating the findings of a study. In doing this we will:

- explore issues to consider when writing up and getting the job done
- consider strategies to avoid the risk of plagiarism
- reinforce the need to disseminate research findings
- explore possible dissemination strategies including writing for publication.

Within this chapter guidance will be given on writing up research, whether this is a piece of academic work, a report for a funding body or an article for publication. The need to adhere to any pre-specified requirements such as assignment briefs or publisher guidelines will be emphasised. Tips will be given to support the task of writing up and strategies will be identified to maximise the likelihood of success. Some of these handy hints may seem obvious. However, they are worth emphasising here to assist completion of the task. One of the most important elements we will explore is strategies to avoid the risk of plagiarism. Different ways of disseminating research findings will be identified and the advantages and disadvantages of the different options will be considered.

WRITING UP FOR ACADEMIC ASSESSMENT

There are a number of different scenarios where a researcher reaches the point when the study must be written up. Given the nature and purpose of this book, it is most likely that the researcher will be an undergraduate nurse or midwife who is writing up their research for academic assessment. We will therefore focus on this scenario here and we will consider other situations later in the chapter. If you are writing up research for academic assessment it is most likely to be a literature review, a research proposal or a small-scale study. For clarity in this section we will use the collective term 'research' and we will provide handy hints to facilitate writing this up.

FOLLOW THE ASSIGNMENT GUIDELINES

Whatever the nature of the work to be written up, the most important advice we can give you is to follow the assignment guidelines for that particular assignment. We will give you some general guidance here, including some tips based on our own experiences of writing up. However, the assignment guidelines that you have been given by your academic institution must take precedence. Therefore, if there is anything that we suggest that appears to contradict these guidelines, you should seek clarification from your lecturers about what is required.

ENSURE EFFECTIVE TIME MANAGEMENT AND FORWARD PLANNING

It is sometimes the case, that so much effort has been put into 'doing' the research, that when it comes writing it up, the researcher has run out of time, energy and perhaps even enthusiasm. Like any assignment, time management and forward planning are crucial. However, for this type of assignment these are even more important because research assignments tend to be bigger pieces of work and may therefore be more influential in determining degree classification. The modules supporting these assignments also tend to be delivered over a longer period of time compared to other modules and consequently there is the risk that students become distracted by other assignments or the clinical component of their course. However, a research assignment will not go away just because it has been 'put on the back burner'. Indeed, for most students the longer the delay in starting the writing up process the more difficult the task is, when it finally begins.

CONSIDER WHETHER THE ASSIGNMENT COULD BE WORKED ON INCREMENTALLY

An advantage of writing up research is that it can often be done incrementally. You could therefore use this to your advantage when juggling the need to complete other assignments or episodes of clinical practice. Working on the assignment incrementally can also be less daunting than attempting a big piece of work all in one go. Getting aspects of the work completed, albeit perhaps in draft form, can build confidence and create a sense of achievement.

A research proposal and a small-scale study can lend themselves to being written up incrementally whereby different aspects of the research process can be written at different times. Clearly the incremental approach presents some challenges and any work produced in this way will need to be revisited and if necessary updated immediately prior to submission. We also are aware that some students may find that this way of working is disjointed and does not suit their learning style (see Box 23.1).

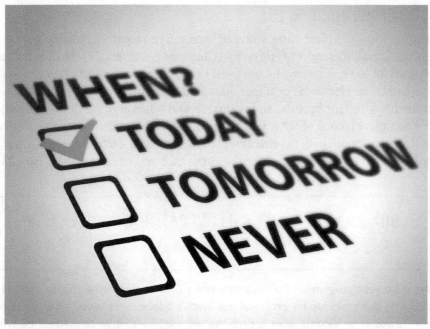

© Aquir / Shutterstock

BOX 23.1   ILLUSTRATION OF TIME MANAGEMENT AND THE WRITING UP PROCESS

Paulette has to write a 6,000-word literature review. The assignment is launched at the beginning of the third year and it must be submitted at the end of the course. In the weeks following the assignment launch, Paulette chooses her topic, develops her research question and conducts a preliminary literature search. She then writes up the parts of her assignment in which she has to explain why she has chosen that particular topic, how she developed her question and how she conducted the preliminary literature search. The latter must include the search terms and criteria she used, the databases she has searched and the number of papers yielded. Paulette then has an eight-week clinical placement. During this time Paulette reads the papers from the search to start the process of deciding which she will use in her review. However, she does not continue the writing up process until her placement has finished.

KEEP A RESEARCH DIARY OR LOG

We have previously explored the value of qualitative researchers keeping a reflective diary and audit trail to support reflexivity (Chapters 8, 20 and 21). However, keeping a research diary or log can be invaluable to all researchers particularly those who are novices. This can be an electronic or paper diary and in it you can log what you have done, when and why. This can become an invaluable tool when writing up, because it should provide a complete record of what you have done and the decisions that you have made. Without it, it may be difficult to remember the reasons why certain decisions were made, the people you have spoken to and the resources that you have used (see Box 23.2).

BOX 23.2   EXAMPLE ILLUSTRATING THE VALUE OF A RESEARCH DIARY

For his third year assignment Ravi has to write a 6,000-word research proposal. He has decided that the topic for his proposal will involve adolescents who self-harm but he is unclear at this stage exactly what aspects he will explore and what method he will use. Whilst on placement at a Child and Adolescent Mental Health Service (CAMHS) unit Ravi has a chance conversation with Darren, a social worker who is working with a particular family. Darren says he feels that fathers of adolescents who self-harm are much less well supported than mothers. Ravi therefore decides that his proposal will focus on fathers. He writes about his conversation with Darren and his thoughts and ideas in his research diary when his shift ends. When he looks at this several months later Ravi recalls that Darren identified a range of resources and literature he could use and the ways in which potential participants could be accessed.

In the diary or log you can also keep copies of all other documentation relating to your work. This could include letters, copies of supervisory meetings and screen-shots of literature searches. Having everything in one place will provide a running commentary that describes the progress of your work.

ACCESS ACADEMIC SUPPORT AND GUIDANCE

Usually research assignments feature in the third year of undergraduate programmes. By this time students may feel more confident about their academic skills such as assignment writing and searching the literature. Nevertheless, for this piece of work we suggest that students take every opportunity to access supervisory meetings or tutorials. Even if you feel that you know what you are doing, confirmation of this will provide reassurance and boost your confidence. In addition, your lecturers may suggest things that you had not thought about. Regular meetings will also help you to keep 'on track' with the work required. Similarly we would advise students to access any other support available, such as searching the literature with library staff.

TALK TO PEOPLE ABOUT THE ASSIGNMENT

A disadvantage of having a larger piece of work to do over a longer period of time is that students feel it is permanently 'hanging over them'. However, you can turn this into an advantage by talking about it to mentors, senior staff, recently qualified staff and fellow students. They may suggest things you had not thought about and identify relevant literature and resources you could use. Sometimes students worry about sharing their ideas with fellow students and we will explore issues pertaining to plagiarism later. However, recently qualified nurses and midwives who completed the same or a very similar assignment may be an invaluable resource. Sometimes lecturers arrange sessions with former students and this may include being able to see their work. Potential risks involving plagiarism may apply; however, hearing the importance of time management and forward planning from someone who has recently 'been there and done it' can be very powerful. They may also have novel tips and hints for getting the job done.

ENSURE YOUR WORK HAS A CLEAR STRUCTURE AND FOLLOW THE RESEARCH PROCESS WHERE APPROPRIATE

An advantage of writing up research is that it has a natural and logical process which can provide a structure for your work. This is particularly the case when writing up a research proposal (see Chapter 25). If you structure your work in accordance with the research process you will reduce the risk of inadvertently omitting an important aspect of the study. However, sometimes when writing up research, particularly a study or a proposal, it can be difficult to decide what should go where. For example, strategies to recruit participants could be discussed either in the 'sampling' or 'ethical issues' sections. Although usually larger assignments, once you start writing you will almost certainly find that you do not have the wordage to discuss the same issues in more than one section. In any case, you should avoid repetition in your work. It may therefore be appropriate to use cross-references in the same way that we have done in this book. When it comes to deciding 'what goes where' you should follow the assignment guidelines and advice from your supervisor or lecturer. The assignment marking criteria may also be helpful in determining the wordage required and the marks available for the different sections.

BE TRUTHFUL TO YOUR WORK

One of the challenges that researchers face when writing up a research study is using an appropriate literary style whilst at the same time being truthful to the research.

For example, verbatim quotes can sometimes appear incoherent and difficult to read when presented as text. This may make the work appear disjointed and lead readers to make inappropriate judgements about participants (Brinkmann and Kvale, 2015). Therefore verbatim quotes have sometimes to be made readable. This can be done by taking out 'ums', 'errs' and repeated words. It is essential, however, that quotes remain faithful to the participant's narrative (Braun and Clarke, 2006). Overall meanings should not therefore be changed. It should also be noted that editing data should only be done *after* data analysis and will not be appropriate if writing up some forms of data analysis such as conversational or discourse analysis (Chapter 20) (see Box 23.3).

BOX 23.3   EXAMPLE ILLUSTRATING THE DIFFERENCE BETWEEN A VERBATIM AND EDITED EXCERPT FROM AN INTERVIEW

The following example gives two versions of the same quote. The first is as it was said by the participant and the second is as presented in the text.

"They spotted that on err, Wednesday night err, if I remember, umm, so to start with err, she was umm, normal, umm, I can't remember the name for it now, umm, but she was head first, umm, but they err, was checking the err, baby's heartbeat, umm, every hour up until the, err, Thursday dinner time."

"They spotted that on Wednesday night, if I remember, so to start with she was normal, I can't remember the name for it now, but she was head first, but they was checking the baby's heart beat every hour up until the Thursday dinner time."

GET THE ABSTRACT RIGHT

If your work requires an abstract (see your assignment guidelines) you will probably find that you cannot write this until the rest of the work has been completed. The abstract provides a summary of the work in a pre-specified format (see your guidelines) in a defined number or words (usually 200–300). You will know from conducting your own literature searches that the abstract should capture the essence of the paper. However, writing an abstract can be a challenge because potentially complex information has to be summarised in a limited number of words. Remember that the abstract will probably be the first thing that the person marking your work will read. It should therefore create a good impression and provide them with all the information they need. Therefore make sure that you allow sufficient time to ensure that you get the abstract right (see below).

ALLOW SUFFICIENT TIME IMMEDIATELY PRIOR TO SUBMISSION TO REVISE, UPDATE AND PROOF READ THE ASSIGNMENT

However well you have planned your work, you need to ensure there is sufficient time immediately prior to submission to revisit aspects of the assignment. For example, the literature search may need to be updated. You should also allow sufficient time for proof reading and making corrections. You need to allow time to do the job properly and do justice to your hard work and the commitment of others such as your supervisor or research participants. Overall, it is important not to underestimate the time needed to write up and the importance of the presentation of your work.

AVOIDING PLAGIARISM

THINK POINT ACTIVITY   23.1

We are assuming here that you understand the meaning of the term plagiarism. If you are unclear about this, please refer to the glossary.

Although we have discussed plagiarism elsewhere, it is particularly pertinent here. One of the pitfalls that students and researchers can fall into when writing a literature review is committing plagiarism. Almost always this is done unintentionally. The way in which this usually occurs is when sections of text from another source are 'copied and pasted' into a draft version of the review with the intention that the reviewer will summarise the text in their own words citing the appropriate reference. However, for whatever reason the reviewer forgets to do this and the literature review is submitted with verbatim excerpts of text from another source that are not referenced. Most academic institutions and publishers now use software which is able to establish if any work has been plagiarised. Any suspicion of plagiarism will be investigated. This can be a lengthy and distressing process for those involved. If plagiarism is confirmed the penalties for students may include a requirement to resubmit the work, receiving a mark capped at a borderline pass, the withdrawal of academic credits already achieved (all of which may affect degree classification), a delay in completing the course or, the worst-case scenario, being withdrawn from the course. For others being found to have committed plagiarism may have a negative impact on their reputation and subsequent career. Plagiarism therefore has serious implications and should be avoided at all costs. However, this can be easier said than done, particularly given workload pressures.

Nevertheless there are strategies that can be employed to reduce the risk of committing plagiarism. Ensure everything that you write, including preliminary drafts, is in your own words. Summarising the key concepts in this way is an invaluable skill to develop. However, this can sometimes be difficult. A strategy that may help is to think to yourself 'if I had to tell to someone what this paper is saying, what would I tell them?' Verbalising the key concepts may help you to summarise the essence of the paper in your own words. Ensure everything that you write including drafts are appropriately referenced. This will also be useful when writing the reference list and using referencing software may help. Ensure verbatim sections from other sources are referenced as a direct quote. If you do need to copy and paste text, ensure when it is pasted into your draft that you use a different colour font (such as red) so that when you return to the draft you can clearly see verbatim sections which you still need to summarise in your own words. Use plagiarism software to check your work before submission. This software is now available for students to use in most academic institutions.

WRITING UP FOR OTHER REASONS

Whilst we have focused on writing up research for academic assessment earlier in this chapter, there may be other reasons why researchers have to write up their work. This may include a report for the funding body or employer, or writing research for publication. Most funding bodies have specific requirements in terms of format and

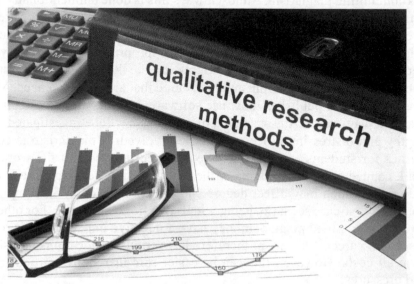

© designer491 / iStock

content which researchers must adhere to, for example, the National Institute for Health Research.

Researchers should treat these requirements in exactly the same way as a student following assignment criteria. In other words, they should be followed to the letter. Most of the other writing up strategies that we have previously outlined will apply. However, for larger studies it is likely that several members of the team will be involved in this process and therefore it will be important to ensure that there is consistency of literary style and that there are no omissions or unnecessary repetitions. It will be important to ensure that sufficient time is available immediately prior to submission to ensure that the whole report is complete.

Website activity 23.1

DISSEMINATING RESEARCH FINDINGS

THINK POINT ACTIVITY 23.2

Make a list of the reasons why researchers should disseminate their research findings.

Nursing and midwifery research findings should be disseminated for a number of reasons. These include:

- to build a body of evidence to ensure practice is evidence-based
- to facilitate the delivery of safe, effective, high quality care
- to enable patients, clients and families to make informed decisions about their care
- to maximise patient and client outcomes
- to facilitate patient and client satisfaction
- to support the development, evaluation and on-going improvement of care
- to support the fulfilment of clinical governance requirements
- to promote the delivery of cost-effective care
- to ensure that the ethical, moral and professional responsibilities of nurses and midwives are addressed
- to reduce the risk of litigation for individual practitioners and the wider service
- to ensure nurses and midwives retain professional identity within the provision of health care
- to facilitate the autonomy of nurses and midwives
- to enable the researcher to fulfil their duty to the participants to disseminate the research findings
- to enable the researcher to fulfil any obligation they may have to the research funder and their employer to disseminate the research findings.

It should be noted here that it is just as important to disseminate the findings of a study where it is demonstrated that an intervention or strategy did not work. This sort of finding will still add to the body of knowledge and sharing information with other health care professionals and possible research funders could save the repetition of equally unsuccessful research in the future. However, it must be acknowledged that some journals place less emphasis on publishing unsuccessful studies.

THINK POINT ACTIVITY   23.3

Make a list of the ways in which the findings of a research study may be disseminated.

Research findings can be disseminated in a number of different ways including:

- publication in journals, including Open Access journals and books
- research reports and summaries
- websites and other forms of social media
- conference presentations
- posters, displayed at conferences and in practice areas
- lunchtime meetings, seminars, workshops and teaching sessions
- newsletters, electronic or paper copy
- mainstream media such as magazines, newspapers, radio and television.

Website activity 23.2

The dissemination methods used are often determined by the time and resources available to the researcher. Sometimes funding for dissemination is included in the costing of the study and increasingly researchers are being advised to budget for publication in Open Access journals. The presentation of the research findings will vary according to the target audience. For example, the style and format of a research report for the participants and user groups may be different from that used for the report to the funding body.

WRITING FOR PUBLICATION

This is probably the most commonly suggested method of disseminating research and yet many nurses and midwives lack the confidence to publish their work (Parker et al., 2010; Richardson and Carrick-Sen, 2011). A key driver in the current agenda is demonstrating the impact of a study (Chapter 26), for example, has the study led to a change in practice or an improvement of patient outcomes? If a literature review or research study has been written for academic assessment, the author has the basis of a paper that could be developed for publication. As we will see in the final chapter, writing for publication is going to become more and more important for nurses and midwives in the future (Clark and Thompson, 2013), so why not start doing it now?

CONFERENCE PRESENTATIONS AND POSTERS

Another method of disseminating research findings is a conference presentation or poster. In most cases, there will be some form of selection process, which usually involves peer review of abstracts submitted a few months prior to the conference. Selected abstracts will usually be published in the conference documentation. As we have indicated earlier in the chapter, writing an abstract can be a challenge, particularly as there will almost certainly be a word limit (usually 200–300 words). The aim is to capture the essence of the work and attract the attention of the selectors. In order to increase your chances of selection ensure the focus of your work matches the conference themes and present the abstract in the exact format specified by the conference organisers. For most conferences abstract submission will be online using a pre-specified template. This usually includes:

- aim and objectives
- background
- methods/methods of data collection
- results
- conclusion.

However, there may be additional sections for description of the 'setting', 'sample' and 'ethics approvals'. Alternatively you may be required to provide this information within the 'methods' section.

Website activity 23.3

THINK POINT ACTIVITY   23.4

Make a list of the benefits for nurses and midwives of having their research published.

There are a number of benefits for nurses and midwives of having their work, and their research in particular, published. These benefits include:

- getting something back for their hard work
- making use of readily available material
- enhancing their CV and career opportunities

- networking
- developing a reputation for an interest and expertise in a particular subject area
- payment, however it would be sensible not to rely on this as a source of income! Not all journals pay to publish work and if payment is offered, this is usually only a token amount.

WHERE SHOULD I PUBLISH MY WORK?

You should be familiar with the most likely journals you could approach to publish your work. Nevertheless it is worth doing some market research. Look at the subject areas and the types of authors that different journals tend to publish. Try to find out the usual length of time between a script being accepted and published. Sometimes this can be several months, even perhaps a year. If your work is 'cutting edge' you should aim to have it published as soon as possible. Journal websites should provide information about the usual length of time to publish.

Whilst a range of nursing and midwifery journals are available it may be worth considering a journal from a related subject area such as psychology, speech therapy or social work. Alternatively, your paper may be suited to a journal that focuses on a particular approach to research such as qualitative research or a specific aspect of research such as ethics.

In deciding which journal to approach, you may also consider the impact factor of the journal (this can also be found on the journal's website). In general terms the higher a journal's impact factor, the greater the esteem in which it is held and the more widely your work will be accessed. However, publication in higher impact factor journals can be more difficult, primarily because editors have a larger pool of work to draw from. Increasingly researchers try to have their work published in an Open Access journal. These journals are, as their name suggests, available electronically to anyone. Wide-scale and international circulation is therefore more likely. However, payment for publication is usually required and this is often beyond the scope of individual researchers and students in particular. If publication in an Open Access journal is not a realistic proposition, you should aim for publication in a peer reviewed journal. This means that your work will have undergone a process of critical review and that two (or more) independent reviewers have considered your work and decided that it is worthy of publication.

Having decided on your target journal, you need to follow the publication guidelines to the letter. You should treat these in exactly the same way as you would assignment guidelines. This is where you may come unstuck if you had assumed you can 'shoe-horn' an assignment into a paper for publication. You must accept that you may have to make some changes such as editing it to meet the word limit, changing the referencing system or taking out any mention of the fact that it was originally written as an assignment. As you revise the work, review your assignment feedback as this may include some useful advice such as clarifying terminology or adding supporting evidence. It may be prudent to invite

Website activity 23.4

your supervisor, personal tutor, module leader or module lecturer to be the second author. This means that you can work on the paper together and they may have prior experience of writing for publication which may prove useful.

You should be aware that before considering the publication of a research study, most journals now ask for evidence of ethics committee approval. If you do not have this, you may find that you are unable to proceed with publication. Most journals have an electronic submission process and this will include running work through software to detect plagiarism.

A range of resources are available to support nurses and midwives through the process of writing for publication (Fahy, 2008; Watson and Holland, 2012). Our advice to you would be to not waste the resources that you have at your finger-tips, in other words your research assignments, proposals or research studies.

Website activity 23.5

SUMMARY

Within this chapter we have explored strategies to support the process of writing up research and minimising the risk of plagiarism. We have emphasised the need to adhere to any pre-specified requirements such as assignment briefs or publisher guidelines. We have considered the different ways of disseminating research including writing for publication.

FURTHER READING

Nygaard, L.P. (2015) *Writing for Scholars* (2nd edn). London: Sage Publications.

This excellent book provides general guidance on developing writing skills and finding your voice for research and publication.

Taylor, D.B. (2013) *Writing Skills for Nursing and Midwifery Students*. London: Sage Publications.

A helpful guide that looks at the specific challenges of writing about research in nursing and midwifery.

Watson, R. and Holland, K. (2012) *Writing for Publication in Nursing and Healthcare: Getting It Right*. Chichester: Wiley-Blackwell.

A useful digital source which includes chapters on writing a journal article, converting an assignment into a paper for publication and avoiding plagiarism.

> Don't forget to visit https://study.sagepub.com/harveyandland to watch videos, take quizzes and to follow specially designed web activities.

24

USING RESEARCH IN CLINICAL PRACTICE

In this chapter we will explore the ways in which research findings can be introduced and used in clinical practice. In doing this we will:

- identify the main challenges to implementing research findings in clinical practice
- explore strategies that can facilitate the use of research findings
- identify practical solutions and resources that can assist the process of research implementation.

This chapter builds upon many of the issues we have explored in this book. Within this chapter, the hurdles that must be overcome when implementing research findings in clinical practice will be identified. We will identify frameworks or models that can be used to conquer these hurdles and facilitate the delivery of care that is evidence-based. We will also identify other practical tips and resources that can be used to promote the use of research in clinical practice. It should be acknowledged that the implementation of research evidence may occur in one of two ways. The first is when individual nurses and midwives use research findings to inform their own personal practice; for example, the way in which they communicate with patients and clients. The other way is the more large-scale implementation of new findings to a practice area which all staff are required to follow. The focus of this chapter will be on the latter scenario.

In Chapters 1, 2 and 3 we identified why midwifery and nursing practice should be evidence-based. The ways in which research can be critically appraised and reviewed were explored in Chapters 10, 14 and 22. Having identified the 'best evidence' to underpin an aspect of practice, nurses and midwives next need to identify ways of ensuring this 'best evidence' is used. It might be considered that the implementation of research findings into practice should be straightforward; the evidence is identified and so is immediately put in to practice. Whilst on some occasions this may be the case, the reality can often be more complex and time consuming.

Hunt, writing in 1981, identified five reasons why nurses did not use research findings in clinical practice:

- they did not know about the research findings
- they did not understand the findings
- they did not believe the findings
- they did not know how to implement the findings
- they were not allowed to implement the findings. (Hunt, 1981: 192)

Website activity 24.1

Of the factors listed by Hunt (1981), hopefully nurses' and midwives' awareness, knowledge and understanding of research have improved over the last few decades. However, it may still be the case that some nurses and midwives do not know how to go about implementing research findings or, indeed, feel that they do not have 'permission' to do so. More recent research has identified other barriers to the implementation of research findings (Hilton et al., 2009; Breimaier et al., 2011; Moreno-Casbas et al., 2011). These include lack of relevant studies for a specific aspect of practice, poor quality research and conflicting evidence. Nurses and midwives may as a consequence be uncertain which findings should be put into practice. As we have discussed in earlier chapters, a key factor in this scenario is establishing the 'best evidence'.

THINK POINT ACTIVITY   24.1

Make a list of the others factors to consider and hurdles to overcome when attempting to implement new research findings in a practice setting.

CHALLENGES TO IMPLEMENTING RESEARCH FINDINGS IN CLINICAL PRACTICE

A nurse or midwife, having identified new research findings or the best evidence to underpin an aspect of practice, must next consider how to go about ensuring it is implemented. This will involve identifying the factors to be considered, the challenges, the hurdles or in some cases the outright barriers to be overcome (see Figure 24.1). These will vary according to the practice setting, the people who work there, the patient/client group and the nature of the findings to be implemented.

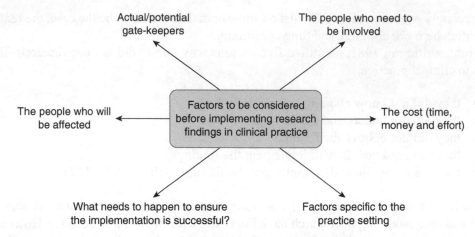

Figure 24.1   Factors to be considered before implementing research findings in clinical practice

THINK POINT ACTIVITY   24.2

Think of a practice area that you know well and make a list of the potential gate-keepers to the implementation of nursing/midwifery research into that setting.

THE GATE-KEEPERS

In most cases, these are the senior nurses and midwives with managerial responsibility for the particular clinical area. It is not necessarily the case that they will block attempts to implement new research findings into clinical practice. Indeed, the very nature of their role and responsibilities will be to ensure that practice is evidence-based. Nevertheless, their approval or agreement will almost certainly be required. In some situations senior personnel representing other health care professional groups may also be gate-keepers. This is likely to be the case if the new way of caring for patients and clients impinges on the work of other groups in a direct way. In some care settings, the culture may be that changes in nursing or midwifery practice must be agreed by a senior health care professional even if the new way of caring does not impact in any way on other groups. Historically, the most common example of this was the need to get the senior doctor's permission for any changes in nursing and midwifery practice. Hopefully, these days have now passed, but it may still be the case in some practice areas (Wilkinson et al., 2011).

In some care settings the gate-keepers may be other nurses and midwives working in that area. The most likely scenario is one or two more senior people who have taken on the self-appointed and unofficial role of gate-keeper. They will influence what does or does not happen in the practice area (see Chapter 3).

Other gate-keepers may include:

- patients, clients and service users
- relatives or carers of patients and clients
- budget holders.

THE PEOPLE WHO NEED TO BE INVOLVED

Some of the people who will be involved in the implementation of the new findings can be easily identified. These will include the nurses and midwives working in the practice setting, patients, clients and their relatives. However, some thinking 'outside the box' may be required in order to identify those who will be involved in perhaps a less direct way. For example, this could include other health care professional groups such as pharmacists, physiotherapists, budget holders or house-keeping staff. Another factor to consider here is who will lead the implementation of the new findings. This could be an individual or a small group of people.

THE PEOPLE WHO WILL BE AFFECTED

The groups of people who will be affected by the implementation are very similar to those identified in the previous group. However, some of those involved will be 'behind the scenes' and will not necessarily be affected by the change in a direct way.

The groups of people who will be affected should be identified and could include:

- patients, clients and service users
- nurses, midwives and other members of the health care team
- relatives or carers of patients and clients
- service user groups
- managers
- budget holders
- commissioners
- policy makers.

THE COST

The cost of implementing new research findings into practice should not be under-estimated. Most often the biggest and yet generally overlooked cost is the time and effort spent ensuring the research findings are implemented. There may be other costs to consider as well, such as the purchase of equipment or training packages and programmes for staff.

FACTORS SPECIFIC TO THE PRACTICE SETTING

In addition to the factors considered above, there may be other issues that are specific to the practice setting that should be considered before new research findings are implemented. These may be factors associated with, for example, the culture of the practice area, staffing levels or the particular patient/client group.

WHAT NEEDS TO HAPPEN TO ENSURE THE IMPLEMENTATION?

The final factor to consider is what needs to happen to ensure the implementation of the research findings is successful. The important message here is the need to think the process through and to make a plan. Unsuccessful attempts to put research findings into practice often occur because someone, albeit enthusiastically, has rushed to implement the new way of working without making a plan. The implementation of the findings will, as a consequence, be hurried and fragmented.

IMPLEMENTING RESEARCH FINDINGS

Various models and frameworks have been devised to support the implementation of research findings into clinical practice (Feldstein and Glasgow, 2008; Damschroder et al., 2009; Rycroft-Malone and Bucknall, 2010). These have common features,

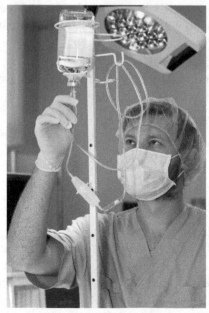

© vzmaze / iStock

many of which are based on the work of Lewin on theories of change management and group dynamics (see Chapter 9).

WHO WILL LEAD THE IMPLEMENTATION?

A key issue is to identify who will lead the implementation of the findings. Recently qualified nurses and midwives and students may feel more comfortable with evidence-based practice because of their recent or current exposure to it in their programmes of study (Gerrish et al., 2008). Conversely, they may not feel sufficiently empowered to ensure that new evidence is put into practice. This will largely be determined by the culture of the practice setting which, in turn, will often be influenced by the philosophy of the senior personnel and gate-keepers. In addition, students will probably feel the length of a placement does not give them sufficient time to implement research findings into that particular area. The nurse or midwife who would be best placed to implement the research may feel reluctant to do so because of professional inertia, lack of confidence or a perceived lack of time. Similarly a nurse or midwife who does take on the task may not be the right person for the job. In some contexts a person external to the practice setting may be appropriate to lead the implementation (Damschroder et al., 2009). Finding the right leader is therefore essential and it has been identified that communication and negotiation skills are integral to this role (van Bekkum and Hilton, 2013).

Website activity 24.2

Alternatively, it may be prudent to identify a group of colleagues who will help to promote the implementation. It may be sensible to ensure this small group includes representation from the groups who will be affected by the new way of working, for example, a dietician and a service user. Whilst ultimately one of the group members may need to take on a leadership role, having like-minded colleagues to share the burden may be a useful strategy.

Website activity 24.3

GAINING SUPPORT FOR THE CHANGE

The next phase in the implementation of research findings is gaining support, particularly from the gate-keepers, those who would be involved and those who would be directly affected. Different approaches may be required in order to inform different groups.

Methods to inform different health care professional groups could include:

- presentation of the new findings at a journal club
- displaying the key research papers on staff notice boards
- one-to-one discussions with key players/gate-keepers
- newsletters
- emails and use of the intranet
- presentations at staff meetings
- posters and leaflets
- developing a business case for managers and budget holders.

Through these various interactions those leading the change will be able to determine the level of health care professional support. Gaining support from patient, clients, relatives, carers and service user groups can also provide a powerful impetus for ensuring the findings are implemented. Therefore, time spent informing these groups will also generally be time well spent. However, informing patients, clients, relatives and carers about research evidence can be challenging, particularly if this indicates that new care strategies are required and previous care strategies are now redundant (van Bekkum and Hilton, 2013).

THINK POINT ACTIVITY   24.3

What strategies could be used to inform patients, clients, relatives, carers and service user groups about the proposed implementation of new research findings? What factors should be considered when deciding which method(s) to use?

Website activity 24.4

Whilst some health care professional and service user groups may be in favour of the implementation, others may feel ambivalent about it or be resistant to the change. A key issue at this stage is therefore managing any lack of support or hostility towards the proposed new way of working. Those who would be affected may be reluctant to embrace the change in practice for a variety of reasons.

For example, health care professionals may find their previous ways of working have been challenged (see Chapter 3 regarding traditional knowledge). Similarly patients, clients, carers and relatives may have to accept new approaches to care. This can be particularly challenging for those who have become used to established care strategies. In addition there may be support amongst those opposing the change for conflicting research evidence which advocates an alternative approach (Hilton et al., 2009). Determining the 'best evidence' is therefore vitally important. The evidence may be considered more credible if it has been identified in a systematic or Cochrane review.

Website activity 24.5

There are two opposing approaches to handling resistance to change amongst health care professionals. Firstly, time could be spent trying to win over those who do not support the change. Conversely, time might be better spent working with those who support the change. The rationale for this latter approach is that in time those who resist it will either accept the new way of working or have to face the consequences of delivering care that does not comply with that of their colleagues or their professional responsibilities and is not evidence-based practice.

THINK POINT ACTIVITY   24.4

Think of a practice area that you know well. Which of the two approaches identified above do you think should be adopted to deal with resistance to a new way of working and why?

ENSURING ADEQUATE PREPARATION

In order to ensure everyone is prepared for the implementation of the research findings, a number of strategies may need to be employed. Teaching sessions for those using the research findings in their practice may be required. This may also necessitate assessment of competence. In order to support staff in their new way of working, practice guidelines, protocols or policies may need to be developed.

Another important factor will be costing because putting the research findings into practice may have financial implications. This might include:

- time spent implementing the findings
- purchase of new equipment or other resources
- staff training
- training for the patient, client or their carers
- the development of practice guidelines or protocols
- maintenance of equipment
- reorganising the provision of care to accommodate the change
- employing new personnel.

If different items to those previously used in the clinical setting need to be purchased, for example, feeding tubes or types of dressing, then contracts may need to be negotiated with the supplier.

PUTTING THE FINDINGS INTO PRACTICE

Rather than implementing the findings as if a permanent arrangement, it may be more appropriate to first trial the new way of working (Damschroder et al., 2009). This provides the opportunity for all those involved to feel they can have some input to the decision about whether to implement the findings permanently. Piloting can also lead to more successful implementation in the long run (Feldstein and Glasgow, 2008).

Putting the findings into practice is in many ways the most straightforward phase. Having been satisfied that all the required preparatory work has been undertaken, a date should be set for the implementation. Strategies should be employed to ensure all those who will be affected by the change are aware of the implementation date. During the early implementation phase, the new way of working should be monitored. Additional teaching, reminders and support for those involved may be required. Having key personnel identified whom others can consult about the new way of working may be a useful strategy. Teething problems should be addressed and as a consequence, practice guidelines, protocols or policies may need minor amendment. Any such changes should be disseminated to all those involved. In some contexts, incentives may be considered but this may present further challenges such as ethical concerns or a negative impact on team-working.

EVALUATION

After a defined period of time the new way of working should be evaluated and the impact assessed (Damschroder et al., 2009; Rycroft-Malone and Burton, 2011). This may involve an audit which will establish the level of compliance amongst all those involved. Patient and staff satisfaction surveys and student placement evaluations may also determine experiences and perceptions of the practice change. More defined evaluation of patient/client outcomes may also indicate the longer term consequences of the practice change. The whole process from conception of the idea, putting the research findings into practice through to the final evaluation should then be disseminated to a wider audience to promote the concept of evidence-based practice and the development of care more widely (Rycroft-Malone and Burton, 2011) (see Chapter 23). Gaining support for a change in practice on a national or international scale can ensure the new way of working is embedded in clinical practice. Ensuring policy makers and service user groups are aware of the change in practice can therefore be vitally important.

HANDY HINTS TO IMPLEMENTING RESEARCH FINDINGS INTO PRACTICE

- Ensure you have identified the 'best evidence'.
- Time spent planning the implementation is time well spent. Do not be tempted to rush the process.
- Consider and carefully select which strategies to use to inform those who will be affected by the change.
- Establish clear leadership either by one person or a small group of people. Ensure someone is always available to provide colleagues with guidance, support and information about the new way of working.
- Develop a strategy to address those who are resistant to the change.
- Engage patients, clients, relatives, carers and students (nurses or midwives) with the change. They can become powerful levers to ensure the changes in practice are implanted and maintained.

THINK POINT ACTIVITY   24.5

Think of a practice area that you know well. Who would be the most appropriate person/people to lead the practice change and why?

The reality of implementing research findings into clinical practice is often more complicated and time consuming than might at first be anticipated. Inevitably some practice areas and the staff working in that setting will be more receptive to change than others. Strategies to overcome some of the potential barriers have been discussed above. The characteristics of the person (or people) leading the implementation, the setting and the culture have been identified as key factors (Sandström et al., 2011; Wilkinson et al., 2011). Ultimately a failed attempt to implement research findings into practice is usually the result of poor preparation, inadequate leadership and support (from those who will be affected by the change or from the organisation) or insufficient resources (time and money).

Website activity 24.6

Website activity 24.7

SUMMARY

In this chapter, we have identified some of the barriers to the implementation of research findings in clinical practice. We have identified a range of frameworks or models that can be used to conquer these hurdles and facilitate the delivery of care that is evidence-based. We have also given other practical tips and resources that can be used to promote the use of research in clinical practice.

FURTHER READING

Appleby, B., Roskell, C. and Daly, W. (2015) What are health professionals' intentions toward using research and products of research in clinical practice? A systematic review and narrative synthesis. *Nursing Open.* http://onlinelibrary.wiley.com/doi/10.1002/nop2.40/epdf (last accessed 9 June 2016).

This article includes a systematic review of the factors influencing the use of research findings in clinical practice.

Rycroft-Malone, J. and Bucknall, T. (2010) *Models and Frameworks for Implementing Evidence-Based Practice: Linking Evidence to Action.* Chichester: Wiley-Blackwell.

This text provides a comprehensive exploration of the implementation of research into clinical practice.

Don't forget to visit https://study.sagepub.com/harveyandland to watch videos, take quizzes and to follow specially designed web activities.

25

WRITING A PROFESSIONAL RESEARCH PROPOSAL

This chapter examines the use of research proposals and how they are developed. You will need to refer to other chapters for more detail about each section. In this chapter we will:

- discuss the need to construct a research proposal before undertaking a piece of research
- describe the process of writing a research proposal
- establish the difference between writing a research proposal for academic purposes and proposals to apply for bid funding.

A research problem often begins with a discrepancy or an uncomfortable feeling about things as they are; this stimulates the researcher to investigate further. For example, at present nursing and midwifery education generally consists of a mix of academic study and assessment, together with periods of observed clinical experience, and all over the world nursing and midwifery education will contain variations of this. How do we know which education programme is best?

Before any research on any topic can begin a well-designed and articulated research proposal is needed. The proposal is a detailed plan of work – a recipe that contains a precise description of all activities that will be undertaken in the research study itself and serves to provide a frame of reference as researchers undertake the study.

DEFINING THE RESEARCH QUESTION

Every piece of proposed research requires a clear question – if the question lacks clarity it cannot be answered with clarity. Research questions should express the substantive nature of the research and need to be reflected in the title of the research. Many students will have experienced frustration when gathering articles for an assignment. Having searched a database we discover a paper which appears ideal for our particular topic, only to find that the content of the article bears no resemblance to its title. Similarly the author of a paper may think it clever to use a catchy title to attract attention but it actually deters people from retrieving it (see Box 25.1).

BOX 25.1   UNACCEPTABLE AND ACCEPTABLE TITLES

Unacceptable

- An investigation of hormone secretion and weight in rats
- Fat rats: are their hormones different?

Acceptable

- The relationship of luteinising hormones to obesity in the Zucker rat.

The unacceptable titles as they stand do not include a real indication of what the article might be about. This means that if we are conducting a key word search on a database the article might not appear in the search results. Alternatively it may appear in search results, when in fact it is not relevant. Electronic library databases classify articles according to key words supplied by the authors and group them under medical subject headings or other codes used to describe areas of research. Ultimately a failure to use the title to represent the content of the article means that it will not be read as widely as it could have been.

The research question and subsequent title are best formed from a PICO, described in Chapters 2 and 10, and it is also vital that the question is 'interrogated'; that is, that questions are asked of the question to ensure that it is both focused and answerable. Defining the research question requires a great deal of thought and some first-time researchers tend to want to find the solution to 'grand' problems which cannot be answered by a single research question. The novice researcher may also make the mistake of thinking that a problem requires research when it only requires change management because they are unfamiliar with previous research. For example, a practitioner may have noticed perceived difficulty in discharging patients and would like to investigate this, but a Cochrane systematic review (Shepperd et al., 2013) suggests that this may be improved by implementing individually tailored discharge plans. Before undertaking research the researcher should make sure that the problem is manageable and that they have the requisite skills to undertake it.

WRITING PROPOSALS FOR FUNDING

Website
activity 25.1

The principles of research proposal development are universal but contain specific variations depending on the purpose of the proposal. Academic research proposals that are submitted in preparation for an undergraduate or postgraduate degree or indeed a PhD studentship will look quite different from a proposal written to obtain funding from a health care funding body, industry sponsor or charitable institution.

Successful applicants plan and prepare well in advance and target their applications carefully. Grant holders look for evidence of suitability in three key areas:

- expertise of the research team demonstrated by previously completed projects
- the scientific quality of the research proposal and its potential to answer the specified research question
- value for money.

It is tempting to adopt a scattergun approach whereby the researcher submits lots of bids in a hope that they'll get lucky eventually. There are three key questions a researcher should always ask before developing a project proposal.

1   Is it deliverable? (That is, can you do what needs to be done in the time specified with the resources you have identified?)
2   Is it winnable? (That is, do you meet the funder's criteria in the first instance, and do you have a strong case that elevates your proposal above others?)
3   Does it meet with your university's criteria for ethical research? (For example, does your university have a policy about not working with certain organisations or countries where human rights are an issue?)

Many bids fail simply because they're not as compelling as others submitted during the same round – it is a competition! Research teams who have a better track record in completion of funded research will always be favoured over 'unknowns' simply because funders will not risk large sums of money on those who are untried and untested. The research proposal needs to be complete and compelling, demonstrating a clear demand for the work. Outcomes must be clear and measurable, management and financial models robust. Overall the research team and their organisation must appear capable and credible with definite aims and objectives.

THE STRUCTURE OF A RESEARCH PROPOSAL

A generic outline for research proposals is illustrated in Figure 25.1 and the proposal should begin by providing an introduction to the topic to be investigated.

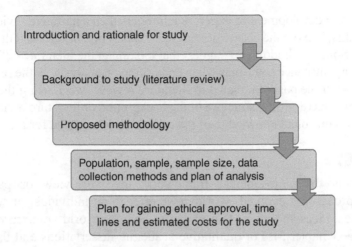

Figure 25.1 The structure of a research proposal

Researchers engage in research activity for a number of reasons, for example, to extend the scope of a research study undertaken earlier, or perhaps to engage in research that develops the practitioner's clinical expertise. Alternatively there may be a strategic imperative to research a topic, for example, global public health issues such as increasing resistance to antibiotics. Whatever the impetus for the research, these reasons should be declared right at the start of the proposal and should be supported by literature such as government reports and key pieces of previous research. By providing a sound rationale for the study the researcher can convince their academic supervisor or funding body that there is a real need to conduct the study.

THINK POINT ACTIVITY   25.1

Read the research proposal provided on the companion website (https://study.sagepub. com/harveyandland) and identify the stages of the research proposal shown in Figure 25.1.

BACKGROUND TO THE STUDY (LITERATURE REVIEW)

A literature review involves organising a process to search the literature described in Chapter 13 and the process of reviewing the literature is described in Chapters 10 and 14. Some methodologies demand systematic literature reviews; others require a narrative approach. If the research proposes to study an intervention such as a new treatment, it would be difficult to justify the use of a narrative review, but if, for example, the research topic concerns the development of expert practitioners then a narrative review might trace the history of this, explore the characteristics of an expert practitioner and their educational requirements. Some methodologies suggest that looking at the literature before embarking on the study may introduce some bias when embarking on analysis, so the researcher needs to be familiar with the position related to literature reviews when using the methodology of choice. Decisions regarding structure of the background or literature review to the study need to be based on sound knowledge of the methodology adopted for the study.

METHODOLOGY

Methodology is the philosophical framework, the worldview or paradigm from which the approach has evolved. Worldviews refer to an individual or society's belief systems, values, ideas and ethics that underpin how the world is interpreted and interacted with (see Chapter 3). For qualitative academic dissertations and theses, students need to demonstrate their understanding of where their methodology is placed and to justify its suitability for the study they are conducting. For quantitative studies such as experiments or cohort studies no justification is required as the standard of the protocol is measured against a recognised standard, for example, the CONSORT 2010 statement. Funding bodies take a pragmatic stance and therefore do not require a philosophical justification, but do want the methodology to have a sound rationale for use. It is important that the methodology reflects the question rather than the other way round. It is tempting to favour one type of methodology over another because we feel we understand it better or to choose a qualitative methodology over a quantitative one to avoid having to deal with statistical analysis. However, the success of a study rests on the collection of appropriate data underpinned by a suitable methodology. Refer to the relevant methodology chapters to understand their principles.

METHODS

Within the methodology section of the proposal the method of conducting the study should be articulated. In this section the researcher needs to maintain congruence between the research question, the research methodology and the methods. Essentially this is the 'how to' of a research proposal and should articulate how the study will be executed as precisely as possible. A clear audit trail allows the reader of the final study to make a judgement about the veracity of the findings.

POPULATION AND SAMPLING

One of the first decisions that needs to be made is who *could* be included in the study and who *should* be included. This is discussed in more detail in Chapter 15 but it is essential that a proposal includes a clear explanation of both the characteristics of the potential participants and a justification of the sample size.

COLLECTION OF DATA

Techniques adopted for the collection of data must align with the chosen methodology. For example, if we were researching post-surgical pain in neonates we wouldn't give a questionnaire to a baby in a special care unit and ask them to complete it! Whilst this example is absurd it is not unknown for researchers to use an inappropriate method of data collection that is not likely to yield data in the form they need to answer the research question. Qualitative researchers may generate data through one-to-one interviews with participants, whilst quantitative researchers are more likely to make a structured observation or measurement. The proposal should describe the method chosen and if there is a different way that data could legitimately be gathered then the researcher needs to justify the preferred method. The use of questionnaires over interviews is the most common dilemma for data collection. See Chapters 16 and 17 on data collection for a more detailed explanation.

ANALYSIS OF DATA

Making sense of the data is the stage of the research process referred to as the analysis phase. As the data collection method should be chosen for its ability to answer the research question most clearly, so the analysis of the data should be congruent with the form the data take. It would defeat the object of a study to conduct an interview in a phenomenological study only to count the number of times a certain theme occurs. With quantitative research mistakes can occur more often if researchers don't understand the type of data they have collected and try to conduct inappropriate statistical analysis. The plan of analysis should be as detailed as possible and justified with regard to its suitability for the study. See Chapter 19 regarding measures of clinical effectiveness and Chapter 20 regarding qualitative data analysis.

ETHICAL CONSIDERATIONS

Every research project contains an ethical dimension and any research study involving human participants, including the introduction of a novel intervention or medication and tissues drawn from human participants, requires clearance from an ethics committee. Consideration needs to be given in the development of a research proposal to potential risks to participants, researchers and others, that may arise during the conduct of the research. Whilst ethical principles need to be understood, the proposal should include the application of these principles to the particular study rather than an essay on the theoretical concepts of beneficence and maleficence. See Chapter 18 and further reading.

TIMELINES

A proposal should include a timetable for each phase of the research: completing the literature review, gaining ethical approval, collecting and analysing the data and

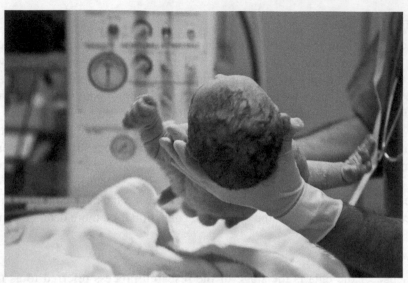

© yarn / iStock

writing up the final report. Researchers need to identify realistic timelines and recognise that each part of the process often takes longer than initially anticipated. This is particularly important if the report is for an external body as they will expect the delivery of the final report on time. Researchers will often utilise a Gantt chart as a tool to capture the estimated timelines (see Figure 25.2). These can be developed using project management software, plotted on a spreadsheet or by inserting a table in a word-processing document.

BUDGET

All research has resource implications. Whilst a definitive budget is usually only made explicit in proposals written for funding bids, it is worth remembering that undertaking research as part of a dissertation might incur travelling costs or transcription services for example. Developing a budget that details the costs for conducting a research study should be included in a proposal if funding is to be sought. Budgets typically include four broad areas of support: personnel, equipment, travel and other.

PERSONNEL

In this section researcher time should be included as a budget item, including a realistic calculation of rates of pay for the researchers, and should reflect time they will dedicate to the project. Administrative support and other specialist assistance such as a statistician and information technologist are included in this budget line. Costings for personnel may

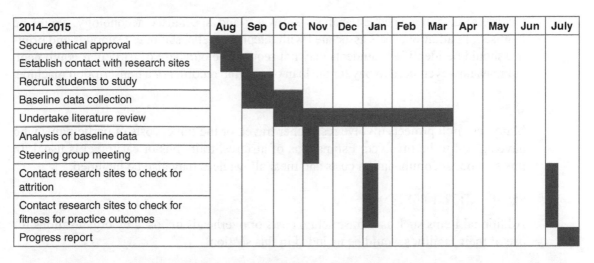

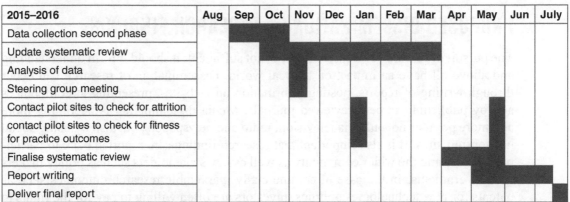

Figure 25.2 Gantt chart: Evaluation of the impact of care experience prior to undertaking NHS funded education and training

be calculated on an hourly, day, monthly or yearly basis, and a justification of what the roles of the personnel will be and each of the other items must be detailed. Depending on the instructions provided by targeted funding bodies, employer costs may also be included. Students might not employ other personnel (research assistants, for example) for their dissertations but they may need someone to translate interviews or perhaps to transcribe recorded interviews.

EQUIPMENT AND MAINTENANCE

Equipment that must be purchased or rented for completion of the research is included and costed in this section. For example, computers and computer tablets, digital voice recorders, data management/analysis software, and specialised technology would be itemised. In addition, costs associated with telephone calls, stationery supplies and printing should be identified. Students may not require the purchase of particular equipment, but may, however, need to pay for the loan of a digital recorder or a transcription machine.

TRAVEL

Many research projects involve researcher travel, or the travel costs of participants who have agreed to be involved. Estimations of airfares, train, bus or car travel is usual. In this section, accommodation costs and meal allowances may also be included.

ORGANISATIONAL COSTS

Additional items such as infrastructure costs or overheads imposed by organisations for use of their facilities would be included in this section.

PROPOSED DISSEMINATION OF RESEARCH FINDINGS

The pursuit of research for research sake is not sufficient; it should inform understanding and above all have an impact on the real world. Dissemination of research can occur through writing of reports, posting information on websites, presenting at conferences and by publishing in peer reviewed journals. Media dissemination is becoming more and more popular not only via television, radio and newspapers, but also by using social networking sites. It is also important that research findings are reported back to participant groups and the wider community as well as key stakeholders such as policy makers and governments. In the case of commercially marketable research outcomes such as patents for new technologies or drugs, investors are often willing to pay for the rights to reproduce these outcomes.

SUMMARY

This chapter has provided a structure for writing a research proposal. Each step of a research project has been discussed and direction given towards other chapters in the book which provide particular detail of what is involved. Undertaking research is an exacting process and one that needs careful and meticulous planning. A sound research proposal is a valuable tool, not just for the researcher who develops it but for other researchers to further study in that particular sphere of research.

FURTHER READING

Dachev, D. and Ross, A. (2013) *Research Ethics for Counsellors, Nurses and Social Workers*. London: Sage Publications.

This provides an in-depth explanation of the theoretical base for a range of ethical demands and approaches in research, together with important resources to support learning. It is a practical, step-by-step guide for all levels of researchers.

Denicolo. P. and Baker, L. (2012) *Developing Research Proposals*. London: Sage Publications.

A short and snappy guide to getting started, this is a good place to begin your research.

Martin, V. (2006) *Managing Projects in Health and Social Care*. Abingdon: Routledge.

This book is about developing the skills to manage and improve health and social care services. Examples from social care and health settings are used to illustrate techniques for managing people, resources, information, projects and change, and the book includes case studies and examples.

Punch, K.F. (2007) *Developing Effective Research Proposals*. London Sage Publications.

Simple-to-follow advice and examples from an international academic.

Don't forget to visit https://study.sagepub.com/harveyandland to watch videos, take quizzes and to follow specially designed web activities.

26

WHERE DO I GO FROM HERE?

In this final chapter we will consider what the future may hold for nurses and midwives regarding research and evidence-based practice. In doing this we will:

- enable the reader to reflect upon their thoughts, feelings and knowledge about research
- identify strategies that nurses and midwives could use to consolidate and further develop their research knowledge
- identify potential research roles and opportunities for nurses and midwives
- consider the ways in which the research agenda may impact upon nursing and midwifery education and practice in the future, with particular reference to the Research Excellence Framework (REF).

The direct nature of the title of this chapter is deliberate. It is predominately about you, the reader. In the first part of the chapter you will be asked to reflect on your thoughts, feelings and knowledge about research and the ways in which these may have evolved. A review of your current knowledge and understanding should also enable you to identify any gaps that still need to be filled. We will explore possible strategies that you could use in order to fill these gaps, consolidate your knowledge and expand your involvement with research. For some nurses and midwives this may include securing a specific research post and we will highlight other possible research opportunities. The book will conclude by considering the ways in which the research agenda may impact upon nursing and midwifery in the future.

WHERE AM I NOW?

THINK POINT ACTIVITY   26.1

Write down your thoughts and feelings about research. Summarise your thoughts by establishing if you regard research in a positive or negative way?

In this book we have explored research methods and processes and evidence-based practice. Now that we are reaching the end of book, this is a useful point to reflect upon your thoughts and feelings about research and what you have learned. It is also an opportunity to identify any gaps in your knowledge about research. The activity that you have just undertaken is the first stage in this process. You may recall that we asked you to undertake a similar activity in Chapter 1.

THINK POINT ACTIVITY   26.2

Compare what you have just written about your thoughts and feelings about research for think point activity 26.1 with what you wrote for think point activity 1.2 in Chapter 1. If you did not undertake this earlier activity or you are unable to access what you wrote previously, try to identify what you would have written then and compare this with what you have written now.

As the authors of this book, we hope that you now feel more comfortable and confident about research and evidence-based practice than you did at the beginning of this book. If you had a tendency to feel negative about research before, we hope that you feel more positive about it now. However, we do acknowledge that research and research theory in particular do not create feelings of overwhelming enthusiasm in everyone. Nevertheless, we reiterate what we said in Chapter 1; research is everyone's business and it should underpin everything that nurses and midwives do. Therefore, whatever your career progression in nursing and midwifery from this point on, research and evidence-based practice should be integral components. In other words, research and evidence-based practice are not going to go away. If you set out on qualification with the intention of using research to support your practice, you are more likely to achieve this (Forsman et al., 2012).

Website activity 26.1

You may well have not read this book cover to cover. However, we hope that the previous activity has enabled you to identify what you have learned. Inevitably there will be some gaps in your knowledge and there may be some aspects of research that you still feel uncertain about (Loke et al., 2014). Indeed there is always something new to learn about research. However, this is the time for you to be honest with yourself. This is particularly the case if the gap in your knowledge relates to a fundamental aspect of the research process (see Box 26.1).

There is also nothing like working with students to identify gaps in your knowledge. If you are not yet qualified, you soon will be. No doubt at some point a student will ask you to explain something related to research, for example, terminology used in a research paper, whether or not unmarried fathers can consent to their child's participation in a study or what grounded theory is. So now is the time to fill any gaps in your

---

BOX 26.1   SCENARIO ILLUSTRATING GAPS IN RESEARCH KNOWLEDGE AND SKILLS

Anna is newly qualified. The ward manager has asked her to work with three other members of staff to update the policy relating to an aspect of practice. Anna is unable to attend the first meeting of the group. It is decided in her absence that as she is newly qualified, she would be the most appropriate person to perform a literature search using relevant databases on the aspect of practice. However, Anna did not take the opportunity to learn how to do this during her course. She 'got by' by searching for information on google, using module reading lists and asking fellow students to share their material.

Website activity 26.2

knowledge. However, identifying what you should know is not always clear cut. This book is primarily aimed at undergraduate students and we believe what is contained in this text amounts to what you should know about research and evidence-based practice on qualification. As you progress to Master's and PhD level study you will find that more detailed understanding of concepts and research methods is required, for which you will need to read more widely.

Whilst there may be some gaps in your current knowledge, we also recognise that it can be difficult to retain comprehensive information about every aspect of research theory. We hope therefore, that this text will be a useful resource to dip back into to clarify information and consolidate your knowledge base. It may be useful to undertake or repeat some of the activities (those in the text and on the companion website) and undertake additional reading using the sources we have identified.

CONSOLIDATING AND DEVELOPING YOUR RESEARCH KNOWLEDGE

There are a number of things you can do to consolidate and further develop your knowledge in order to keep yourself 'research-aware'. We have some suggestions here, but this is by no means an exhaustive list.

The first and probably the most obvious, is to read research and evidence-based practice papers. You may subscribe to a journal or receive one as part of your membership of a professional organisation. Alternatively you may be able to access journals that your practice area subscribes to, or electronically via your place of work or local academic institution. However, reading research and evidence-based practice papers can sometimes be rather laborious. There are, however, a number of strategies that could help provide the motivation. This could include challenging yourself to read a paper once a week, setting up a journal club or having a notice board in the practice area which displays the latest publications. Staff could take it in turns to identify a paper to display, summarising the key points in bullet points alongside the paper.

Other things you could do to consolidate and develop your research knowledge include:

- Mentor students, as we have previously identified there is nothing like an enthusiastic student to keep you on your toes.
- Display the research/evidence-based practice work of colleagues and students such as posters in the practice area.
- Organise workshops, seminars, teaching sessions or research meetings for colleagues and students.
- Spend time with research nurses or midwives working in your area of practice. You may be able to spend a day, perhaps a week with them seeing what they do whilst also gaining a more 'hands on' understanding of research and the research process.
- Talk to patients and clients who are research participants. This may provide an insight into why they agreed to take part and their perspective of the study.
- Join a standard or policy writing group or get involved with bench-marking.
- Get involved in teaching nurses and midwives at your local academic institution. Preparing sessions or lectures will require you to ensure that your material is relevant and current.
- Attend conferences and consider submitting an abstract for the presentation of a poster or a paper.
- Join the special interest group that relates to your specific area of practice if there is one. If there isn't one, then set one up.
- Join the research interest group of your professional organisation.
- Undertake further study such as an MSc, MA, MPhil, PhD or EdD.

THINK POINT ACTIVITY   26.3

Which of the suggestions do you think you could realistically achieve? Think about the barriers to the unachievable suggestions, are they real or self-imposed? What could you or your place of work do to overcome these barriers?

Later in this chapter will be considering possible research roles and opportunities that you could pursue. Increasing the chances of securing these will be facilitated by networking with relevant individuals and organisations and developing a credible curriculum vitae. Getting your name in print can help you to build a network and it will also strengthen your CV. As getting your name in print can be such an important factor, we will explore this in more detail here.

GETTING YOUR NAME IN PRINT

In Chapter 23 we discussed writing up your research or research related assignments for publication. However, there are other ways that you can get your name in print. This could help to establish you in a particular subject area and could be the first step towards a career in research.

   In addition to publishing research related assignments, other ways of getting your name in print include writing about what you do in practice. For example, have you been involved in implementing a practice change, carrying out an audit, benchmarking or writing a protocol, policy or procedure? You could write about this and if you prefer you could co-author the paper with other colleagues to share the workload. Presenting a poster or paper at a conference is another way of getting your name in print because the abstract will almost certainly be published in a relevant journal or the conference documentation. Alternatively, most professional journals have a letters section, so you could write a letter or a response

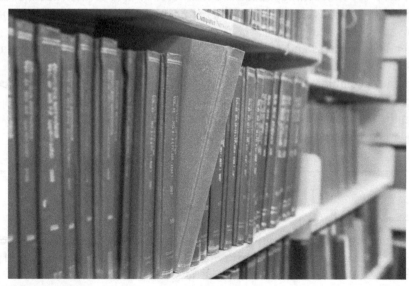

© Shutterstock

to someone else's previously published letter. Periodically journal editors put out a call for reviewers to write reviews of conferences, books, DVDs, teaching materials and other resources for journals. Not only is writing the review a way of getting your name in print, you are also usually able to keep the resource and may receive a small payment. Some journals, in addition to publishing a study will publish a critique of the research alongside it (see www.midirs.org). Whilst journal editors may approach specific people to undertake a critique, they may also put out a call for reviewers to add to their pool of nurses and midwives with a particular area of interest. Similarly you could undertake peer reviews of papers being considered for publication. Again, look out for calls for peer reviewers made by journal editors. Many practice settings now have 'in house' journals or newsletters for which you could write a piece. This is a good way of developing your writing skills before perhaps writing for more widely disseminated publications. Another option is to join the editorial board of a journal. Although it depends somewhat on the target audience, most nursing and midwifery journals endeavour to ensure that the editorial board membership includes a student and/or newly qualified practitioner. Finally you could write a chapter in a book. You may be approached by the publisher or the book editor to do this. In the longer term you could consider writing or editing a book yourself. If you have an idea, particularly if you think there is a gap in the market, contact a publisher and this could be the start of your career in print.

PURSUING POSSIBLE RESEARCH ROLES AND OPPORTUNITIES

Whilst there may be an element of being in the right place at the right time, in most cases if you want to pursue research opportunities, maybe a career in research, then there are things that you can do to help make it happen. Such opportunities rarely fall out of the sky and land at your feet. If you feel that your future lies somewhere in the realms of research and evidence-based practice, then you need to make it known to others, for example, during your appraisal or performance review with your manager. If they are aware of your interest then they may be able to direct opportunities your way. Also talk to research nurses and midwives about their career pathway. They will almost certainly be able to give you some advice to facilitate the achievement of your goals. There are other things you can do to help set you on your way to a career in research:

- Undertake further study such as an MSc, MA, MPhil, PhD or DEd and ensure your research is disseminated through publication and conference presentations.
- Look out for early career researcher training opportunities. Places may include funding or a bursary.

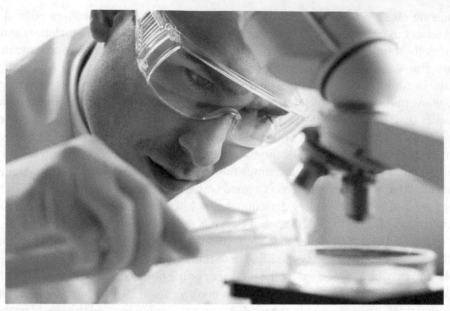

© Pressmaster / Shutterstock

- Ask if a research nurse or midwife in your practice area would act as a mentor or 'buddy' for you.
- Make links with user groups and support groups that relate to your specific area of practice. This will give you an insight to their research priorities. It will also enable you to network with organisations and individuals who you may be able to collaborate with in the future.
- Undertake further research training. Look at the website for training opportunities run by your local Clinical Research Network (CRN). The Good Clinical Practice training, which is free, is a good place to start. See www.crn.nihr.ac.uk.
- Join a research ethics committee either at your local academic institution or an NHS research ethics committee. Look out for a call for members, which is usually located on the university or NRES website.
- Take responsibility for some aspect of a study being undertaken in your practice area. This may be a formalised arrangement whereby you are allocated a specific amount of time per week, for example, to monitor the recruitment of participants or ensuring data collection is undertaken in accordance with standard operating procedures (see Chapter 21).
- Look for funding opportunities for you to undertake a small-scale study in your practice area. Speak to your manager and Trust Research and Development department about a study you would like to undertake.

Website activity 26.3

- Make contact with expert researchers in your area of interest. Look at their websites or websites for the studies they are undertaking. These may identify special interest groups you could join or employment opportunities.
- Look for secondment opportunities. This might be for a set amount of hours or days per week for a defined period of time such as two days a week for six months or a full-time secondment for a defined period of time, for example, one year. The advantage of a secondment is your employer is reimbursed your salary for the agreed period of time so that they can employ staff to cover your work. The secondment also provides you with a level of security whereby you can return to your previous post on completion of the secondment or sooner if, for whatever reason, it does not work out. A secondment is therefore a good way of 'putting your toe in the water'.
- Secure a permanent clinical research post. In order to do this, you may have to move further afield than your current place of work.

Website
activity 26.4

RESEARCH, EVIDENCE-BASED PRACTICE, NURSING AND MIDWIFERY: THE LONGER TERM

Most of this chapter has been about you and the ways in which you can consolidate your research knowledge and perhaps pursue a career in research. We want to conclude the book by putting this into the wider context and explore what the future may hold for nursing and midwifery research and researchers.

THINK POINT ACTIVITY   26.4

Reread the section 'Nursing and midwifery research: where we started and where we are now' in Chapter 1.

If you consider where nursing and midwifery has come from in relation to research, it is clear we have travelled a long way. However, we still have further to go. Some of this will be determined by external forces such as governmental pressure and the availability of funding but it should also be shaped by the nursing and midwifery professional organisations, academic institutions and individual practitioners. Having a clear research strategy should set the agenda for nursing and midwifery research in the future (Kenke et al., 2013). So now is the time for some 'blue-sky thinking' both in terms of your longer term goals but also for the professions of nursing and midwifery.

Website
activity 26.5

Website
activity 26.6

The professions of nursing and midwifery need to ensure that in the context of research and evidence-based practice they not only have a voice but they also establish a body of expert researchers who are leading research rather than following it. However, a study conducted by Loke et al. (2014) identified that nurses are still generally engaged in low-level research activity. So there is still work to be done and the most effective way of increasing research capacity, competence and engagement is, as yet, unclear (O'Byrne and Smith, 2010). Nevertheless research and evidence-based practice are at the forefront of national guidelines, directives and strategies regarding the future development of nursing and midwifery (Chief Nursing Officers for England, Northern Ireland, Scotland and Wales, 2010; Department of Health, 2010). Research and evidence-based practice will continue to have a central role in the development of new nursing and midwifery knowledge and the provision of a rationale for practice.

Inevitably securing funding is always going to be a challenge. It is probably the case that over time an increasing number of researchers will be trying to secure funding from an ever-shrinking pot. However, success breeds success and having won one bid, a researcher will be more likely to secure further bids in the future as they become more skilled at bid writing and establish their reputation in a particular field. However, nurses and midwives need to be vigilant for funding opportunities, particularly those that whilst health related are not specific to nursing and midwifery. There is also a need to work more collaboratively with other disciplines and service user organisations (Clark and Thompson, 2013). To raise the profile of nursing and midwifery research, researchers should also strive to publish their work in high impact and Open Access journals (Clark and Thompson, 2013).

Website
activity 26.7

THE RESEARCH EXCELLENCE FRAMEWORK

The research outputs of UK academic institutions are measured periodically. The first such assessment was undertaken in 1986 and was called the Research Assessment Exercise (RAE). This has now been replaced by the Research Excellence Framework, the most recent outcome of which was published in 2014. Academic institutions are required to provide a range of information relating to a defined period of time including, for example, the number of successfully completed PhDs, funding awarded and conference presentations by staff. A key aspect of the data collected about an institution is the number and quality of research papers published by staff. This is sometimes referred to as REF-returnable outputs. The publications that attain the highest rating in the REF are those published in high impact, peer reviewed, international academic journals and staff are required to submit their four best papers to the REF. Based on the overall REF assessment, institutions and departments within those institutions are given a credit rating. This rating influences future funding and the institution's reputation. Nursing and midwifery are relatively new players in the REF arena. As might be anticipated, other health care professions, particularly medicine, are more established and score more highly.

You may be thinking, 'what has this got to do with me?' However, if you secure some sort of academic post in the future, it is very likely that you will be required to participate in the next REF assessment (at the time of writing expected to be REF 2021), which will be taking publication in Open Access journals into consideration for the first time. Therefore, the sooner you start publishing your work, preferably in high impact, peer reviewed, Open Access and international academic journals, the better. This will contribute to the institution's/department's rating. A person's REF-returnable outputs are also increasingly being used as a means of determining promotion and securing senior academic and research posts.

Website activity 26.8

LONGER TERM RESEARCH ROLES

On qualification, most nurses and midwives want to secure a clinical post and consolidate their training. Some might have longer term career plans which may include research. For others their career may evolve as experiences and opportunities arise, and other factors such as family circumstances dictate. So whilst you may not be thinking right now about having a career in research in the longer term, we anticipate, indeed we hope that this will be the case for some of you. In order to make this happen you will almost certainly need to undertake further study such as an MSc, MA, MPhil, PhD or EdD. You may also need to specialise in a particular research method or a specific aspect of practice such as pain management or mentorship. However, others establish a successful career as more generic researchers. In some ways it is difficult to predict what these future roles may include because we do not know how the arena of nursing and midwifery research will evolve. However, these roles could include:

- chief investigator/lead researcher for a nursing, midwifery or health related study
- leading a programme of research
- leading a research network
- clinical academic researcher (Finlay, 2012)
- teaching, most academic institutions now require academics to be research-active; this specifically relates to the REF as discussed above
- joint appointments between an academic institution and clinical practice
- a senior research governance role such as chair of an indemnity insurance or ethics committee

Website activity 26.9

- reader or associate professor or professor.

SUMMARY

Within this chapter we have encouraged you to reflect upon the ways in which your thoughts, feelings and knowledge about research have evolved. The chapter has also explored the ways in which you can consolidate and further develop your knowledge and potential research roles and opportunities that you may wish to pursue. We have also looked to the future to try to get a glimpse of the place that research will have in the context of nursing and midwifery practice and education in the future.

FURTHER READING

Gerrish, K. and Lathlean, J. (2015) *The Research Process in Nursing* (7th edn). Chichester: Wiley-Blackwell.

See especially Chapter 40, 'Future trends in nursing research'.

Loke, J.F.C., Laurenson, M.C. and Wai Lee, K. (2014) Embracing a culture in conducting research requires more than nurses' enthusiasm. *Nurse Education Today*, 34(1): 132–137.

This paper explores some of the issues that have the potential to impact upon the conduct of nursing research.

> Don't forget to visit https://study.sagepub.com/harveyandland to watch videos, take quizzes and to follow specially designed web activities.

AFTERTHOUGHT

We hope that this book has supported your first steps into the world of research and evidence-based practice. For some of you this may lead to a career in research. However, we end where we began by emphasising that in the context of your career in nursing or midwifery, research and evidence-based practice should underpin everything that you do whether this is clinical practice, mentorship, teaching, leadership or management.

GLOSSARY

Accidental sampling (convenience or opportunistic sampling)

A non-probability sampling strategy whereby the researcher recruits the most readily available participants who meet the study's inclusion criteria.

Action research (participatory research)

A research method which uses a problem-solving approach. Action research usually takes a qualitative approach to evaluate the impact of an intervention.

After-only design (post-test only design)

A design of experimental research in which the only measurement that takes place is of the impact of the experimental and control interventions, which are measured after the manipulation of the independent variable.

After the fact design (ex post facto or retrospective design)

A non-experimental research design which involves the collection of data retrospectively whereby the dependent variable has already been affected by the independent variable.

Analytical survey (explanatory survey)

Aims to establish cause and effect relationships or associations between variables without the use of experimental manipulation.

Anonymity

The identity of participants is unknown, possibly also to the researcher.

Audit

Measurement of aspects of care, data or clinical outcomes against previously agreed local, national or international standards in order to make judgements about service provision.

Audit trail

Documentation, usually in the form of a research diary, which details all aspects of the research process from beginning to end.

Before and after design (pre-test, post-test design)

A design of experimental research which involves the collection of dependent variable data before and after the independent variable is introduced.

Between-participants design

A design of experimental research which involves two separate groups of participants.

Bias

When the findings are distorted. This can be due to random error, poor study design or deliberate manipulation.

Blended methods research (mixed methods research)

Research that involves both qualitative and quantitative methods in one study.

Boolean operators

Literature search operators which allow the inclusion of multiple words and concepts searches.

Bracketing

Before a study begins, the researcher sets aside their knowledge, assumptions, beliefs, attitudes and prejudices about the topic under investigation to minimise the impact of these on data collection and data analysis.

Case-control study

A quantitative research method in which cases with a condition or problem are compared with people without that condition or problem. This is done retrospectively after the condition or problem occurred or has been diagnosed.

Case studies

Detailed exploration, usually of a small number of cases, for example, people, institutions or groups of people.

Chain sampling (snowball, network or nominated sampling)

A non-probability sampling strategy which involves the identification of potential participants through referrals from earlier participants.

Clinical effectiveness

An analysis which is directly relevant to a patient's situation.

Cluster sampling

A type of probability sampling. The study total population is divided into sub-groups or clusters. The clusters are then selected randomly. Either the whole cluster participates in the study or participants may be randomly selected from the cluster.

Cohort study

A quantitative research method involving the prospective comparison of groups: participants who have been exposed to the presumed cause of a problem or condition and participants who are similar in every other way except that they have not been exposed to the presumed cause.

Combined methods research (mixed methods research)

Research that involves both qualitative and quantitative methods in one study.

Confidence interval

The numerical range of the observed effect.

Confidentiality

Protecting participants by not divulging data or information which would identify them or cause them to be at risk of harm.

Constant comparison

A strategy used in qualitative data analysis whereby the researcher compares data that they have collected from different sources and looks for confirmations and contradictions, similarities and differences.

Construct validity

The outcome measure of a study which has previously been confirmed or established in another study.

Content analysis (template analysis)

A method of analysis whereby the researcher devises a coding framework before data analysis begins. The data are then coded in accordance with the framework.

Content validity

The extent to which a data collection tool encompasses all aspects of the variables being measured.

Control

In the context of research, control can have two meanings. It is the control group against which the findings of the experimental group are compared. It is also the control that the researcher exerts over the study to minimise the impact of other variables which may otherwise influence the findings.

Control event rate

A measure of how often an event (such as response to a drug) occurs within the control group of an RCT.

Control group

Participants who receive the conventional (usual) or placebo intervention in a randomised controlled trial.

Controlled clinical trial

A term sometimes used to describe an RCT which test treatments in the real world.

Convenience sampling (accidental or opportunistic sampling)

A non-probability sampling strategy whereby the researcher recruits the most readily available participants who meet the study's inclusion criteria.

Conversation analysis

Method used to analyse naturally occurring everyday conversation between individuals whereby the researcher is not only interested in what the participant says but also how they say it.

Correlation

Link or association.

Correlational design

A non-experimental research design which involves the collection of data in order to determine links or associations between variables.

Counter intervention

In the context of a PICO question, the counter intervention is the comparison intervention.

Covert observation

Observation carried out when participants do not know that they are being observed.

Credibility

A term used in the context of qualitative data analysis whereby consideration is given to whether or not the findings are realistic or believable.

Critical appraisal (critique)

Identifying a study's strengths, weaknesses and limitations in an objective and balanced way to determine whether it is valid and reliable or trustworthy.

Critique (critical appraisal)

Identifying a study's strengths, weaknesses and limitations in an objective and balanced way to determine whether it is valid and reliable or trustworthy.

Cross-over design (within-participants or repeated measures design)

An experimental research design in which participants act as their own control. During the course of the study each participant is exposed to both the experimental and control treatment.

Cross-sectional design (one-hit or one-shot design)

A non-experimental research design which involves data collection at one point in time from a cross-section of a defined population.

Data (single – datum)

Pieces of information collected in a research study.

Data saturation

When data collection and analysis does not reveal any new findings and so the recruitment of further participants is unnecessary.

Data sources

A term used in grounded theory research to describe participants.

Deductive reasoning

Testing a theory or hypothesis.

Delphi design

A non-experimental research design which involves a panel of experts recruited with the aim of reaching consensus about the topic under investigation through rounds of data collection.

Dependent variable

The presumed effect, caused by the independent variable.

Descriptive phenomenology

A qualitative approach which aims to describe an individual's perception or account of their lived experiences.

Descriptive statistics

Statistics used to describe and summarise variables.

Descriptive survey

Aims to describe as accurately as possible the situation as it is.

Diaries

A method of data collection in which participants record information about aspects of their daily lives.

Discourse analysis

A method of qualitative analysis which incorporates elements of conversation analysis but aims to understand any communication between people. It can therefore also include the analysis of written and non-verbal communication.

Double-blind study or trial

When the researcher and the participant do not know which intervention or treatment the participant has received.

Embedded model

A model of mixed methods research in which one component (qualitative or quantitative) is embedded or 'nested' within the other component. The embedded component is intentionally secondary to the component into which it is nested.

Emic perspective

A term used in relation to ethnographic research, meaning the insider's perspective.

Epistemology

Beliefs about the nature of knowledge and how knowledge is acquired.

Ethnography

A qualitative research method used when researchers wish to explore the cultures, customs, language, interactions, actions and behaviours of groups of people.

Evidence-based practice

A structured and objective approach to determine the best evidence upon which care should be based. The four elements of evidence-based practice are the best research evidence, the values and preferences of the patient or client, the knowledge and expertise of the practitioner and the resources available.

Exclusion criteria

The characteristics or features which preclude potential participants from taking part in a study.

Experimental event rate

A measure of how often an event (such as response to a drug) occurs within the experimental group of an RCT.

Experimental group

Participants who receive the new treatment or intervention in a randomised controlled trial.

Explanatory survey (analytical survey)

Aims to establish cause and effect relationships or associations between variables without the use of experimental manipulation.

Ex post facto design (after the fact or retrospective design)

A non-experimental research design which involves the collection of data retrospectively whereby the dependent variable has already been affected by the independent variable.

External validity

The extent to which the findings can be generalised to the total population and other settings.

Face validity

The extent to which a data collection tool appears to measure what is intended.

Fair test

A fair test of treatments is undertaken in an RCT to determine which is the most effective. This is done by controlling the research environment as much as possible to minimise the occurrence of bias.

Feasibility study (pilot study)

A small-scale version of the larger planned study undertaken to ensure the proposed research process and procedures will be successful. The findings of the pilot study may indicate that aspects of the proposed larger study need to be refined.

Feminism

In the context of research, a research paradigm that advocates empowering participants by working collaboratively with them in an atmosphere of cooperation, trust and mutual respect.

Fidelity

In the context of research, this is evaluation of the way in which a study was conducted to determine the validity, reliability and generalisability of the findings.

Field notes

Data in documentary format collected by the researcher in the setting in which events occur.

Focus group

A method of data collection whereby a group of participants discuss issues. The discussion is facilitated by the researcher.

Follow-up design (longitudinal, panel or trend design)

A non-experimental research design which involves the repeated collection of data at pre-specified intervals from the same sample over a set or on-going period of time.

Generalise (generalisability)

The study findings can be applied to the wider population.

Grey literature

Literature not published in conventional journals and books. Grey literature may include reports, working papers, theses, dissertations, newsletters, official and governmental publications and conference papers.

Grounded theory

A research method that is usually qualitative in approach, which is used to explore phenomena by developing a theory.

Hawthorne effect

Changes in participant behaviour when they become aware that they are being observed.

Historical research

Involves the collection and analysis of data that relate to people, places and events in the past.

Hypothesis

A statement that predicts a relationship between the variables measured during a study.

Inclusion criteria

The characteristics or features that participants have which enable them to take part in a study.

Independent variable

The presumed cause that causes the effect, the dependent variable.

Inductive reasoning

Development of a theory based on the study's findings.

Inferential statistics

Statistical tests which enable inferences to be made from the sample to the wider population.

Intention to treat analysis

The process by which the researcher makes sure that data from all the participants are analysed according to the trial protocol and according to the groups to which they were randomly assigned, regardless of their adherence with the entry criteria, regardless of the treatment they actually received and regardless of subsequent withdrawal from treatment or deviation from the protocol.

Internal validity

The extent to which other possible explanations of the findings can be excluded.

Interpretative phenomenological analysis

Analysis used in phenomenological studies whereby the researcher actively draws on their prior knowledge and experiences when interpreting data.

Interpretive phenomenology

A qualitative approach which attempts to interpret, analyse or explain an individual's lived experiences.

Interpretivism (naturalism)

A school of thought which believes that reality is subjective and that there is no universal truth.

Inter-rater reliability

Achieving consistency between two or more data collectors or data analysts.

Intervention

In the context of a PICO question, the intervention is a treatment or care option used in an attempt to solve the problem.

Interview

A method of data collection whereby a researcher asks the participants questions.

Iterative process

A term used in relation to qualitative research, particularly grounded theory, whereby the data are constantly reviewed and revisited until the researcher feels that the analysis has been completed.

Judgement sampling (purposive or purposeful sampling)

A non-probability sampling strategy whereby the researcher decides which potential participants to invite to take part in a study.

Life histories

A biography, a narrative about a participant's life experiences.

Likert scale

A scale with a range of response options (usually an odd number)

List sampling (systematic sampling)

Combines probability and non-probability sampling whereby a list is made of all participants in the population. The first participant is selected randomly and from then on, every nth participant is selected.

Literature review

A review of the current literature, usually undertaken at the beginning of a study to establish what is already known, to identify gaps in the knowledge and to support the development of the research hypothesis/research question(s).

Longitudinal design (panel, trend or follow-up design)

A non-experimental research design which involves the repeated collection of data at pre-specified intervals from the same sample over a set or on-going period of time.

Macroethnography

Ethnographic studies which involve large groups such as a whole community.

Manipulation

A term used in the context of RCTs. The researcher's intention is to isolate the cause (ruling out any other possible causes), and so manipulates the situation to try to demonstrate its effect.

Matched pairs design

An experimental design in which participants in the experimental and control groups are matched as closely as possible.

Mean

The average, calculated by adding all of the scores or cases and dividing the total by the number of scores (or the cases).

Median

The middle value when all the scores or cases are placed in numerical order.

Meta-analysis

Combining and integrating the statistical data from a number of studies.

Microethnography (focused ethnography)

Ethnographic studies which focus on a small group of people.

Mixed methods research

Research that involves both qualitative and quantitative methods in one study.

Mixed strategy research (mixed methods research)

Research that involves both qualitative and quantitative methods in one study.

Mode

The most commonly occurring score or case.

Multiple methods research (mixed methods research)

Research that involves both qualitative and quantitative methods in one study.

Multi-strategy research (mixed methods research)

Research that involves both qualitative and quantitative methods in one study.

Narrative review

A scholarly analysis and summary of several papers relating to a particular topic.

Naturalism (interpretivism)

A school of thought which believes that reality is subjective and that there is no universal truth.

Network sampling (snowball, chain or nominated sampling)

A non-probability sampling strategy which involves the identification of potential participants through referrals from earlier participants.

Nominated sampling (snowball, chain or network sampling)

A non-probability sampling strategy which involves the identification of potential participants through referrals from earlier participants.

Non-participant observation

A method of data collection whereby the researcher observes a group and does not participate in group activities during episodes of data collection.

Non-probability sampling methods

A sampling strategy which means that participants are recruited because they have on-going or prior experience of the phenomena the researcher is exploring.

Number needed to harm

A calculation which determines how harmful a treatment might be.

Number needed to treat

The number of patients/participants who must be treated in order to achieve a result.

Objectivity

Measurement or observation made without bias, influence or prejudice.

Observation

A method of data collection whereby the researcher observes the activities and behaviours of individuals or groups of participants.

Observational studies

A term used to describe quasi experiments.

Odds ratio

A measure of treatment effectiveness determined by the ratio between exposure and outcome.

One-hit design (cross-sectional or one-shot design)

A non-experimental research design which involves data collection at one point in time from a cross-section of a defined population.

One-shot design (cross-sectional or one-hit design)

A non-experimental research design which involves data collection at one point in time from a cross-section of a defined population.

Ontology

Beliefs about the nature of being and the characteristics of reality.

Opportunistic sampling (convenience or accidental sampling)

A non-probability sampling strategy whereby the researcher recruits the most readily available participants who meet the study's inclusion criteria.

Order effect (practice effect)

When whatever is done first influences the final findings of the study.

Outcome

In the context of a PICO question, the outcome should be as close as possible to the anticipated solution.

Overt observation

Observation carried out when participants are fully aware that they are being observed.

Panel design (longitudinal, trend or follow-up design)

A non-experimental research design which involves the repeated collection of data at pre-specified intervals from the same sample over a set or on-going period of time.

Parallel model (triangulation model)

A model of mixed methods research in which the qualitative and quantitative components are carried out at the same time but the findings are not synthesised until both sets of data have been analysed separately.

Participant observation

A method of data collection whereby the researcher observes a group whilst at the same time participating in the group's activities.

Participant reactivity

This is when participants change their behaviour because they know they are being observed by a researcher.

Participants

People who take part in a study, in the past sometimes referred to as subjects.

Participatory research (action research)

A research method which uses a problem-solving approach. Participatory research usually takes a qualitative approach to evaluate the impact of an intervention.

Phenomena (single – phenomenon)

Events, experiences or attributes investigated in a study that can be perceived by the senses.

Phenomenology

A qualitative research method which aims to gain insight to the lived experience of participants.

Pilot study (feasibility study)

A small-scale version of the larger planned study undertaken to ensure the proposed research process and procedures will be successful. The findings of the pilot study may indicate that aspects of the proposed larger study need to be refined.

Placebo

A mock or dummy treatment.

Plagiarism

When someone takes someone else's work, words or ideas and passes them off as their own.

Population

In the context of a PICO question, the population is the group of people that we are interested in and want to find research studies about.

Positivism

A school of thought which advocates that reality is objective and measurable.

Post-positivism

A research paradigm which advocates that reality is multifaceted. Whilst researchers strive to remain objective, post-positivists accept that the researcher will to some extent influence the generation of probabilistic knowledge.

Post-test only design (after-only design)

A design of experimental research in which the only measurement that takes place is of the impact of the experimental and control interventions, which are measured after the manipulation of the independent variable.

Power calculation

A calculation which identifies the minimum number of participants required to measure the impact of the independent variable.

Practice effect (order effect)

When whatever is done first influences the final findings of the study.

Pragmatism

A school of thought which takes a practical approach to research advocating the use of mixed methods.

Pre-test, post-test design (before and after design)

A design of experimental research which involves the collection of dependent variable data before and after the independent variable is introduced.

Probabilistic knowledge

Knowledge that probably explains phenomena.

Probability sampling methods

A sampling strategy which means that potential participants have an equal or random chance of being invited to take part or being allocated to groups (experimental or control group).

Purposeful sampling (purposive or judgement sampling)

A non-probability sampling strategy whereby the researcher decides which potential participants to invite to take part in a study.

Purposive sampling (purposeful or judgement sampling)

A non-probability sampling strategy whereby the researcher decides which potential participants to invite to take part in a study.

Q-sort

A quantitative approach whereby participants are given predetermined statements about a particular topic on individual cards. They are then asked to sort or rank the cards, usually on a continuum that ranges between strongly agree and strongly disagree.

Qualitative research

Aims to understand the meaning individuals give to their experiences, thoughts and feelings. The key features include gaining insight to multiple realities, subjectivity and evolving, flexible designs.

Quantitative research

Aims to test a theory or prediction or explain cause and effect relationships. The key features of quantitative research include explaining universal truths, measurement, objectivity and structured fixed designs.

Quasi experiments

A research method which is similar to a true experiment but either the randomisation or control element is missing.

Questionnaires

A method of data collection consisting of open and/or closed questions.

Quota sampling

A non-probability sampling strategy whereby the researcher pre-specifies the required characteristics of a sample to ensure the final sample includes a certain number with each characteristic.

Random error

The impact of uncontrollable factors on the findings that occur in an arbitrary way.

Randomised controlled trial (true experiment)

A quantitative research method which involves randomisation of participants to the experimental or control groups, manipulation and control of the independent variable.

Random sampling

All of the cases in a study's total population have an equal chance of being included in the sample. They are selected using random sampling methods.

Random selection

Selection in an unbiased way, study participants have an equal chance of being selected.

Reflexivity

A term commonly used in relation to qualitative studies whereby the researcher reflects upon the impact of their knowledge, experience and beliefs in the conduct of the research.

Relative risk

The ratio of the likelihood of an event occurring in an experimental group to the likelihood of the event occurring in the control group.

Reliability

The uniformity and accuracy of the data collection tool used and the researcher using it.

Repeated measures design (within-participants or cross-over design)

An experimental research design in which participants act as their own control. During the course of the study each participant is exposed to both the experimental and control treatment.

Representative (representativeness)

A term used to describe the sample, whereby the study participants represent or reflect the wider population.

Research

A study that is carried out in a systematic and credible way in order to answer questions, find solutions to problems, generate new knowledge or confirm existing knowledge.

Research design

The overall plan which identifies the way in which a study will be carried out.

Research method

The specific way in which a study is conducted.

Research methodology

The principles, philosophy or science of a method.

Research paradigm

A framework that encompasses ideas and beliefs about reality, the ways in which knowledge is acquired and the way in which research should be carried out.

Response rate

The number of participants who respond, a term usually used in relation to participants returning completed questionnaires in a survey.

Retrospective design (ex post facto or after the fact design)

A non-experimental research design which involves the collection of data retrospectively whereby the dependent variable has already been affected by the independent variable.

Rigour

The extent to which a study has been conducted in a thorough, consistent and meticulous way, in accordance with the principles of the particular method and design used.

Sample

The sample is part of, a selection from, a sub-group or a sub-set of the total population who actually take part in the study.

Sequential model

A model of mixed methods research in which the qualitative and quantitative components are undertaken separately and one leads to and informs the other.

Simple random sampling

The most basic type of probability sampling. Sample selection is usually done using a computer programme or a random table. Each potential participant has an equal chance of being included in the sample.

Single-blind study

When either the researcher or the participant does not know which intervention or treatment the participant has received.

Snowball sampling (chain, network or nominated sampling)

A non-probability sampling strategy which involves the identification of potential participants through referrals from earlier participants.

Solomon Four design

An experimental research design which is a variation of the pre-test, post-test design. The Solomon Four design determines the impact of the pre-test through comparison of the groups who did and did not undertake the pre-test.

Standard operating procedure

Detailed documentation of each aspect of a research study, for example, participant recruitment, data collection, procedures for maintaining contact with participants, etc.

Stratified random sampling

A type of probability sampling. The total population is divided into strata or sub-groups from each of which the sample is selected randomly.

Subjectivity

Measurement or observation influenced to some extent by individual interpretation.

Survey

A research method which can be quantitative or qualitative in approach. Surveys gather information about attitudes, beliefs, behaviours and the prevalence, distribution and incidence of a variable usually using questionnaires, diaries or observation.

Systematic review

Studies that address the same research question are collated and analysed to see if they could provide a clearer or definitive answer to the research question.

Systematic sampling (list sampling)

Combines probability and non-probability sampling whereby a list is made of all participants in the population. The first participant is selected randomly and from then on, every nth participant is selected.

Tacit knowledge

Knowledge about activities and behaviours which has not previously been discussed or openly acknowledged but is recognised when reported.

Template analysis (content analysis)

A method of analysis whereby the researcher devises a coding framework before data analysis begins. The data are then coded in accordance with the framework.

Thematic analysis

A method of qualitative data analysis in which data are coded into broad themes each of which usually contains a number of sub-themes.

Theoretical framework

Literature about a theory that provides a perspective or context for a study or the findings of a study.

Theoretical sampling

A non-probability sampling strategy used in grounded theory research whereby the researcher specifically recruits participants who will help them to refine or challenge the theory they are developing.

Thick description

A detailed description of the context of a study and the participants.

Total population (wider population)

The entire population from which the sample is drawn.

Transferability

The extent to which the findings can be applied to other similar populations in other similar settings.

Trend design (longitudinal, panel or follow-up design)

A non-experimental research design which involves the repeated collection of data at pre-specified intervals from the same sample over a set or on-going period of time.

Triangulation

The use of two or more different theoretical frameworks, research methods, data sources or methods of data analysis to compare and corroborate the findings to gain more accurate understanding.

Triangulation model (parallel model)

A model of mixed methods research in which the qualitative and quantitative components are carried out at the same time but the findings are not synthesised until both sets of data have been analysed separately.

True experiment (randomised controlled trial)

A quantitative research method which involves randomisation of participants to the experimental or control groups, manipulation and control of the independent variable.

Trustworthiness

A term used in the appraisal of the quality of a study. Trustworthiness incorporates: credibility, transferability, dependability, confirmability and authenticity.

Validity

The extent to which what was intended to be measured, actually has been and the findings are therefore accurate.

Variable

The characteristics or entities that the researcher observes or measures during a study.

Vignettes

These are scenarios describing a hypothetical situation or event which can be used to elicit participant responses about how they would respond in that situation or their thoughts and feelings about the scenario.

Wash-out period

A length of time incorporated between the first and second phases of a study to allow the effect of the first phase to diminish.

Wider population (total population)

The entire population from which the sample is drawn.

Within-participants design (cross-over or repeated measures design)

An experimental research design in which participants act as their own control. During the course of the study each participant is exposed to both the experimental and control treatment.

REFERENCES

Alcock, J. and Iphofen, R. (2007) Computer-assisted software transcription of qualitative interviews. *Nursing Research*, 15(1): 16–26.

Alise, M.A. and Teddlie, C. (2010) A continuation of the paradigm wars? Prevalence rates of methodological approaches across the social/behavioural sciences. *Journal of Mixed Methods Research*, 4(2): 103–126.

Allotey, J., Nuttall, A., Lynch, M., Mander, R., Reid, L., Allison, J., Jenkins, L., Tully, S. and Ebenezer, C. (2012) Mothers and midwives, 1952–2012. *MIDIRS Midwifery Digest*, 22(2): 143–152.

Anderson, G. (2011) Students as valuable but vulnerable participants in research: getting the balance right using a feminist approach and focus group interviews. *Evidence Based Midwifery*, 9(1): 30–34.

Anderson, V., Chaboyer, W., Gillespie, B. and Fenwick, J. (2014) The use of negative pressure wound therapy dressing in obese women undergoing caesarean section: a pilot study. *Evidence Based Midwifery*, 12(1): 23–28.

Andrews, S. (2006) A framework for evaluation of scientific research papers. *Midwives*, 9(8): 306–309.

Angen, M.J. (2000) Pearls, pith and provocation. *Qualitative Health Research*, 10(3): 378–395.

Ashworth, P. (2008) Conceptual foundations of qualitative psychology. In J.A. Smith (ed.), *Qualitative Psychology: A Practical Guide in Research Methods* (2nd edn). London: Sage Publications, pp. 4–25.

Attewell, A. (2005) Of lamps and lanterns: throwing light on Florence Nightingale. *Kai Tiaki Nursing New Zealand*, 11(3): 28–29.

Aveyard, H. (2014) *Doing a Literature Review in Health and Social Care* (3rd edn). Maidenhead: Open University Press.

Azzopardi, D.V., Strohm, B., Edwards, A.D., Dyet, L., Halliday, H., Juszczak, E., Kapellou, O., Levene, M., Marlow, N., Porter, E., Thoresen, M., Whitelaw, A. and Brocklehurst, P. for the TOBY Study Group (2009) Moderate hypothermia to treat perinatal asphyxia encephalopathy. *New England Journal of Medicine*, 361(14): 1349–1358.

Baker, K. (2014) How to … make critiquing easy. *Midwives*, 17(2): 34–35.

Baker, L. (2006) Ten common pitfalls to avoid when conducting qualitative research. *British Journal of Midwifery*, 14(9): 530–531.

BBC News (2011) Laughing 'better than latest technology for leg ulcers'. www.bbc.com/news/health-12699016 (last accessed 27 May 2016).

Bench, S., Day, T. and Metcalfe, A. (2013) Randomised controlled trials: an introduction for nurse researchers. *Nurse Researcher*, 20(5): 38–44.

Besen, J. and Gan, S.D. (2014) A critical evaluation of clinical research study designs. *Journal of Investigative Dermatology*, 134(3). doi:10.1038/jid.2013.545.

Bird, C.M. (2005) How I stopped dreading and learned to love transcription. *Qualitative Inquiry*, 11(2): 226–248.

Birks, M., Chapman, Y. and Francis, K. (2008) Memoing in qualitative research: probing data and processes. *Journal of Research in Nursing*, 13(1): 68–75.

Bishop, F.L. and Homes, M.M. (2013) Mixed methods in CAM research: a systematic review of studies published in 2012. *Evidence-Based Complementary and Alternative Medicine*, vol. 2013, Article ID 187365, doi:10.1155/2013/187365.

Bohman, D.M., Ericsson, T. and Borglin, G. (2013) Swedish nurses' perception of nursing research and its implementation in clinical practice: a focus group study. *Scandinavian Journal of Caring Sciences*, 27(3): 525–533.

Booth, R.G. (2014) Happiness, stress, a bit of vulgarity, and lots of discursive conversation: a pilot study examining nursing students' tweets about nursing education posted to Twitter. *Nurse Education Today*, 35(2): 322–327.

Bradbury-Jones, C., Sambrook, S. and Irvine, F. (2009) The phenomenological focus group: an oxymoron? *Journal of Advanced Nursing*, 65(3): 663–671.

Braun, V. and Clarke, V. (2006) Using thematic analysis in psychology. *Qualitative Research in Psychology*, 3(2): 77–10.

Breakwell, G.M. (2012) Diary and narrative methods. In G.M. Breakwell, J.A. Smith and D.B. Wright (eds), *Research Methods in Psychology* (4th edn). London: Sage Publications, pp. 391–410.

Breimaier, H.H., Halfens, R.J.G. and Lohrmann, C. (2011) Nurses' wishes, knowledge, attitudes and perceived barrier on implementing research findings into practice among graduate nurses in Austria. *Journal of Clinical Nursing*, 20(11–12): 1744–1756.

Brinkmann, S. and Kvale, S. (2015) *Interviews: Learning the Craft of Qualitative Research Interviewing* (3rd edn). Los Angeles: Sage Publications.

Broom, A. and Willis, E. (2007) Competing paradigms and health research. In M. Saks and J. Allsop (eds), *Researching Health: Qualitative, Quantitative and Mixed Methods*. London: Sage Publications, pp. 16–30.

Broussard, L. (2006) Understanding qualitative research: a school nurse perspective. *Journal of School Nursing*, 22(4): 212–218.

Brunstad, A. and Hjälmhult, E. (2014) Midwifery students learning experiences in labor wards: a grounded theory study. *Nurse Education Today*, 34(12): 1474–1479.

Bryman, A. (2012) *Social Research Methods* (4th edn). Oxford: Oxford University Press.

Caldwell, K. and Atwal, A. (2005) Non-participant observation: using tapes to collect data in nursing research. *Nurse Researcher*, 13(2): 42–54.

Casey, D. and Devane, D. (2010) Sampling. *The Practising Midwife*, 13(1): 40–43.

Chapman, G.E. (1983) Ritual and rational action in hospitals. *Journal of Advanced Nursing*, 8(1): 13–20.

Charmaz, K. (2008) Grounded theory. In J.A. Smith (ed.), *Qualitative Psychology: A Practical Guide in Research Methods* (2nd edn). London: Sage Publications, pp. 81–110.

Chief Nursing Officers for England, Northern Ireland, Scotland and Wales (2010) *Midwifery 2020: Delivering Expectations*. London: Department of Health.

Clamp, C.G.L., Land, L. and Gough, S. (2004) *Resources for Nursing Research: An Annotated Bibliography*. London: Sage Publications.

Clark, A.M. and Thompson, D.R. (2013) Succeeding in research: insights from management and game theory. *Journal of Advanced Nursing Research*, 69(6): 1221–1223.

Coates, V. (2011) Research and diabetes nursing. Part 3: Quantitative designs. *Journal of Diabetes Nursing*, 15(3): 113–117.

Connelly, R. and Platt, L. (2014) Cohort profile: UK Millennium Cohort Study (MCS). *International Journal of Epidemiology*, 4(6): 1719–1725.

CONSORT (2010) CONSORT 2010 Statement. www.consort-statement.org/consort-2010 (accessed 15 March 2016).

Corbin, J. and Morse, J.M. (2003) The unstructured interactive interview: issues of reciprocity and risks when dealing with sensitive topics. *Qualitative Inquiry*, 9(3): 335–354.

Corbin, J. and Strauss, A. (2015) *Basics of Qualitative Research* (4th edn). Thousand Oaks: Sage Publications.

Coughlan, M., Cronin, P. and Ryan, F. (2007) Step-by-step guide to critiquing research. Part 1: Quantitative research. *British Journal of Nursing*, 16(11): 658–663.

Council for International Organizations of Medical Sciences in collaboration with the World Health Organization (2008) *International Ethical Guidelines for Epidemiological Studies*. Geneva: Council for International Organizations of Medical Sciences in collaboration with the World Health Organization.

Coyle, A. (2007) Introduction to qualitative psychological research. In E. Lyons and A. Coyle (eds), *Analysing Qualitative Data in Psychology*. London: Sage Publications, pp. 9–30.

Creswell, J.W. (2014) *Research Design: Qualitative, Quantitative and Mixed Methods Approaches* (4th edn). London: Sage Publications.

Creswell, J.W. and Plano Clark, V.L. (2011) *Designing and Conducting Mixed Methods Research* (2nd edn). London: Sage Publications.

Crossan, F. (2003) Research philosophy: towards an understanding. *Nurse Researcher*, 11(1): 46–55.

Crowther, J.L. and Lloyd-Williams, M. (2012) Researching sensitive and emotive topics: the participant's voice. *Research Ethics*, 8(4): 200–211.

Cruz, E.V. and Higginbottom, G. (2013) The use of ethnography in nursing research. *Nurse Researcher*, 20(4): 36–43.

Cullum, N., Al-Kurdi, D. and Bell-Syer, S.E.M. (2010) Therapeutic ultrasound for venous leg ulcers. *Cochrane Database of Systematic Reviews*, Issue 6, Art. No.: CD001180. DOI: 10.1002/14651858.CD001180.pub3.

Daly, J., Willis, B., Small, R., Green, J., Welch, N., Kealy, M. and Hughes, E. (2007) A hierarchy of evidence for assessing qualitative health research. *Journal of Clinical Epidemiology*, 60(1): 43–49.

Damschroder, L.J., Aron, D.C., Keith, R.E., Kirsh, S.R., Alexander, J.A. and Lowery, J.C. (2009) Fostering implementation of health services research findings into practice: a consolidated framework for advancing implementation science. *Implementation Science*, 4(50). doi:10.1186/1748-5908-4-50.

Darawsheh, W. (2014) Reflexivity in research, promoting rigour, reliability and validity in qualitative research. *International Journal of Therapy and Rehabilitation*, 21(12): 560–568.

Dearnley, C. (2005) A reflection on the use of semi-structured interviews. *Nurse Researcher*, 13(1): 19–28.

Deery, R. (2011) Balancing research and action in turbulent times: action research as a tool for change. *Evidence Based Midwifery*, 9(3): 89–94.

DeMauro, S.B., Cairnie, J., D'Ilario, J., Kirpalani, H. and Schmidt, B. (2014) Honesty, trust, and respect during discussions in neonatal clinical trials. *Pediatric Perspectives*, 134(1): e1–e3.

Denscombe, M. (2010) *The Good Research Guide* (4th edn). Maidenhead: Open University Press.

Denzin, N.K. and Lincoln, Y.S. (2011) Introduction: the discipline and practice of qualitative research. In N.K. Denzin and Y.S. Lincoln (eds), *The Sage Handbook of Qualitative Research* (4th edn). Thousand Oaks: Sage Publications, pp. 1–20.

Department of Health (2005) *Research Governance Framework for Health and Social Care* (2nd edn). London: Department of Health.

Department of Health (2010) *Advanced Level Nursing: A Position Statement.* London: Department of Health.

Department of Health and Social Security (1972) *Report on the Committee of Nursing* (The Briggs Report). London: DHSS.

Doll, R. and Hill, A.B. (1950) Smoking and carcinoma of the lung. *British Medical Journal*, 2(4682): 739–748.

Dove, S. and Muir-Cochrane, E. (2014) Being safe practitioners and safe mothers: a critical ethnography of continuity of care midwifery in Australia. *Midwifery*, 30(10): 1063–1072.

Doyle, L., Brady, A.-M. and Byrne, G. (2009) An overview of mixed methods research. *Journal of Research in Nursing*, 14(2): 175–185.

Driessnack, M. and Furukawa, R. (2012) Arts based data collection techniques used in child research. *Journal for Specialists in Pediatric Nursing*, 17(1): 3–9.

Dunne, C.L., Fraser, J. and Gardner, G.E. (2014) Women's perceptions of social support during labour: development, reliability and validity of the Birth Companion Support Questionnaire. *Midwifery*, 30(1): 847–852.

Dyas, J.V., Togher, F. and Siriwardena, A.N. (2014) Intervention fidelity in primary care complex intervention trials: qualitative study using telephone interviews of patients and practitioners. *Quality in Primary Care*, 22(1): 25–34.

Dykes, F. (2004) What are the foundations of qualitative research? In T. Lavender, G. Edwards and Z. Alfirevic (eds), *Demystifying Qualitative Research in Pregnancy and Childbirth*. Salisbury: MA Healthcare Ltd, pp. 17–34.

Earl-Slater, A. (2002) *The Handbook of Clinical Trials and Other Research*. Oxford: Radcliffe Medical Press.

Edwards, P., Roberts, I., Clarke, M., DiGuiseppi, C., Pratap, S., Wentz, R. and Kwan, I. (2002) Increasing response rates to postal questionnaires: systematic review. *British Medical Journal*, 324(7437): 1183–1192.

Elton, M. (2014) Mill owners falsified data in bid to preserve child labour. *BBC History Magazine*, 6(6): 11.

Endacott, R. (2005) Clinical research 4: qualitative data collection and analysis. *Intensive and Critical Care Nursing*, 21(2): 123–127.

Endacott, R. and Botti, M. (2005) Clinical research 3: sample selection. *Intensive and Critical Care Nursing*, 21(1): 51–55.

English, I. (1994) Nursing as a research-based profession: 22 years after Briggs. *British Journal of Nursing*, 3(8): 402–406.

Engward, H. and Davis, G. (2015) Being reflexive in qualitative grounded theory: discussion and application of a model of reflexivity. *Journal of Advanced Nursing*, 71(7): 1530–1538.

Evans, G., Duggan, R. and Boldy, D. (2014) An exploration of nursing research perceptions of registered nurses engaging in research activities at a metropolitan hospital in Western Australia. *Collegian*, 21(3): 225–232.

Fahy, K. (2008) Writing for publication: the basics. *Women and Birth*, 21(3): 86–91.

Farchaus Stein, K., Sargent, J.T. and Rafaels, N. (2007) Intervention research: establishing fidelity of the independent variable in nursing clinical research. *Nursing Research*, 56(1): 54–62.

Farrelly, P. (2013) Selecting a research method and designing the study. *British Journal of School Nursing*, 7(10): 508–511.

Fealy, G., Kelly, J. and Watson, R. (2013) Legitimacy in legacy: historical scholarship published in *Journal of Advanced Nursing* 1976–2011. *Journal of Advanced Nursing*, 69(8): 1881–1894.

Fealy, G.M., McNamara, S. and Geraghty, R. (2010) The health of hospitals and lessons from history: public health and sanitary reform in the Dublin hospitals, 1858–1898. *Journal of Clinical Nursing*, 19(23–24): 3468–3476.

Feher Waltz, C., Strickland, O.L. and Lenz, E.R. (1991) *Measurement in Nursing Research* (2nd edn). Philadelphia: F.A. Davis Company.

Feldstein, A.C. and Glasgow, R.E. (2008) A practical, robust implementation and sustainability model (PRISM) for integrating research findings into practice. *Joint Commission Journal on Quality and Patient Safety*, 34(4): 228–243.

Finlay, V. (2012) *Developing the Role of the Clinical Academic Researcher in the Nursing, Midwifery and Allied Health Professions*. London: Department of Health.

Forsman, H., Wallin, L., Gustavsson, P. and Rudman, A. (2012) Nursing students' intentions to use research as a predictor of use one year post graduation: a prospective study. *International Journal of Nursing Studies*, 49(9): 1115–1164.

Foss, C. and Ellefsen, B. (2002) The value of combining qualitative and quantitative approaches in nursing research by means of method triangulation. *Journal of Advanced Nursing*, 40(2): 242–248.

Foster, J.P., Richards, R., Showell, M.G. and Jones, L.J. (2015) Intravenous in-line filters for preventing morbidity and mortality in neonates. *Cochrane Database of Systematic Reviews*, Issue 8, Art. No.: CD005248. doi: 10.1002/14651858.CD005248.pub3.

Fothergill, A. and Lipp, A. (2014) A guide to critiquing a research paper on clinical supervision: enhancing skills for practice. *Journal of Psychiatric and Mental Health Nursing*, 21(9): 834–840.

Fraser, A.G. and Dunstan, F.D. (2010) On the impossibility of being expert. *British Medical Journal*, 341: 6815.

Freer, Y., McIntosh, N., Teunisse, S., Anand, K.J.S. and Boyle, E.M. (2009) More information, less understanding: a randomized study on consent issues in neonatal research. *Pediatrics*, 123(5): 1301–1305.

Gardner, L. (2008) Memoing in qualitative research. *Journal of Research in Nursing*, 13(1): 76–77.

Geertez, C. (1993) *The Interpretation of Cultures*. London: Fontana Press.

Gelling, L. (2014) Complexities of ethnography. *Nurse Researcher*, 22(1): 6–7.

Gelling, L. and Munn-Giddings, C. (2011) Ethical review of action research: the challenges for researchers and research ethics committees. *Research Ethics*, 7(3): 100–106.

Gergett, B. and Gillen, P. (2014) Early pregnancy loss: perceptions of healthcare professionals. *Evidence Based Midwifery*, 12(1): 29–34.

Gerrish, K., Ashworth, P., Lacey, A. and Bailey, J. (2008) Developing evidence-based practice: experiences of senior and junior clinical nurses. *Journal of Advanced Nursing*, 62(1): 62–73.

Gibson, W.J. and Brown, A. (2009) *Working with Qualitative Data*. London: Sage Publications.

Giorgi, A. and Giorgi, B. (2008) Phenomenology. In J.A. Smith (ed.), *Qualitative Psychology: A Practical Guide in Research Methods* (2nd edn). London: Sage Publications, pp. 26–52.

Goelz, R., Meisner, C., Bevot, A., Hamprecht, K., Kraegeloh-Mann, I. and Poets, C.F. (2013) Long-term cognitive and neurological outcome of preterm infants with postnatally acquired CMV infection through breast milk. *Archives of Disease in Childhood Fetal and Neonatal Edition*, 98(5): F430–F433.

Greene, D.A. and Naughton, G.A. (2011) Calcium and vitamin-D supplementation on bone structural properties in peripubertal female identical twins: a randomised controlled trial. *Osteoporosis International*, 22(2): 489–498.

Greenhalgh, T. (1997a) Statistics for the non-statistician I: different types of data need different statistical tests. *British Medical Journal*, 315(7104): 364–366.

Greenhalgh, T. (1997b) Statistics for the non-statistician II: 'significant' relations and their pitfalls. *British Medical Journal*, 315(7105): 422–425.

Greenwood, D.J. and Levin, M. (2011) Revitalizing universities by reinventing the social sciences: *Bildung* and action research. In N.K. Denzin and Y.S. Lincoln (eds), *The Sage Handbook of Qualitative Research* (4th edn). Thousand Oaks: Sage Publications, pp. 27–42.

Grove, S., Gray, J. and Burns, N. (2014) *Understanding Nursing Research: Building an Evidence-Based Practice*. New York: Elsevier.

Grubs, R.E. and Piantanida, M. (2010) Grounded theory in genetic counseling research: an interpretive perspective. *Journal of Genetic Counseling*, 19(2): 99–111.

Guba, E. and Lincoln, Y. (1994) Competing paradigms in qualitative research. In N. Denzin and Y. Lincoln (eds), *Handbook of Qualitative Research*. Thousand Oaks: Sage Publications, pp. 105–117.

Gupta, S.K. (2011) Intention to treat concept: a review. *Perspectives in Clinical Research*, 2(3): 109–112.

Hall, D. (2001) Reflecting on Redfern: what can we learn from the Alder Hey story? *Archives of Disease in Childhood*, 84(6): 455–456.

Harder, M., Christensson, K. and Söderbäck, M. (2015) Undergoing an immunization is effortlessly, manageable or difficult according to five-year-old children. *Scandinavian Journal of Caring Science*, 29(2): 268–276.

Hart, C. (1998) *Doing a Literature Review*. London: Sage Publications

Harvey, M.E. (2010) The experiences and perceptions of fathers attending the birth and immediate care of their baby. Unpublished PhD Thesis, Aston University.

Harvey, M.E. and Pattison, H.M. (2012) Being there: a qualitative interview study with fathers present during the resuscitation of their baby at delivery. *Archives of Disease in Childhood – Fetal and Neonatal Edition*, 97(6): F439–F443.

Harvey, M.E., Athi, R. and Denny, E. (2014) Exploratory study on meeting the health and social care needs of mothers with twins. *Community Practitioner*, 87(2): 28–31.

Hilton, S., Bedford, H., Calnan, M. and Hunt, K. (2009) Competency, confidence and conflicting evidence: key issues affecting health visitors' use of research evidence in practice. *BMC Nursing*, 8(4). www.biomedcentral.com/1472-6955/8/4 (last accessed 20 May 2016).

Holloway, I. and Galvin, K.T. (2015) Grounded theory. In K. Gerrish and A. Lathlean (eds), *The Research Process in Nursing* (7th edn). Chichester: Wiley-Blackwell, pp. 185–198.

Holloway, I. and Wheeler, S. (2013) *Qualitative Research in Nursing and Health* (3rd edn). Chichester: Wiley-Blackwell.

Holme, A. (2015) Why history matters to nursing. *Nurse Education Today*, 35(5): 635–637.

Houghton, C., Hunter, A. and Meske, P. (2012) Linking aims, paradigm and method in nursing research. *Nurse Researcher*, 20(2): 34–39.

Houghton, C., Casey, D., Shaw, D. and Murphy, K. (2013) Rigour in qualitative case-study research. *Nurse Researcher*, 20(4): 12–17.

Hull, A. with Jones, A. (2012) Nursing, 1920–2000: the dilemmas of professionalization. In A. Borsay and B. Hunter (eds), *Nursing and Midwifery in Britain Since 1700*. Basingstoke: Palgrave Macmillan, pp. 74–105.

Hunt, J. (1981) Indicators for nursing practice. *Journal of Advanced Nursing*, 6(3): 189–194.

Hunter, B. (2007) 'The art of teacup balancing': reflections on conducting qualitative research. *Evidence Based Midwifery*, 5(3): 76–79.

Hunter, B. and Borsay, A. (2012) Nursing and midwifery: an uneasy alliance or natural bedfellows? In A. Borsay and B. Hunter (eds), *Nursing and Midwifery in Britain Since 1700*. Basingstoke: Palgrave Macmillan, pp. 205–223.

Jacelon, C.S. and O'Dell, K.K. (2005) Analyzing qualitative data. *Urologic Nursing*, 25(3): 217–220.

Jayasekara, R.S (2012) Focus groups in nursing research: methodological perspectives. *Nursing Outlook*, 60(6): 411–416.

Jennings, B.M. (1986) Nursing science: more promise than threat. *Journal of Advanced Nursing*, 11(5): 505–511.

Johnson, B. and Macleod Clarke, J. (2003) Collecting sensitive data: the impact on researchers. *Qualitative Health Research*, 13(3): 421–434.

Johnson, M.E. (1992) A silent conspiracy? Some ethical issues of participant observation in nursing research. *International Journal of Nursing Studies*, 29(2): 213–223.

Johnson, M.E. (2000) Heidegger and meaning: implications for phenomenological research. *Nursing Philosophy*, 1(2): 134–146.

Jolley, M. (1987) The weight of tradition: an historical examination of early educational and curriculum development. In P. Allan and M. Jolley (eds), *The Curriculum in Nursing Education*. London: Chapman and Hall, pp. 1–14.

Kandola, D., Banner, D., O'Keefe-McCarthy, S. and Jassal, D. (2014) Sampling methods in cardiovascular nursing research: an overview. *Canadian Journal of Cardiovascular Nursing*, 24(3): 15–18.

Kanthimathinathan, H.K. and Scholefield, B.R. (2014) Dilemmas in undertaking research in paediatric intensive care. *Archives of Disease in Childhood*, 99(11): 1043–1049.

Keeney, S., Hasson, F. and McKenna, H. (2006) Consulting the oracle: ten lessons from using the Delphi technique in nursing research. *Journal of Advanced Nursing*, 53(2): 205–212.

Keeney, S., Hasson, F. and McKenna, H. (2011) *The Delphi Technique in Nursing and Health Research*. Chichester: Wiley-Blackwell.

Kelly, J. and Watson, R. (2014) Instrument development and validation of a quality scale for historical research papers (QSHRP): a pilot study. *Journal of Advanced Nursing*, 70(12): 2964–2967.

Kenke, J., Wallace, C., Davies, R., Bale, S. and Thomas, S. (2013) Developing and implementing a Community Nursing Research Strategy for Wales. *British Journal of Community Nursing*, 18(11): 561–566.

Kenyon, S., Sears, J. and Reay, H. (2013) The development of a standard training toolkit for research studies that recruit pregnant women in labour. *Trials*, 14: 362. www.trialsjournal.com/content/14/1/362 (last accessed 27 May 2016).

Keyzer, D.M. (1988) Challenging role boundaries: conceptual frameworks for understanding the conflicts arising from the implementation of the nursing process in practice. In R. White (ed.), *Political Issues in Nursing: Past, Present and Future*, Volume 3. Chichester: John Wiley and Sons, pp. 95–119.

Kingdon, C. (2004) Why carry out qualitative research? In T. Lavender, G. Edwards and Z. Alfirevic (eds), *Demystifying Qualitative Research in Pregnancy and Childbirth*. Salisbury: MA Healthcare Ltd, pp. 1–16.

Koch, T. (1995) Interpretive approaches in nursing research: the influence of Husserl and Heidegger. *Journal of Advanced Nursing*, 21(5): 827–836.

Kumpunen, S., Shipway, L., Taylor, R.M., Aldiss, S. and Gibson, F. (2012) Practical approaches to seeking assent from children, *Nurse Researcher*, 19(2): 23–27.

Kvale, S. (2007) *Doing Interviews*. Thousand Oaks: Sage Publications.

Lalor, J.G., Begley, C.M. and Devane, D. (2006) Exploring painful experiences: impact of emotional narratives on members of a qualitative research team. *Journal of Advanced Nursing*, 56(6): 607–616.

Larkin, V. (2013) Encounters in the field, challenges and negotiations in midwifery research. *Evidence Based Midwifery*, 11(3): 99–106.

Lawton, J., Jenkins, N., Darbyshire, J.L., Holman, R.R., Farmer, A.J. and Hallowell, N. (2011) Challenges of maintaining research protocol fidelity in a clinical care setting: a qualitative study of the experiences and views of patients and staff participating in a randomized controlled trial. *Trials*, 12: 108. www.trialsjournal.com/content/12/1/108 (last accessed 27 May 2016).

Letourneau, N., Duffett-Leger, L., Dennis, C.-L., Stewart, M. and Tryphonopoulos, P.D. (2011) Identifying the support needs of fathers affected by post-partum depression: a pilot study. *Journal of Psychiatric and Mental Health Nursing*, 18(1): 41–47.

Lincoln, Y.S. and Guba, E.G. (1985) *Naturalistic Inquiry*. Thousand Oaks: Sage Publications.

Lindgren, B.-M., Enmark, A., Bohman, A. and Lundström, M. (2015) A qualitative study of young women's experiences of recovery from bulimia nervosa. *Journal of Advanced Nursing*, 71(4): 860–869.

Lingard, L., Albert, M. and Levinson, W. (2008) Grounded theory, mixed methods, and action research. *British Medical Journal*, 337(39602): 337–461.

Lipp, A. and Fothergill, A. (2015) A guide to critiquing a research paper: methodological appraisal of a paper on nurses in abortion care, *Nurse Education Today*, 35(3): e14–e17.

LoBiondo-Wood, G. and Haber, J. (2014) *Nursing Research: Methods and Critical Appraisal for Evidence-based Practice* (8th edn). St Louis: Elsevier Mosby.

Loke, J.F.C., Laurenson, M.C. and Wai Lee, K. (2014) Embracing a culture in conducting research requires more than nurses' enthusiasm. *Nurse Education Today*, 34(1): 132–137.

Loke, Y.K. (2014) Use of databases for clinical research. *Archives of Disease in Childhood*, 99(6): 587–589.

McCourt, C. (2005) Research and theory for nursing and midwifery: rethinking the nature of evidence. *Worldviews on Evidence-Based Nursing*, 2(2): 75–83.

McDougall, G.J., Oliver, J.S. and Scogin, F. (2014) Memory and cancer: a review of the literature. *Archives of Psychiatric Nursing*, 28(3): 180–186.

McNeill, J. and Nolan, A. (2011) Midwifery research by midwifery researchers: challenges and considerations. *Evidence Based Midwifery*, 9(2): 61–65.

Mahon, P.Y. (2014) Internet research and ethics: transformative issues in nursing education research. *Journal of Professional Nursing*, 30(2): 124–129.

Manning, D. (2004) What are ethical considerations? In T. Lavender, G. Edwards and Z. Alfirevic (eds), *Demystifying Qualitative Research in Pregnancy and Childbirth*. Salisbury: MA Healthcare Ltd, pp. 35–47.

Mapp, T. (2008) Understanding phenomenology. *British Journal of Midwifery*, 16(5): 308–311.

Markey, K., Tilki, M. and Taylor, G. (2014) Reflecting on the challenges of choosing and using a grounded theory approach. *Nurse Researcher*, 22(2): 16–22.

Mason, S.A. (1993) Employing quantitative and qualitative methods in one study. *British Journal of Midwifery*, 2(17): 869–872.

Maz, J. (2013) Employing a grounded theory approach: core characteristics. *British Journal of Cardiac Nursing*, 8(9): 453–458.

Melia, K.M. (2013) *Ethics for Nursing and Healthcare Professionals*. London: Sage Publications.

Miles, M.B., Huberman, A.H. and Saldaňa, J. (2014) *Qualitative Data Analysis: A Methods Sourcebook* (3rd edn). Thousand Oaks: Sage Publications.

Ministry of Health and Scottish Home and Health Department (1966) *Report of the Committee on Senior Nursing Staff Structure* (The Salmon Report). London: HMSO.

Moreno-Casbas, D.L., Fuentelsaz-Gallego, C., de Miguel, A.G., González-Marìa, E. and Clarke, S.P. (2011) Spanish nurses' attitudes towards research and perceived barriers and facilitators of research utilisation: a comparative survey of nurses with and without experience as principal investigators. *Journal of Clinical Nursing*, 20(13–14): 1936–1947.

Morgan, D.L. (2007) Paradigms lost and pragmatism regained. *Journal of Mixed Methods Research*, 1(1): 48–76.

Morse, J.M. (2006) The critique of research. *Qualitative Health Research*, 16(2): 171–172.

Murtagh, M. and Folan, M. (2014) Women's experiences of induction of labour for post-date pregnancy. *British Journal of Midwifery*, 22(2): 105–110.

Naughton, M. and Nolan, M. (1998) Developing nursing's future role: a challenge for the millennium: 1. *British Journal of Nursing*, 7(16): 983–986.

Needle, J.S., O'Riordan, M. and Smith, P.G. (2009) Parental anxiety and medical comprehension within 24 hrs of a child's admission to the pediatric intensive care unit. *Pediatric Critical Care Medicine*, 10(6): 668–674.

Noble, H. and Smith, J. (2014) Qualitative data analysis: a practical example. *Evidence Based Nursing*, 17(1): 2–3.

Northway, R., Howarth, J. and Evans, L. (2015) Participatory research, people with intellectual disabilities and ethical approval: making reasonable adjustments to enable participation. *Journal of Clinical Nursing*, 24(3–4): 573–581.

Nursing and Midwifery Council (2015a) *The Code: Professional Standards of Practice and Behaviour for Nurses and Midwives*. London: NMC.

Nursing and Midwifery Council (2015b) *Raising Concerns: Guidance for Nurses and Midwives*. London: NMC.

O'Byrne, L. and Smith, S. (2010) Models to enhance research capacity and capability in clinical nurses: a narrative review. *Journal of Clinical Nursing*, 20(9/10): 1365–1371.

O'Leary, Z. (2014) *The Essential Guide to Doing Your Research Project* (2nd edn). London: Sage Publications.

Östlund, U., Kidd, L., Wengström, Y. and Rowa-Dewar, N. (2011) Combining qualitative and quantitative research within mixed method research designs: a methodological review. *International Journal of Nursing Studies*, 48(3): 369–383.

Papastavrou, E. and Andreou, P. (2012) Exploring sensitive nursing issues through focus group approaches. *Health Science Journal*, 6(2): 185–200.

Parker, V., Giles, M., Parmenter, G., Paliadelis, P. and Turner, C. (2010) (W)riting across and within: providing a vehicle for sharing local nursing and midwifery projects and innovation. *Nurse Education in Practice*, 10(6): 327–332.

Patton, M.Q. (2015) *Qualitative Research and Evaluation Methods* (4th edn). Thousand Oaks: Sage Publications.

Peat, J. (2002) *Health Science Research: A Handbook of Quantitative Methods* (3rd edn). London: Sage Publications.

Phillips, R. and Davies, R. (1995) Using diaries in qualitative research. *British Journal of Midwifery*, 3(9): 473–493.

Ploeg, J. (2008) Identifying the best research design to fit the question. Part 2: Qualitative research. In N. Cullum, D. Ciliska, R.B. Hayes and S. Marks (eds), *Evidence-based Nursing: An Introduction*. Oxford: Blackwell, pp. 53–57.

Plummer-D'Amato, P. (2008) Focus group methodology. Part 2: Considerations for analysis. *International Journal of Therapy and Rehabilitation*, 15(3): 123–129.

Polit, D.F. and Beck, C.T. (2014) *Essentials of Nursing Research* (8th edn). Philadelphia: Wolters Kluwer Health, Lippincott Williams & Wilkins.

Préau, M., Bouhnik, A.D., Rey, D., Mancini, J. and the ALD Cancer Study Group (2009) Two years after cancer diagnosis, which couples become closer? *European Journal of Cancer Care*, 20(3): 380–388.

Punch, K.F. (2014) *Introduction to Social Research* (3rd edn). London: Sage Publications.

Pushpa-Rajah, A., Bradshaw, L., Dorling, J., Gyte, G., Mitchell, E.J., Thornton, J. and Duley, L. on behalf of the Cord Pilot Trial Collaborative Group (2014) Cord pilot trial – immediate versus deferred cord clamping for very preterm birth (before 32 weeks gestation): study protocol for a randomized controlled trial. *Trials*, 15: 258. www.trialsjournal.com/content/15/1/258 (last accessed 27 May 2016).

Rafferty, A.M. and Wall, R. (2010) Historical research. In K. Gerrish and A. Lacey (eds), *The Research Process in Nursing* (6th edn). Chichester: Wiley-Blackwell, pp. 321–330.

Rager, K.B. (2005) Compassion stress and the qualitative researcher. *Qualitative Health Research*, 15(3): 423–430.

Rees, A., Beecroft, C. and Booth, A. (2015) Critical appraisal of the evidence. In K. Gerrish and A. Lathlean (eds), *The Research Process in Nursing* (7th edn). Chichester: Wiley-Blackwell, pp. 105–118.

Rees, C. (2012) *An Introduction to Research for Midwives* (3rd edn). Edinburgh: Churchill Livingstone Elsevier.

Richards, L. (2009) *Handling Qualitative Data: A Practical Guide* (2nd edn). London: Sage Publications.

Richardson, A. (1994) The health diary: an examination of its use as a data collection method. *Journal of Advanced Nursing*, 19(4): 782–791.

Richardson, A. and Carrick-Sen, D. (2011) Writing for publication made easy for nurses: an evaluation. *British Journal of Nursing*, 20(12): 756–759.

Robson, C. (2011) *Real World Research* (3rd edn). Chichester: John Wiley and Sons.

Roethlisberger, F.J., Dickson, W.J. and Wright, H.A. (1939) *Management and the Worker*. Cambridge, MA: Harvard University Press.

Rogers, K. (2008) Ethics and qualitative research: issues for midwifery researchers. *British Journal of Midwifery*, 16(3): 179–182.

Rolfe, G. (2006) Validity, trustworthiness and rigour: quality and the idea of qualitative research. *Journal of Advanced Nursing*, 53(3): 304–310.

Ryan, F., Coughlan, M. and Cronin, P. (2007) Step-by-step guide to critiquing research. Part 2: qualitative research. *British Journal of Nursing*, 16(12): 738–744.

Rycroft-Malone, J. and Bucknall, T. (eds) (2010) *Models and Frameworks for Implementing Evidence-Based Practice: Linking Evidence to Action*. Chichester: Wiley-Blackwell.

Rycroft-Malone, J. and Burton, C.R. (2011) Is it time for standards for reporting on research about implementation? *Worldviews on Evidence-based Nursing*, 8(4): 189–190.

Sackett, D.L., Straus, S.E., Richardson, W.S., Rosenberg, W. and Haynes, R.B. (2001) *Evidence Based Medicine: How to Practice and Teach* (2nd edn). Edinburgh: Churchill Livingstone.

Sadler, G.R., Lee, H.-C., Lim, R.S.-H. and Fullerton, J. (2010) Recruitment of hard-to-reach population sib-groups via adaptations of the snowball sampling strategy. *Nursing and Health Sciences*, 12(3): 369–374.

Sandström, B., Borglin, G., Nilsson, R. and Willman, A. (2011) Promoting the implementation of evidence-based practice: a literature review focusing on the role of nursing leadership. *Worldviews on Evidence-based Nursing*, 8(4): 212–223.

Scottish Intercollegiate Guidelines Network (2012) *Management of Perinatal Mood Disorders*. Edinburgh: Scottish Intercollegiate Guidelines Network.

Shaha, M., Wenzel, J. and Hill, E.E. (2011) Planning and conducting focus group research with nurses. *Nurse Researcher*, 18(2): 77–87.

Shepperd, S., Lannin, N.A., Clemson, L.M., McCluskey, A., Cameron, I.D. and Barras, S.L. (2013) Discharge planning from hospital to home. *Cochrane Database of Systematic Reviews*, Issue 1, Art. No.: CD000313. doi: 10.1002/14651858.CD000313.pub4.

Shirvani, M.A. and Ganji, J. (2014) The influence of cold pack on labour pain relief and birth outcomes: a randomised controlled trial. *MIDIRS Midwifery Digest*, 24(4): 484–485.

Silverman, D. (2015) *Interpreting Qualitative Data* (5th edn). London: Sage Publications.

Sinclair, M. (2015) Accessing data from safe havens and warehouses: pinnacles and pitfalls. *Evidence Based Midwifery*, 13(4): 111.

Skirton, H., Stephen, N., Doris, F., Cooper, M., Avis, M. and Fraser, D.M. (2012) Preparedness of newly qualified midwives to deliver clinical care: an evaluation of pre-registration midwifery education through an analysis of key events. *Midwifery*, 28(5): e660–e666.

Sleep, J. (1992) Research and the practice of midwifery. *Journal of Advanced Nursing*, 17(12): 1465–1471.

Sleep, J. and Grant, A. (1988) Relief of perineal pain following childbirth: a survey of midwifery practice. *Midwifery*, 4(3): 118–122.

Smith, J.A. (1996) Beyond the divide between cognition and discourse: using interpretative phenomenological analysis in health psychology. *Psychology and Health*, 11(2): 261–271.

Smith, J.A. and Osborn, M. (2008) Interpretative phenomenological analysis. In J.A. Smith (ed.), *Qualitative Psychology: A Practical Guide in Research Methods* (2nd edn). London: Sage Publications, pp. 53–80.

Stevenson, A. and Waite, M. (2011) *Concise Oxford Dictionary* (12th edn). Oxford: Oxford University Press.

Stewart, M. (2014) A look at life. *Midwives*, 17(2): 43.

Stockwell, F. (1972) *The Unpopular Patient*. RCN Research Project, Series 1, Number 2. London: Royal College of Nursing.

Stringer, E., Tierney, S., Fox, J., Butterfield, C. and Furber, C. (2010) Pregnancy, motherhood and eating disorders: a qualitative study describing women's views of maternity care. *Evidence Based Midwifery*, 8(4): 112–121.

Suntharalingam, G., Perry, M.R., Ward, S., Brett, S.J, Castello-Cortes, A., Brunner, M.D. and Panoskaltsis, N. (2006) Cytokine Storm in a Phase 1 Trial of the Anti-CD28 Monoclonal Antibody TGN1412. *New England Journal of Medicine*, 355(10): 1018–1028.

Tarabulsy, G.M., Provost, M.A., Larose, S., Moss, E., Lemelin, J.-P., Moran, G., Forbes, L. and Pederson, D.R. (2008) Similarities and differences in mothers' and observers' ratings of infant security on the Attachment Q-sort. *Infant Behavior and Development*, 31(1): 10–22.

Teague, G.B., Mueser, K.T. and Rapp, C.A. (2012) Advances in measurement for mental health services research: four measures. *Psychiatric Services*, 63(8): 765–771.

Teddlie, C. and Tashakkori, A. (2009) *Foundations of Mixed Methods Research*. Thousand Oaks: Sage Publications.

Thorne, S. (2008) Data analysis in qualitative research. In N. Cullum, D. Ciliska, R.B. Hayes and S. Marks (eds), *Evidence-based Nursing*. Oxford: Blackwell, pp. 93–100.

Tuckett, A.G. (2005) Rigour in qualitative research: complexities and solutions. *Nurse Researcher*, 13(1): 29–42.

Välimäki, T., Vehviläinen-Julkunen, K. and Pietilä, A.-M. (2007) Diaries as research data in a study on family caregivers of people with Alzheimer's disease: methodological issues. *Journal of Advanced Nursing*, 59(1): 68–76.

Van Bekkum, J.E. and Hilton, S. (2013) The challenges of communicating research evidence in practice: perspectives from UK health visitors and practice nurses. *BMC Nursing*, 12(17). www.biomedcentral.com/1472-6955/12/17 (last accessed 27 May 2016).

Van der Zalm, J.E. and Bergum, V. (2000) Hermeneutic-phenomenology: providing living knowledge for nursing practice. *Journal of Advanced Nursing*, 31(1): 211–218.

Vernon, W. (2009) The Delphi technique: a review. *International Journal of Therapy and Rehabilitation*, 16(2): 69–76.

Wakefield, A.J., Murch, S.H., Anthony, A., Linnell, J., Casson, D.M., Malik, M., Berelowitz, A.P., Dhillon, A.P., Thomson, M.A., Harvey, P., Valentine, A., Davies, S.E. and Walker-Smith, J.A. (1998) Ileal lymphoid nodular hyperplasia, non-specific colitis, and pervasive developmental disorder in children [retracted]. *Lancet,* 351(9103): 637–641.

Walby, S., Greenwell, J., Mackay, L. and Soothill, K. (1994) *Medicine and Nursing: Professions in a Changing Health Service*. London: Sage Publications.

Walker, W.M. (2014) Emergency care staff experiences of lay presence during adult cardiopulmonary resuscitation: a phenomenological study. *Emergency Medicine Journal*, 31(6): 453–458.

Waller, S. (1998) Clarifying the UKCC's position in relation to higher level practice. *British Journal of Nursing*, 7(16): 961–964.

Walsh, D. and Baker, L. (2004) How to collect qualitative data. In T. Lavender, G. Edwards and Z. Alfirevic (eds), *Demystifying Qualitative Research in Pregnancy and Childbirth*. Salisbury: MA Healthcare Ltd, pp. 63–86.

Walsh, D. and Downe, S. (2006) Appraising the quality of qualitative research. *Midwifery*, 22(2): 108–119.

Wangensteen, S., Johansson, I.S., Björkström, M.E. and Nordström, G. (2011) Research utilisation and critical thinking among newly graduated nurses: predictors for research use. A quantitative cross-sectional study. *Journal of Clinical Nursing*, 20(17–18): 2436–2447.

Watson, R. and Holland, K. (2012) *Writing for Publication in Nursing and Healthcare: Getting it Right*. Chichester: Wiley-Blackwell.

Way, S. (2011) The combined use of diaries and interviewing for the collection of data in midwifery research. *Evidence Based Midwifery*, 9(2): 66–70.

Weaver, K. and Olson, J.K. (2006) Understanding paradigms used for nursing research. *Journal of Advanced Nursing*, 53(4): 459–469.

Wilkes, L., Cummings, J. and Haigh, C. (2015) Transcription saturation: knowing too much about sensitive health and social data. *Journal of Advanced Nursing*, 71(2): 295–303.

Wilkinson, J.E., Nutley, S.M. and Davis, H.T.O. (2011) An exploration of the roles of nurse managers in evidence-based practice implementation. *Worldviews on Evidence-based Nursing*, 8(4): 236–246.

World Health Organization (2011) *Standards and Operational Guidance for Ethics Review of Health-Related Research with Human Participants*. Geneva: World Health Organization.

Yardley, L. (1997) *Material Discourses of Health and Illness*. London: Routledge.

Yardley, L. (2008) Demonstrating validity in qualitative psychology. In J.A. Smith (ed.), *Qualitative Psychology: A Practical Guide in Research Methods* (2nd edn). London: Sage Publications, pp. 235–251.

Yardley, L. and Bishop, F. (2008) Mixed qualitative and quantitative methods: a pragmatic approach. In C. Willing and W. Stainton-Rogers (eds), *The Sage Handbook of Qualitative Research in Psychology*. London: Sage Publications, pp. 352–370.

Yuill, O. (2012) Feminism as a theoretical perspective for research in midwifery. *British Journal of Midwifery*, 20(1): 36–40.

INDEX